With an excellent blend of inforn.
Dr. Ellison's book provides a rare look at the wide diversity of pleasures
and problems that women experience in their sexual lives. This is a
user-friendly book—respectful, gentle, comprehensive and encouraging.

> —Linda Perlin Alperstien, M.S.W., L.C.S.W., Certified Sex
> Therapy Supervisor, American Association of Sex
> Educators, Counselors and Therapists, and Associate
> Clinical Professor, Department of Psychiatry, University
> of California San Francisco

Every woman will find herself in this book. Dr. Ellison's work offers a
great endorsement of each woman's individuality, as well as a sense of
inclusiveness in the great sisterhood. Her gentle guidance is a welcome
tool for helping women increase their sexual self-esteem as they struggle
to claim their sexuality, own it and celebrate it.

> —Janice M. Epp, Ph.D, Founding Fellow, American Board
> of Sexology, Director of Specialized Graduate, Academic
> and Professional Training, The Institute for Advanced
> Study of Human Sexuality

Women's Sexualities offers an in-depth look at seventy women who
reveal the details of their sex lives—stories that inform and fascinate.

> —Betty Dodson, Ph.D., author of *Sex for One*

Carol Ellison lights the way towards a new model of women's sexuality.
Her insight, compassion, and broad experience are finally available
to a wide audience. Every woman, whatever her situation, will learn
something of lasting value from this book. I will strongly recommend
it both to patients and colleagues.

> —Leonore Tiefer, Ph.D., author, *Sex is Not a Natural Act*

Any woman could benefit from reading Dr. Carol Ellison's Women's
Sexualities. *If she needs to transition into a deeper, richer, more
self-accepting and exciting sex life, this book will facilitate that passage.
Ellison has provided a travelogue that educates and gives women
permission to truly eroticize their love lives!*

> —Diana Wiley, Ph.D., host of "Fifty-Plus and Fabulous: A
> Show About Successful Aging," and board-certified sex
> therapist and gerontologist

At last, here is every woman's story. Women's Sexualities *fills the
void in our understanding of women's experiences and is an important
book for all women—young, middle aged, or older. The best practical
guide ever published for women who are seeking validation of themselves
as women.*

> —Sandra L Caron, Ph.D., Associate Professor of Family
> Relations and Human Sexuality, University of Maine

*Dr. Ellison's ambitious book illuminates the diversity of female sexuality.
She allows the participants to speak for themselves, giving voice to the
richness of women's sexual experience throughout the lifespan and across
generations. The respondents' comments reveal the wealth of sexual
curiosity, shame, excitement, pleasure, disappointment and longing that
women seldom share.*

> —Peggy J. Kleinplatz, Ph.D., School of Psychology,
> University of Ottawa

*Carol Ellison's book offers new insights into women's sexualities.
A must read for students of female sexuality and sexuality in general.*

> —Ruth Sherman, Ph.D., LMFT, AASECT Certified Sex
> Therapist

Women's Sexualities

Generations of Women Share Intimate Secrets of Sexual Self-Acceptance

Carol Rinkleib Ellison, Ph.D.

Foreword by Beverly Whipple, Ph.D., R.N.

New Harbinger Publications, Inc.

Publisher's Note

This publication is designed to provide accurate and authoritative information in regard to the subject matter covered. It is sold with the understanding that the publisher is not engaged in rendering psychological, financial, legal, or other professional services. If expert assistance or counseling is needed, the services of a competent professional should be sought.

Distributed in the U.S.A. by Publishers Group West; in Canada by Raincoast Books; in Great Britain by Airlift Book Company, Ltd.; in South Africa by Real Books, Ltd.; in Australia by Boobook; and in New Zealand by Tandem Press.

Copyright © 2000 by Carol Rinkleib Ellison
New Harbinger Publications, Inc.
5674 Shattuck Avenue
Oakland, CA 94609

Cover design by Blue Design
Cover art from a detail of Cool, Cool Water by Zanne Christensen © 1999
Edited by Kayla Sussell
Text design by Tracy Marie Powell

Library of Congress Catalog Card Number: 99-75291
ISBN 1-57224-196-9 Paperback

New Harbinger Publications' Web site address: www.newharbinger.com

02   01   00
10   9   8   7   6   5   4   3   2   1
First printing

Dedication

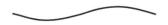

To my mentor, the late Richard Olney, developer of Self-Acceptance Training. His teachings honored and celebrated feminine sensibilities.

Contents

Foreword   vii

Acknowledgments   xi

Introduction   1

Part 1   The Sexualities of Women

1   Our Sexual Selves   13

Part 2   Development:
The Path to Sexual Womanhood

2   Sexual Discoveries: Childhood and   25
    Beyond

3   Thinking About Sex: Attitudes and   51
    Values

4   Love, Sexuality, and Sexual Boundaries   77

5   The First Time   101

Part 3 Sexual Partners:
Licit and Illicit

6 Partners and Contexts   **145**

7 Consensual Nonmonogamy and Affairs   **155**

Part 4 Erotic Pleasures

8 Solo Eroticism: Masturbation and   **181**
       Fantasy

9 Sexual Satisfaction and Partnered Sex   **197**

10 One Hundred+ Years of Women's   **213**
        Orgasms

11 The Infinite Variety of Women's   **231**
        Orgasms

12 Sexual Concerns and Problems of   **255**
        American Women

13 Sexual Choreography: Creating   **293**
        Pleasure in Partnered Sex

14 Sexual Self-Acceptance   **321**

        References   **331**

        Resources   **337**

        Index   **345**

Foreword

In *Women's Sexualities*, Dr. Carol Rinkleib Ellison helps women to "find their way" by helping them discover and learn about the variety of their sexualities. And she does this in a very affirming and gentle manner. Her information comes from women of all ages; women born between the years of 1905 and 1977, and who come from all walks of life.

Dr. Ellison began by conducting in-depth interviews with seventy women, ages twenty-three to ninety, about how sexuality fit into their lives at each stage of their development. After conducting the interviews, Dr. Ellison and her colleague, Dr. Bernie Zilbergeld, developed a 16-page questionnaire to survey women throughout the United States about how they experienced and expressed their sexuality. The data from 2,632 completed questionnaires and the data from the initial in-depth interviews provide the supporting material for this powerful book.

Dr. Ellison's data confirm my belief that we are all sexual beings from the moment we are born until the time we die. (And we may be sexual beings before and after that. Male fetuses have been photographed in utero with erections. Admittedly, it is difficult to visualize vaginal lubrication in utero, but then, it is also difficult to visualize lubrication in an adult woman. I don't know what happens after we die, but I do have faith that we continue to be sexual beings.)

There are many ways in which we, as women, can choose to express our sexuality. The data from the women in Dr. Ellison's study support what she has called "the infinite variety of ways" women can and do experience their sexual expression. In her book, sexuality is presented as an essential aspect of a healthy life because it enhances the total quality of life, fosters personal growth, and contributes to human fulfillment.

When the term "sexuality" is viewed holistically, it refers to the totality of a being. It refers to human qualities, not just to the genitals and their reproductive functions. It includes all the qualities—biological, psychological, emotional, cultural, social, and spiritual—that make people who they are. And people can express their sexuality in any of these areas, not just through their genitals (Whipple 1995).

I have spent the past few decades in a human physiology laboratory, validating women's reported sexual experiences and measuring their responses. However, whenever I talk or write about our research, I always present it in terms of a pleasure-oriented as opposed to a goal-oriented model. That is, I don't want people to use our research findings as a goal that they have to achieve. My purpose in conducting physiological research has been to validate women's actual experiences, not to set new goals.

To conceptualize this concept, I use Timmers et al.'s (1976) model that there are two commonly held views of sexual expression and sexual experiences. The first is goal-oriented and the second is pleasure- or nongoal-oriented. The more common view, goal-oriented, can be compared to climbing a flight of stairs. The first step is touch, the next step is kissing, the next steps are caressing, then vagina/penis contact, which leads to intercourse and the top step of orgasm. One or both partners has a goal in mind, and that goal is orgasm. If the sexual experience does not lead to the achievement of that goal, then the goal-oriented couple or person is not satisfied with all that has been experienced.

The second view of sexual experience is pleasure-oriented, which can be conceptualized as a circle with each sexual expression on the perimeter of the circle considered as an end in itself. Whether the experience is kissing, holding, caressing, oral sex, and so forth, each is an end in itself and each is satisfying to the person and/or the couple. There is no need for any particular form of expression to lead to anything else. If one person in a couple is goal-oriented (typically the male) and the other person is pleasure-oriented (typically, but not always, the female), problems may occur if the goals are not achieved or if the person does not communicate his or her goals to the partner (Whipple, Richards, Tepper, et al. 1996).

It was with this concept of pleasure-oriented sexual expression that John Perry and I (1981) listened to—and heard—what women described as pleasurable to them. Listening to the reports of women led to the re-discovery of a sexually sensitive area felt through the front or anterior wall of the vagina, which we called the Grafenberg spot or "G spot." In presenting our findings in *The G Spot and Other Recent Discoveries About Human Sexuality* (Ladas, Whipple, and Perry 1982) we stated that "sex is for pleasure, and when it becomes goal-oriented, the pleasure is often diminished. The facts we have presented indicate that there are many dimensions to the way people experience sexual orgasm and sexual pleasure (p. 170).

In a later book, *Safe Encounters: How Women Can Say Yes to Pleasure and No to Unsafe Sex,* Dr. Gina Ogden and I focused on pleasure-oriented sexual expression (Whipple and Ogden 1989). We emphasized that the whole body can be sexual and gave many examples of how people can enjoy sexual pleasure from "outercourse," behaviors that do not involve the exchange of body fluids. We offered an extragenital matrix to help people to map their bodies to discover which kinds of touch feel pleasurable to each part of their body.

As Dr. Ellison stresses, each woman is unique and, as such, each woman has the capacity of responding sexually in a variety of ways. All women have the potential to experience sexual pleasure from their thoughts, feelings, beliefs, fantasies, and dreams, as well as from physical stimulation. In my physiology laboratory, we documented the report of pleasure and orgasm resulting from imagery alone (Whipple, Ogden, and Komisaruk 1992). For the women in this study, there were no significant differences in the increases in physiological and perceptual correlates of orgasm from genital self-stimulation and from imagery alone. The reports of all the women in Dr. Ellison's study support and validate our findings that women can experience sexual pleasure in a variety of ways.

One of the most valuable experiences for me in reading *Women's Sexualities* was the affirmation I received. My husband and I were married in 1962 and we were both very naive about sexuality. As I wrote in *How I Got into Sex* (1997), although I loved to read, I had just never put it all together and I couldn't ask anyone. My friends in high school and college did not talk about sexuality and I certainly couldn't talk to my mother about it. I didn't realize how common this inability to talk about sexuality was until I read *Women's Sexualities.*

Clearly, I wasn't the only one in the 1950s and 1960s who had no idea what was going on, and I had no one to talk to about it. At that time, I really believed everyone but me had it all together. I have often wondered if this is why I have conducted so much research, published over eighty papers, and given hundreds of interviews and presentations. I didn't want other women to be as naive as I was. I want to give them the information about the wonderful choices that are there for them, and to provide scientific data for the variety of ways women are capable of experiencing sexual pleasure.

Dr. Ellison, thank you for providing this validation for me and for the millions of women who will read your book and benefit from the information you share with them. It is so affirming to know that I am not alone and that other women share the same experiences and feelings. And I loved it when you said, "The sexual self doesn't have to retire; your sexual self can be a lifelong work-in-progress."

—Beverly Whipple, Ph.D., RN, FAAN, President, American Association of Sex Educators, Counselors and Therapists; Professor, College of Nursing, Rutgers, The State University of New Jersey. Co-author of *The G Spot* and *Other Recent Discoveries about Human Sexuality* and *Safe Encounters: How Women Can Say Yes to Pleasure and No to Unsafe Sex.*

Acknowledgments

The idea to do the research—interviews and a national question-naire—on which *Women's Sexualities* is based came from the Survey's co-author Dr. Bernie Zilbergeld. While I did the majority of the inter-views (seventy), Dr. Zilbergeld also recruited other women to do interviews with my schedule of questions. These included Dr. Linda Banner, Barbara Cerf-Majors, Michaelle Davis, Dr. Maria Flaherty, Dr. Suzanne Fraser, Dr. Susan Hennings, and Michele Katz Their contri-butions were helpful to us in construction of the questionnaire.

The Survey

A national survey requires the collective energy and efforts of many people. The following are among those deserving of my thanks and acknowledgment for their roles.

Design

Drs. Joan Sieber and Douglas Wallace, who served as survey consultants; in addition, Dr. Wallace set up the data entry and contin-ues to serve as my statistical consultant; he has been invaluable in helping me interpret and understand the Survey results. Drs. Diane Binson of the University of California, San Francisco, Norma McCoy of California State University, San Francisco, Beverly Whipple, and other members of the International Academy of Sex Research also gave me advice based on their vast experience with survey research.

Pretesting and Questionnaire Development

Dr. Nancy Fugate Woods, then president of the Society for Menstrual Cycle Research, and the board members who allowed me to pretest the questionnaire at the Society's 1993 national meeting in Boston. I am also grateful to the twenty-five women who completed the pilot questionnaires there and offered their feedback. Their comments, plus feedback from colleagues and friends, were invaluable to us in development of the questionnaire; others assisting us with their feedback included Dr. Jackie Hackel, Dr. Susan Hennings, Patricia Laveroni, Dr. Karen Rinkleib, Monica Rinkleib Rogers, Teri Rinkleib Verdooner, Alexander Weiss, Dr. Robyn Young, and Claire Zilbergeld.

Typesetting and Printing

Jo-Anne Rosen of Wordrunner in San Francisco, who put forth heroic efforts in formatting and typesetting the questionnaire, and Christie Ahlf of Hunza Graphics in Berkeley, California, who coordinated the final design, printing and delivery of the questionnaires and return envelopes; the contributions of her colleagues also are appreciated.

Questionnaire Distribution

The volunteers in almost every state who collectively distributed approximately 6,000 questionnaires. Questionnaires were given out by, among others, our relatives, friends, friends of friends, teachers, professors, physicians, nurses, and therapists. Their names are listed below:

Valerie Adinolfi, Christie Ahlf, Sandy Allen, Linda Alperstein, George Alschuler, Mary Ann Alschuler Yuan, Stan Althof, Pam Amato, the women at American Ink Products, Deborah Anapol, Linda Andrist, Kristen Armstrong, the women at Arvey's Office Supplies, Martha (Mary) Backstrom, Lori Badzin, Kathy Balint, Andrea Ballez-Barlam, Shelley Norden Barnes, Nancy Barnett, Stephen Batoff, Carole Beck, Debra Bercuvitz, Bettykay, Judy Blaisdell, Elaine Blake, Dawn Block, Kay Boll, Marcia Bowen, Gloria Buckhalter Brown, Jane Forsyth Brown, Kim Brown, Mary Buxton, Seyma Calihman, Ariel Cannon, Alice Cannon, Linda Caratti, Paula Carvajal.

Jo Chaffee, Ruth Chriss, Amy Christopherson, Joan Cole, Peter Cole, Ann Collentine, Joan M. Collier, Gail Collins, Olga Perez-Stable Cox, Hali Croner, Angela Curiale, Barbara Davis (who invited me to her class at Sacramento City College to talk about the Survey), Dottye Dean, Aubrey Dent, Sherri DiFranza, Gloria Dunn, Marian Dunn, Jill Ellison, Waynette Ellison, Annie Esterson, Pam and Kim Fitzgerald-Wermes, Maria Flaherty, Toni Flynn, Kate Forrest, Suzanne Frayser, Blanche Freund, Joan Friedman, Carrie Fromm, Ellie Gilbert, Jennifer Glanville, Eric Golanty, Aleida Gonzalez, Cynthia (Cindy) Goodwin, Debbie Gore, Diana Gore, Linda Gore, Marianna Greenwood, Betty Guice.

Jackie Hackel, Carolyn Hally, Robin Fautley Hayes, Susan Hennings, Susan Hetherington, Barbara Hillinger, Emily Hoon, Jacqueline Hott, Julia Hsiao, Elizabeth Hughes, Melissa Johannes, Carol Kahn, Joanne Knapp, Susan Knight, Brundhild Kring, the staff at the Lambda Center in Sacramento, California, Carolyn Latier, Chris Lauderbach, Leslie Laveroni, Lori Laveroni Mahoney, Patricia Laveroni, Cecilia Lee-Hiraoka, Marilyn Leigh, Linda Leslie, Amy Linn, Wilhemina Loree, Jennifer Lovejoy, Marilyn Lovell, Carol Luchetti, Kathleen Madden, Eileen Mager, Nick Malone, Susan Maltase, Darlene Mar, Susan Marks, Linda Martin, Barry McCarthy, Ruth McConnell, Norma McCoy, Michele Walker Meyer, Gloria Molica, Chris Molnar, Cecile Moochnek, Colleen Moreno, Michelle Morse, Marie Morse, Richard Mountain, Denise Murray, Jane Mycue.

Cynthia Neill, Cynthia Nelson, Joan Nelson, Joe Nelson, Susan Nelson, Stewart Nixon, Chris Nyirati, Richard Olney, Gabrielle Pereira, Jane Terker Perelman, Marcia Perlstein, Linda Perry, Raymond Pisano, Pamela Pollack, Noelle Poncelet, Marilyn Ramberg, Faye Randle, Ellen Rapp, Liz Raymer, Katherine Renfield, Joan Rhoades, Harry Rice, Karen Rinkleib, Monica Rinkleib, Jacqueline Rose Hott, Jo-Anne Rosen, Marjorie Rosen, Marcia Rosen, Corinne Rovetti, Sally Schumacher, Syndi Seid, Mary Selna, Kathy Shands, Jeanne Shaw, Jean Sieber, Diane Shinberg, Angela Sklavounas, Al Sutton, Jane Swim, Bill Talmadge, Vincent Talotta, Paul Tamminen, Dawn Taylor, Suzan Theriault, Virginia Theriault, Gay Thrower, Leonore Tiefer, Trish Torruella.

Roseanne Umanu, Helen Valdez, Fieni Verdooner, Teri Verdooner, Carol Wade, Liz and Sam Walker, Pamela Walker, Douglas and Sandy Wallace, Cynthia Wallin, Judyth Weaver, Lynne Weisenfels, Alexander Weiss, Jessica Weiss, Beverly Whipple, Amanda Whiting, Henrietta Wiley, Debra Wilson, Cristy Wilson, Jerry Yanuck, Estella Yeung, Robyn Young, Claire Zlbergeld, and others for whom I have only first names. To those whose names were inadvertently omitted from this list, I apologize. Your contributions, too, are appreciated.

Questionnaire Respondents

The women who took the time to anonymously fill out the questionnaires and pen marginal comments. I do not know your names, but you have my gratitude. You made this book possible.

Questionnaire Return

Hugh Kindle, my mailman, who cheerfully delivered over 2,000 return envelopes containing questionnaires.

Data Entry

My daughter, Monica Rinkleib Rogers, who coordinated the data entry and offered many helpful suggestions and interpretations; she was assisted by Jessica Weiss and Estella Yeung.

Financial Support

The Foundation for the Scientific Study of Sexuality, which provided a contribution toward the cost of the Survey. I thank them for their support.

The Interviews

I am grateful to the women who so graciously told me their most intimate secrets and allowed me to share them with you. I also thank Michaelle Davis, who has granted me permission to quote material from the interviews she did, and the women who shared life stories with her.

Readers

Among those who read chapters-in-progress and offered much helpful feedback in the development and writing of this book were Marilyn Abbas, Linda Alperstein, Shelley Norden Barnes, Dr. Karla Baur, Dr. Kenneth Deitchman, Dr. Betty Dodson, Marcia Goodman, Saskia Kleinert, Dr. Edward Laveroni, Patricia Laveroni, Dr. Sandra Leiblum, Wendy Maltz, Dr. Gina Ogden, Dr. Harry Rice, Donna Rinkleib, Dr. Karen Rinkleib, Monica Rinkleib Rogers, Dr. Paul

Rogers, Dr. Randy Rinkleib, Alan Rinzler, Dr. Joan Sieber, Dr. Sara Socher, Ron Sullivan, Dr. Al Sutton, Steven Verdooner, and Alexander Weiss. I thank you all. And an extra-special thank you to my daughter Teri Rinkleib Verdooner and to my sister-in-law Waynette Ellison who gave me the gift of a twelve-hour day spent reading virtually the entire manuscript.

Other Important People

Others who contributed in their own unique ways include Alexander Weiss, my life partner; Dr. Eric Golanty, with whom I've taught many courses, written an advice column, and exchanged and developed many ideas about sex and sexuality; Saskia Kleinert, my masseuse; my mother, Margaret Ellison; my grandchildren, Michael and Elise Verdooner, who represent the next generation finding their way; Alice and John Glaese; Ralph Sutton, my attorney; the representatives of the National Writers Union who gave me excellent advice; George Alschuler; Dr. Al Sutton; Carole Honeychurch for inviting me to publish with New Harbinger, Kristin Beck for her vision of what this book could be, and my New Harbinger editor, Kayla Sussell, who with intelligent wisdom gently and respectfully shaped this book.

I offer my deepest apologies to anyone I've omitted from this list. In a project of this complexity, some contributors will be overlooked. If your name should be here but is not, I apologize; your part in this project is no less valuable or appreciated.

Introduction

─────────

I wish there was some way I could talk to other women about sex and the things that happened to me when I was growing up.

—Susan, a client

Who are you? How does your sexuality fit into who you are? These are the questions with which I began my interviews of the women who contributed their sexual life histories to *Women's Sexualities*. I invite you to consider them now as a first step toward deepening your understanding of how you experience and express your sexuality.

Sexuality is more than sex. When you create and experience erotic pleasure, you are having sex, but you are also experiencing your sexuality, an aspect of yourself that has grown with you throughout your life. In your lifetime you've gone through many changes in how you experience your body, your emotions, your values, and all aspects of your being. Each sexual experience you have can be likened to a hologram that gathers in all of your previous experiences of having sexual feelings, engaging in sex, having and losing relationships, acquiring sexual skills, making sexual decisions, and changing in countless other ways.

It is through your sexuality—your sexual self—your sexual self-image—that you determine with whom you will have sex, the gender and kinds of people you are attracted to, and your values about when, where, with whom, and how you will express this aspect of yourself. Your sexuality encompasses much more than your qualities of femaleness and maleness. It includes not only what you do sexually, but the reasons for what you do and the meanings your sexual behaviors have for you and for others. Your sexuality also involves the sensations and emotions you have during sex and afterwards, whether you are satisfied, and a myriad of other physical, relational, and spiritual outcomes.

What Is Women's Sexualities?

Women's Sexualities is a guide to self-understanding and self-acceptance. With it you can thoughtfully consider your own sexuality and compare your experiences of sex and sexuality with the experiences of many other women, including some older than you are now—unless you've reached age ninety. In this book you will find narratives from interviews with women aged twenty to ninety and responses and comments from 2,632 women born between 1905 and 1977 who participated in a national survey on how women experience and express their sexuality. As you read this book, you will find yourself recognizing some of the same influences on your own sexual development as those described by the women who took part in the Survey.

Women's Sexualities is a source of information that will deepen your understanding of pleasurable lovemaking and enhance your lovemaking skills. The Survey has much to tell us about how women create their own erotic pleasure and sexual satisfaction. Furthermore, in this book, I share some of the secrets of sexual choreography that I have learned working as a psychologist with individuals and couples on issues of sexuality and intimacy for more than twenty years.

Women's Sexualities is a facilitator for sexual decision making. As you will see, women of all ages, even in their eighties, still have decisions to make about their sexuality. Also, Women's Sexualities is a valuable resource for the guidance of others, of any age, whose sexuality you may influence.

Finally, Women's Sexualities is also a stimulus for discussion. You may want to organize or join a women's Sexual Self-Acceptance (SEXSA) Circle in which to talk with other women about sex, sexuality, and each member's unique sexual development. In the Resource section you will find questions to use for such discussions. Some topics, such as sexual development in childhood or sexual trauma, could generate a series of discussions. SEXSA Circles can be peer groups or intergenerational.

Getting the Most Out of This Book

While you are reading, you will find it useful to keep a blank notebook or looseleaf binder nearby in which to write your thoughts, responses, and impressions as they occur. Or you may want to draw or express yourself in poetry. Express yourself anyway that suits you. We tend to think we'll remember our thoughts and feelings later, but they change form, so I recommend that you record them when they arise.

At the end of each chapter there is a section entitled "What Does This Mean to You?" There you will find specific questions relevant to that chapter. You may want to answer some of those in your notebook or binder. If you take the opportunities I suggest to record your thoughts and feelings as you proceed through *Women's Sexualities*, I think you will find yourself surprised when, in response to my suggestion in the final chapter of the book, you review the record you have created.

My intention is to get you thinking about a lot of questions without imposing judgments, either on yourself or on the women who so generously contributed their histories to this project. A stance of acceptance without judging is not always easy to maintain, particularly with those we are closest to and love the most. For many of us it is easiest with strangers, more difficult with intimate others or our children, and most difficult of all with ourselves.

Self-Acceptance

With self-acceptance, you experience what is happening in the moment, right now, without being distracted by regret or resentments about the past or worries and catastrophic expectations about what might happen or not happen in the future. In sex, self-acceptance might mean that you enjoy what happens in the moment, without being distracted by thoughts about the argument with your partner in the morning or concern that you might not reach orgasm. With respect to our sexuality, and, for that matter, anything else we do in our lives, we do the best we can given what we know and what the situation is at the time.

Finding Our Way

Each sexual self is a lifelong work-in-progress. We constantly change because we constantly have new experiences and continue to mature. I call the entire process in which words, images, ideas and experiences lead each of us, step by step, to a clearer understanding of how our sexuality fits into who we are and to fuller acceptance of our sexual selves *finding our way*.

Throughout our lives we find our way. Over and over we make choices and live out the consequences. And, with changes in our cultural values, our age, and our state in life, the rules keep changing. If today you are a young woman deciding when, where, and with whom to engage in your first sexual intercourse, or whether to have your first intimate encounter with another woman, you will experience your sexuality quite differently than if you are forty-five and contemplating an extrarelationship affair. But in each instance, you will be finding your way.

Whatever our age, and whatever decisions we are making, we do the best we can. If no one has shown us or told us what we need to know for it to be otherwise, our process is likely to be primarily one of trial and error. Part of finding our way to sexual self-acceptance is learning not to be too hard on our younger self, who did the best she could, given what she knew. We can all say: *If I knew then what I know now . . .* But we didn't. We had to find our way.

Intergenerational Dialogue

In finding our way, we can learn from others who have found their way and walked the path before us. *Women's Sexualities* is an intergenerational dialogue. It is filled with examples of how women of all ages have, over time, found their way. It contains statements that illuminate the wisdom these women have gleaned from their experiences.

Here you will find what your mother and big sister—or your daughter—didn't, or couldn't, tell you. You will hear from women who had positive experiences and those who did not. Because so many women are represented here, you will begin to see that certain conditions seem to support women feeling good about themselves, in general, and about various aspects of their sexuality and sexual experiences. Patterns emerge and by paying attention to those patterns you can learn from these women's collective experiences how to enhance your own sexuality and accept your sexual self more completely.

Caution

This book may evoke powerful images from your childhood and your life up to the present. If you have a history of sexual trauma, and you think that those memories may be a problem for you, read *Women's Sexualities* and answer the questions posed *only* when someone is available with whom you can discuss your responses. That person could be a therapist, a trusted friend, or a SEXSA Circle member— what is essential is it must be someone you trust. Writing about your thoughts and feelings can help too. You may find it useful to consider parts of your own past as if you were watching them in a movie or on a TV screen. You also can skip sections you do not feel ready to read. Developing a stance of self-acceptance will be most helpful. With respect to a history of some kind of trauma, a stance of self-acceptance begins with *That's what I experienced. That's how it is. Where I am right now is my starting place as I go on to create the kind of life and experiences I want to have.*

Researchers Who Led My Way

Shortly after I began the research for *Women's Sexualities*, I discovered a 1929 book by Katharine Bement Davis (1860-1935) called *Factors in the Sex Life of Twenty-Two Hundred Women*. This 430-page book is a report of 2,200 questionnaires collected in the early 1920s by a "cooperating committee" of women under the auspices of the U.S. Bureau of Social Hygiene. One thousand of the questionnaires were from married women, 1,200 from unmarried women. The married women ranged in age from twenty-one (born about 1901) to eighty-three (born about 1839); the unmarried women ranged in age from twenty-two to sixty-eight. Almost all of the respondents had attended college, a third had done additional graduate work, and 19 percent had earned graduate degrees.

When I discovered this exciting book, it became my goal that, almost exactly seventy years after Davis and her colleagues collected their data, we would have at least 2,200 questionnaires returned in our Survey. I was delighted when we not only reached that number, but found the questionnaires continuing to arrive. Davis' study was the largest scale sex survey done in America before Kinsey's work of the 1940s and '50s, yet who today has ever heard of it? I couldn't help but wonder: If this study had been done by men, would it be well known? Although we did not ask identical questions, some of our questions are similar, as is our predominantly college-educated group of respondents, who are more likely than women in the general population to be working as professionals. I will sometimes compare our data to the data of Davis and her colleagues, something they hoped would happen with future studies.

> We are content to present the data in as clear a form as possible for the use of others. The difficulty and often the impossibility of securing comparable data lead us to hope that these studies of the sex life of so large a group of intelligent women will furnish a way-mark with which future studies may be compared.
>
> —Katharine Bement Davis, *Factors in the Sex Life of Twenty-Two Hundred Women*, p. xvii.

I hope our study, too, will be a way-mark with which future studies may be compared.

Another early woman researcher I discovered at about the same time I was discovering Katharine Bement Davis is Clelia Mosher, a physician whose career overlapped the nineteenth and twentieth centuries. Over the course of twenty-eight years, from 1892 to 1920, Dr. Mosher interviewed and verbally administered a questionnaire to at least forty-five married women about their sexuality. Most of these women spent their formative and early adult years in the nineteenth century; seventeen were born before the Civil War and only one was born after 1890. Mosher's and Davis' surveys are the only ones known to have been done of Victorian-era women in America. Unfortunately, Mosher's work was not published in her lifetime. Among her contemporaries its benefit seems to have been limited to her patients, the students she advised, and those who heard her lectures. The interview-questionnaire forms were discovered in the Stanford University Archives in 1973 and were later transcribed and published (C. Mosher 1980).

Mosher's and Davis' studies challenge almost all of the stereotypes we have of Victorian inhibition and prudery. Although reproduction was considered the primary purpose of sex in that era, over half of Mosher's sample said that the pleasure involved was a worthy purpose in itself. And at least thirty of the women used some form of birth control.

We owe a great deal to the largely unacknowledged work of these women whose research preceded my own. Their research laid the groundwork for mine.

A Note About the Ellison/Zilbergeld Survey

Like Davis and her colleagues, we primarily surveyed women who had attended at least some college. Thirty-two percent had some college or a two-year degree; 21 percent had a four-year degree; and 40 percent had done some graduate work or had a graduate degree. The 2,632 women who responded to our questionnaire were born between 1905 and 1977; 556 were age fifty or older. Although we had planned for and attempted to have greater ethnic diversity, 83 percent were Caucasian. With respect to sexual orientation, 7 percent described themselves as lesbian, 5½ percent as bisexual, the remainder as heterosexual. As you read further, please keep in mind that our statistics and other research findings describe the particular group of women we surveyed, not American women in general.

Women's Narratives

The Survey directions invited women to write their comments directly on the questionnaire or on a separate page and told them: "If a question doesn't accurately describe your experience, please tell us so. We want to know how *you* experience *your* sexuality." And did these women write comments—thousands of them! Some wrote only a few words and some attached several pages of thoughtful musings.

Women's Sexualities is brimming with quotations from the interviews and the comments the survey respondents added to their questionnaires. As a rule, I present these quotes chronologically, beginning with the oldest woman. (The year each woman was born is in parentheses beside her name.) Sometimes, you will find the comments clustered to include women born over a several-year span; these are still in chronological order. I have protected the identities of the women I interviewed by giving each one (and anyone she talks about) new names. Occasionally, I left out a birth year and/or changed a few irrelevant details, also in the interests of anonymity.

As I gathered an enormous mountain of data, I was struck by the great variability with which women experience and express their sexuality. This tremendous variability is an important ongoing theme throughout this book. It has been very rewarding to receive comments like the following from women who completed the Survey questionnaire:

- The choices gave me the message that it is okay to feel one way or another. There is no one right way.

- The questionnaire was comforting because it made me look at my sexual experiences longitudinally rather than just at the recent ending of my marriage.

- It was thought-provoking, it created a kind of *mindfulness* about these issues.

- It helped me clarify some difficulties I was having with my partner.

- Even if you experience something uncomfortable, you are not alone. There are other women out there to share these things with you. Even if you've never told anyone.

- It spurred me to imagine sexual lives different from my own. What if I'd given up a baby for adoption? What if I'd had sex for money? What if a primary concern during sex was a fear of STD? In this way the questionnaire encouraged recognition of and fantasies about a range of sexualities.

I hope that reading about these women's responses will have the same impact on you.

For More Information

Most of the tables and statistics from the questionnaire Survey are not included in this book. To view the entire questionnaire and to learn how you can obtain the statistical data, please visit my website at www.WomensSexualities.com. You can also enter www.womens-sexualities.com. (There is no apostrophe or hyphen.)

Questioning Curiosity

I hope you bring a *questioning curiosity* to your reading and discussions of *Women's Sexualities*. Most important will be your curiosity about your own sexuality. Here are some questions for you to consider:

- Who are you ? How does your sexuality fit into who you are? How is that different now than at other times in your life?

- What is your first memory of yourself as sexual (perhaps you were too young to even have the knowledge or words to describe what you experienced as sexual)?

- What were the influences of your parents, playmates, siblings, cousins, and others on your sexual development?

- What did you read and hear—from your parents, peers, church, school, and the media about sex?

- What absolutely wonderful sexual memories do you have? What experiences do you cherish?

- What sexual scars do you carry? What choices were taken from you, either directly by others or indirectly by others failing to educate or protect you? What choices were you able to make? Did you sometimes find strength and self-efficacy in difficult situations?

- What aspects of your sexuality are—or have been—most important to you? Self-fulfillment? Physical expression? Emotional sharing? Attraction, bonding, nurturance? Realization of your fertility? Sex as a path to spiritual awareness? How have these themes varied throughout *your* life? Which have been the most important aspects of *your* sexuality?

These questions are similar to those I asked the women I interviewed, and they will be addressed throughout this book. You will find your answers becoming more detailed as reading *Women's Sexualities* stimulates you to recall, and perhaps to write about, your own sexual experiences.

Of course, your answers to these and the other questions I will pose about sex and sexuality will be intensely personal. Even though we all have a great deal in common with other women, we find our way to sexual adulthood through experiences and influences uniquely our own. We reach adulthood with a unique *sexual self* through which we experience and express our sexuality. Our singular sexual self-image is made up of beliefs, attitudes, values, and images that link our body, mind, and spirit, all of which contribute to this aspect of who we are.

You are beginning a journey of discovery. I hope the path you take will lead you always in the direction of enhanced self-acceptance. I wish you well.

Part 1

The Sexualities of Women

1

Our Sexual Selves

Out of an exquisitely personal set of life experiences each of us forms a unique sense of a sexual self. When women are asked, *Who are you? How does your sexuality fit into who you are?*, no two responses are ever alike. All women have distinctively personal answers to these questions because each of us has a unique sexual self. We may have a tremendous amount in common with others, but we have found our way to sexual adulthood through experiences and influences uniquely our own.

Our sexual self is that aspect of who we are through which we experience and express our sexuality. One's sexual self-image is made up of the beliefs, attitudes, values, and images linking body and mind that contribute to this aspect of the self or personality. The foundations for healthy and fulfilling expressions of sexuality in adulthood are set down when we are very young. Even before we can walk and talk we learn the language of touch. As babies and toddlers we seek answers to important questions we are too young to articulate, but which, nevertheless, shape our self-image. Among these are "Am I wanted? Is my world protected and secure? Can I make my needs understood? Can I get those needs satisfied? Is it okay to have my own feelings? To be independent? To ask for help? Can I act from my own will and still be loved and accepted?" (Marcher 1991).

The answers to those questions come through early life experiences and shape our bodies and our psychological selves.

Sexuality Is More Than Sex

Your sexual self encompasses much more than your biologically female or male attributes and it involves much more than having or experiencing sex. Sexuality is embedded in many larger contexts, including, among others, intimate relationships, family, and society.

A woman's sexuality is a quality of her being that can be expressed at many levels in her life. Every woman has the potential to positively experience and pleasurably express her sexuality. How she does this—self-pleasuring, with a female or male partner, with more than one partner, with or without genital contact—will vary with her stage of life and the contexts that are available to her. It is impossible to separate a woman's sexuality from the different contexts of her life, and, of course, each life is different.

When I use the word "sexuality" I usually will be referring to the aspect of self I have been describing here. When I use the word "sex" I will be referring to the *doing* of sex, to *having* sex. You may notice, however, that some of the women I quote use these two words interchangeably.

Sexuality Is Multidimensional

Our sexual feelings and experiences are affected by the many threads that link the various aspects of our lives. Experiences of having sex are part of this tapestry. Having sex involves not only a woman's sexual behavior but the reasons for the behavior, the meaning it has for her and for others, with whom she has sex and when, the sensations and emotions she has during sex and afterwards, whether she is satisfied, and what the other physical, relational, and sometimes spiritual outcomes are.

There are many sexualities. Sexuality varies, sometimes dramatically, from woman to woman. Women define, experience, and enjoy their sexuality in many ways. They consider different dimensions of sexuality more or less important, and differ on almost every aspect of their sexual expression.

The narratives that follow clearly demonstrate some of the many dimensions of sexual experience. The women I interviewed described sex as physical and mental attraction, an enjoyable activity, the most intimate and private way of expressing feelings, an unparalleled way to a sense of connection, and as a means to pleasure, love, bonding, and fun that encompasses being a woman, sexual orientation, and body image. They alluded to physical, mental, emotional, relational, and transpersonal dimensions of sexuality and sexual expression.

For **Eleanor (1912):** "Sex is a deep, not only physical, but mental attraction between two people. Your feeling is deep enough for this one person so that you make your own desires and feelings a little subordinate trying to keep this person happy. And the person should do the same for you, so that it can be mutual. A feeling like that between—in my case, a man and a woman—is probably one of the best things you can have in life."

For **Donna (1949):** "Sex is an enjoyable activity that is perhaps the most intimate and private way of expressing feelings and being with someone else. It's a part of life you just can't get away from. It's a part of me. I am a woman."

For **Katy (1970):** "Sex means different things at different times. Sometimes it's pleasure—a way to gain pleasure and to give pleasure. Other times it's a real expression of my love for the other person—a bonding, joining thing. Sometimes it's just fun. It's a game, we're playing together by engaging in sex. It really varies."

The Personal Sexual Comfort Zone

When it comes to personally acceptable sex, each of us has a unique constellation of characteristics and preferences, a *sexual comfort zone*. This is the range of behaviors and partners that we include in what we define as erotic, as sex, or as the kind of sex that is personally okay.

Lucille (1921) told me: "I don't like kinky stuff, like with a third partner. I did that once with a partner of mine and another woman. That was a real strange thing to me. I did not enjoy it at all. It was just ridiculous. It just made me laugh. So that's not sex to me, that's some crazy thing."

Mary Jo (1947) said: "During the sexual revolution it would have been fun to at least once do something in a group-sex situation—just for the hell of it. For the physical fun. And I can't do that anymore. It's like I don't want to do that anymore. But it would have been fun to have had that experience."

For **Vickie (1957),** sex means a lot of different things: "When I'm in a positive mood about sex, I could say, ideally, it's a way of life, or it's living. But then I see something about people wearing leather and getting tattoos or having nipple rings or stuff like that. And it's like, *that's* enhancing their sex life? Is that sex? What is going on?"

Karen (1957) thinks "celibacy is a totally boring concept. My feeling is that I was born with a body; to deny it seems crazy." On the other hand, **Susan (1958)**, who was celibate from late 1981 until August 1983, said: "My celibacy was a conscious choice; after I had a relationship with a woman, before my first marriage. I was a little concerned that I had been with a woman, and I just wanted to take a break and see how I felt about sex. I dated and had relationships but I just didn't have sex. And it felt like I was suppressing it. A piece of me wanted to have sex and another piece just wanted to take a break. When I would tell someone that, it felt good, sort of power-ful. Actually, the first person I had sex with again was my husband, when I first met him, in Acapulco. I was with my mom and he was there with a friend. I think I had a feeling I would be having sex again, because I had brought my diaphragm along, which I thought was strange because I hadn't had sex in over a year. Anyway, it was nice."

Maggie (1965) read some lesbian S-M stories for a course paper: "As I was reading, I was like, *Ah-h-h.* I gave my partner copies and she was like: *I can't do this.* But we started to experiment. The most far-out we ever got was some pretty hard spanking, some vaginal fisting, light bondage. A lot of it was verbal. So we were both coming into this with each other. It was the first time that I ever owned my own sexuality very profoundly. I needed to articulate my desires. Even as a *bottom*, I was really the one in control. And she would make me say what I wanted her to do to me. And it was really hard. And I felt a lot of shame, not about what I was asking for, but just needing to say it. Even something like *I want you to fuck me*, or *I want you to poke me up against a wall*, or whatever it might be. It was the first time I had to say *I'm the sexual person.* This went on for about six months. The issue of power, or control in sex was always there. The level of trust it built between us was incredible. Gradually, it tapered off, also some of my childhood abuse stuff started to get triggered. Sex has not been the same since our relationship ended a year ago."

Most of us tend to accept a range of other people's choices in partners and forms of sexual expression that we wouldn't be comfort-able with for ourselves. And most of us have some experiences in our fantasy lives that we don't plan to live out. But even here there is a comfort zone. Almost certainly there is still a range of sexual acts and contexts that do not fit our sexual self-image. As Lucile said about a threesome: "That's not sex to me, that's some crazy thing." And Vickie wondered about wearing leather, "Is that sex? What is going on?" Yet, Vickie may be able to imagine very comfortably turning her partner on by wearing lacy lingerie that someone who dresses in leather might find totally unappealing. No matter how *normal* we think our own sexual lifestyle is, someone else is likely to say, "That's not sex to me."

Both Maggie's partner and Mary Jo demonstrate that the sexual comfort zone is not as constant as it usually seems. Presented with images of something she had never previously considered doing, Maggie's partner said *I can't do this*. Yet she apparently got used to the idea of lesbian S-M and she joined Maggie in experimenting with this sexual variation.

Mary Jo's statement demonstrates that what we might be comfortable doing at a youthful time in our lives may no longer seem fitting when we become older. And society's mores change, too. There has, for example, been a dramatically changed perspective on sexually transmitted diseases since the advent of AIDS in the 1980s. Mary Jo wistfully regrets she did not have an opportunity to engage in group sex in the 1970s when she was younger and society was more supportive of that kind of experimentation, but she acknowledges that such an experience would not fit into how she views herself now.

She told me, too, about other ways in which she has changed: "In the days when I was experimenting around—I was twenty-three, twenty-two—I once had three guys in one day. But they were three relationships that I was exploring and I did it intentionally because I was feeling wild. They were all relationships that lasted a long time. And two got weeded out and I ended up with one of them. But, at the time, I was seeing all three men and it was very erotic." But twenty years later, Mary Jo reflects: "Unwise, unwise, I don't know why I never caught anything."

Are You Normal?

What is normal, anyway? This question reflects the impossibility of knowing what is *really* going on with other people sexually. What do they *really* do in bed? How do they feel about what they do there? One meaning of normal is: Are you statistically normal? Are you like most other people? Or, at least, are you like most of the people you know? Do you fit into the comfort zone of your peers? Of society? But some of us are slightly rebellious. We want to be *outside* our peers' comfort zone—or, perhaps, outside of our parents' comfort zones or our church's.

Feeling normal, that is, *experiencing* ourselves as normal, has much to do with the norms of our peers. For those in the "leather crowd," wearing tight, black leather corsets may be experienced as normal; but for those who subscribe to the *Victoria's Secret Catalogue*, "normal" might be wearing a flowing negligee of rose-colored silk.

The Importance of Sexuality as a Life Theme

The research underlying this book demonstrates the tremendous range of variation in what may be considered *normal* in how women experience and express their sexuality. There is also a huge variation in the priority women place on sexuality in their lives. For some women, their sexuality is a core life theme. It shapes their lives and often commands nearly all of their attention. For others, such issues as home, school, job security, social relationships, or a spiritual life influence their lives more strongly and occupy their attention more frequently than do sex and their sexuality. Here seven women address the importance of sex in their lives.

Lillian (1905): "My husband and I, surprisingly, had a very good sex relationship. We were both satisfied, and it was very good. I was lucky. I never felt guilty or ashamed or anything as my mother had expected me to. I thought that if you loved your husband, that's what you wanted to do. And luckily I enjoyed it. I looked forward to sex, and so did my husband. We were married fifty-six years, and that continued until about three years before he died. And then he wasn't well. My husband was a wonderful man. And he always thanked me afterwards. And if I didn't feel good, he wouldn't bother me. But I never turned him down, and I never faked an orgasm or anything like that. Sex was maybe three times a week, maybe more often, depending on how he felt. He was a hard worker. In some respects, our sex would be boring to anybody else. But I was happy. And so was my husband."

Katherine (1938): "To me, sex is fun, excitement, love. And it's pretty important to me. I mean, you want to be satisfied, and you also want your partner satisfied. Sex feels good. It relaxes you. And it's good for you. But it's not the ultimate important thing in a marriage. I think it's one of the things. Like, another thing is money."

It's been ten years since **Linda (1940)** has had "any truly sexual involvement, but," she said, "my understanding of sexuality is very different than it was years ago. Today I wouldn't participate in a sexual relationship for the sake of sexual relationship. I see sex in the Taoist way as a way to feed the spirit. A sexual relationship is spiritual. If we use sex in a banal way, a way that is not respectful of the body and one another and the creative gift we're given, then that only takes away from our vital energy. If I evolve to a place where I have sex again, it will be sex in a different way."

Kathy (1949) described herself as "a woman in my mid-forties. I'm a bisexual woman. I'm physically disabled. I use a power wheel-chair. I'm a video producer and editor and performance artist and I have my hands in all kinds of creative stuff. My sexuality fits into just about everything I do. It's a very important part of who I am. I'm considered to be a very flamboyant person. A lot of that is because I'm very sensual in my interactions with people and in the way I dress and in my mannerisms. I think sexuality is a very big part of who I am and I see it as integrated into everything I am. It all over-laps for me, creativity and sexuality and self-expression. I have done a performance show which was specifically about sensuality and dis-ability where I recite poetry I've written. One time I performed on a bed in lingerie and read some of my sensual poetry."

Barbara (1954) said: "I don't know what sex means to me. Sex is there but it doesn't seem to mean as much as it used to. It's not my major concern anymore. Probably there are other things that I want to accomplish. I've been out of a job since March and I'm just kind of getting myself together since then to go on to do something else."

For **Jessica (1970)**, "Sex is not the most important thing in a rela-tionship, but it might be the second or the third. Sex means nice things, because I've had good experiences. Emotions are involved. I like sharing something with another person, the closeness, the physi-cal gratification that you get. Also, I like knowing that person in a dif-ferent way rather than just through talking."

Marybeth (1972) is a student who has not yet engaged in sexual intercourse. She said: "Sexuality doesn't really fit into who I am too much at all, actually. I come from a semi-conservative Roman Catho-lic family. Although I don't go to church all the time, a lot of Roman Catholic beliefs are my beliefs. So I'm a conservative person. And I don't drink and I don't smoke and I don't do drugs. That's me in a nutshell. I've never really dated. I wasn't a particularly dating kind of person in high school because I was a science nerd, or I was always busy, or guys just never asked me out. So I haven't really explored that facet of my life yet; hopefully, in the future I will. I'm waiting to date first, and then fall in love, and then get married, and then do whatever follows that."

These seven women illustrate some of the tremendous variation in what is normal. For women like Kathy, the realm of sexuality is where they live. Kathy's sexuality plays a large part in shaping her life and frequently occupies her attention. Others, like Barbara, rele-gate their sexuality to the back burner when home, school, or job security become issues and need their attention. Linda is primarily concerned with the interrelationship between her spirituality and her sexuality. You will hear more from some of these women in the chapters that follow.

The Sexual Self Is a Lifelong Work in Progress

Sexualities vary not only from person to person, but also over time within the same woman. A woman's sexuality has different meanings for her and is integrated into her life in varying ways as she moves through life's various stages. A woman will experience and express her sexuality differently both throughout her periodic cycles of fertility and at different phases in her life.

In my research I have been particularly interested in these variations and in how they fit within the context of women's lives. I have looked for milestones on the path to sexual womanhood that contribute to a positive sexual self-image, the kinds of things that make sex meaningful and satisfying for some women, and those that detract from sexual well-being and a woman's sense of self. As a result of interviewing women in their eighties and nineties, I now understand that one's sexual self continues to be a work-in-progress throughout our lives. The next four chapters are about the path to sexual womanhood—how we become the sexual women we are. These chapters address the development of the sexual self in childhood and beyond.

What Does This Mean to You?

Now, if you wish, pick up your notebook and express the thoughts and feelings you're having about your sexual self. Here are some questions to consider after you've done that. There are no right or wrong answers. There are only *your* answers. You may wish to respond with just a few words or write page after page. You may feel like drawing or writing poetry. Create a record that expresses what is true for you.

- What is your sexual comfort zone? For example, does it matter to you if your sexual partner is male or female? What about age? Ethnicity? Monogamy? Lovemaking styles? Contraception? Safe-sex practices?

- For most people, their typical personal comfort range is actually fairly narrow relative to the wide range of possibilities that exist. Based on your own responses to these questions, is this true for you?

- What does *feeling* normal mean to you personally? Is that the same as *being* normal?

- How important is the realm of sexuality to you as a life theme?

- If you are recalling experiences that you now regret, consider the circumstances, the roles of others, and how you saw your options at the time. Then, sit quietly with your eyes closed and imagine what you could now gently and lovingly tell your younger self that would be healing and lead to greater self-acceptance.

Part 2

Development: The Path to Sexual Womanhood

2

Sexual Discoveries: Childhood and Beyond

What was your earliest awareness of yourself as sexual? At the time, you may have been too young to have the language and knowledge to call it "sexual." In response to that question the women I interviewed recalled many childhood incidents of experimentation and discovery. Some described solo experiences, some described experiences involving one or more others. For **Ellen (1910)** this question evoked images of a party and the dress she wore: "It was some kind of a party at the high school. I must have been fourteen. And, I had this new dress, red with white polka dots all over." **Ruth (1943)** didn't remember feeling sexual as a child but answered, "I do remember having boyfriends, from when I was in the first grade. I still remember their names." **Sharon (1962)** recalled solo experiences: "I think I've been aware of the sexual part of myself since I was four. I remember waking up and finding myself fondling myself."

Unfortunately, some women were robbed of opportunities to make their own discoveries. **Sara (1949)** told me: "I can't really tell you when I discovered my own sexuality, because it was introduced to me. Because my father was sexual with me when I was very young." But Sara, too, discovered her own capacity for pleasure, although, as she said, "I was a late bloomer."

This chapter is about consensual sexual exploration and experimentation. See chapter 4 for a discussion of the experiences of women who were subjected to early sexual experiences to which they did not consent.

Caution

Unfortunately, few of us have had only pleasant sexual experiences. If you find yourself becoming upset or anxious while recalling some of your experiences, put the sexual questions aside temporarily and consider the following ideas: You may be releasing long-stored feelings. Can you comfortably handle those feelings? If not, would it be better for you to read this book or answer these questions at a time when you can talk about your feelings with a trusted friend, family member, or therapist?

If your distress is related to only one or two incidents, you may find that you will feel more comfortable as you move on to other topics. If you don't begin to feel more comfortable, stop reading and write about your feelings instead. Then, write about what you would need to resolve these issues so at a future time you can return to thinking about these aspects of your sexuality.

Self-Discovery in Childhood

What are your earliest memories of body awareness and self-stimulation for pleasure? For some girls, the first awareness of pleasurable sensations "down there"—of having wonderful, magical, special genital feelings—involved totally innocent discovery uncolored by any parental or social prohibitions. Even if this was not your experience, take a moment now to imagine what it might have been like for you if it had been. How would this have affected your life?

Carole (1930) said: "My first experience of myself as sexual was feeling turned on by my bicycle seat and sitting on fences when I was about six or seven. I remember the feeling and thinking, *Ooooo, this feels good!*

Connie (1956) said: "The first crush I ever had on a man was on Moe of the Three Stooges. I saw him on TV and was just in love with him and his long hair with the bangs. I had this big teddy bear, almost as big as me, and I remember humping this teddy bear at night thinking it was Moe. I remember rubbing my genitals against it. I don't recall if I had orgasms, but it felt great. That's a very clear memory. I couldn't have been more than three years old."

Without words to label the experience, there is no judgment, only curiosity and acceptance. The typical girl, however, develops a sense of privacy around sensuality/sexuality at an early age. For example, **Joan (1944)** recalls: "I used to always like to play with myself. I think the first sexual experience I had was with my dog—a little beagle. I allowed my dog to lick me. *I would lock my door.* So, that was my first masturbation. Or actually sex with something else. I can guess I was five or six."

Awareness of prohibitions alters experience. When a child becomes aware—through the words, facial expressions, and body language of adults—that grown-ups aren't always comfortable with the child's explorations of pleasure, doors are closed, and sometimes impulses are inhibited. This move toward privacy is developmental. It is a normal aspect of a child developing a separate self who can act independently, that is, a normal aspect of individuation.

Finding Our Way Through Shame and Guilt

What do you remember of feeling shame, embarrassment, and guilt in your early childhood? It is likely that these feelings were important in the formation and emergence of your sexual self. Emotions are body reactions that we perceive and label with meaning. Our emotions prepare us to act, or keep us from acting, and they provide us with vital information for our survival and development. None of the emotions—e.g., anger, fear, joy, grief, shame—is inherently bad. We need access to all of them.

Shame and guilt are social emotions. They provide us with awareness of social limits and generate the reluctance or reticence to act outside of those limits. As we are growing up, feelings of shame and of embarrassment (a related feeling) play a significant role in our socialization.

When she is one year old, a little girl begins to walk and move around on her own. She begins to have a sense of—"I"—of self. Consequently, she needs to learn and conform to social rules. She needs to sort out what is okay to do and what is not okay. She is drawn toward autonomy, discovery, and self-esteem, so she tests the limits of the boundaries that parents and others establish. The body-mind responses of doubt and shame mark the *edge* for her. She has to invoke her will to cross that edge. The psychosocial issue of *autonomy* versus *shame* and *doubt* is one of the biggest challenges for the child between one and three years old, as described by developmental psychologist Erik Erikson in the 1950s.

As a girl moves on through childhood, she must confront and resolve over and over again the tensions between her *wish to do* on the one hand and *prohibitions against doing* on the other. Children anticipate adult roles in their fantasies and play and they actively pursue the rules of adulthood.

A predominant psychosocial issue of the three- to six-year-old, as described by Erikson, is the tension between her initiative and the experience of guilt. If her independence is validated, she moves confidently forward. If her autonomy and initiative are denied and her "I" behavior too often punished, doubt and feelings of shame may hold her back. For example, **Sandra (1949)** remembered, "When I was like four to six to eight years old, waking up in the morning and having my genitals feeling tingly and I thought that felt neat. But I didn't touch myself because I remember having that strong message inside, *You can't touch yourself there.*"

That internalized message did not stop Sandra from developing an appreciation of the pleasure to be found in her genital sensations; she did, however, learn to keep her appreciation secret. "Another time when I was six or seven, my younger sister and I got all sandy and dirty at the beach, and so we had to go into the showers and rinse off quick. It was freezing cold. We put on our jeans without any underwear and I remember how the rough fabric felt against my genitals. I had never felt that before and I thought it was *neat.* It was really special and it was a secretive type of feeling."

It was Sandra's *secret*, a secret almost all of us discover at some time or another. Sandra was, of course, not doing anything "bad" or "naughty." She was discovering the wonderful, *neat*, secret place of pleasure that was hers—a part of her self-ness. She was acquiring another bit of knowledge of her sexual self, although she did not realize it at the time. She also probably did not realize that those apparently disapproving adults had their own wonderful, neat, secret places of pleasure, too.

Can I act from my own will and still be loved and accepted? This is one of the dilemmas of the young child. Some girls perceive the reactions of important adults as so negative that their impulses to self-stimulate for pleasure are completely squelched—at least for a time, as they were for the woman who noted on her Survey questionnaire: "I remember masturbating at four or five, but I probably stopped because of my mother scolding. I don't remember doing it after that until I was twenty-four." Her urge to explore was inhibited, for a time. But later, it reemerged. Her path to knowledge of her sexual self took a very different route than Sandra's.

Self-Acceptance

As adults, when we experience shame or guilt, we can understand that these emotions mean that we are breaking some internalized rule. As adults we can consider: Whose rule is it? Where did I get it? Does it make sense for me to follow it? The young child is too limited in experience to have such a vantage point. Consider how **Roberta (1943)** changed her view over time: "When I was real young—I think we were between four and seven—my brother and some neighborhood kids played doctor and stuff. I remember we explored each other's bodies. At the time that I did it, it was just exploratory, but, over time, I was ashamed of it. Now, I think it's just part of growing up."

In this very brief description, Roberta leads us through the critically important process of finding one's way to self-acceptance. From the young girl's perspective, she engaged in innocent exploration. Later, she became aware of social prohibitions and felt shame. Still later, she understood that body exploration is just part of growing up and she felt okay about what had occurred. That's just how it was.

Many of us grow up with a sense of shame about our curiosity-driven early experiences of sexual exploration and experimentation, because we have no way of knowing that so many others are having these experiences, too. The many, many examples in this chapter demonstrate how typical—how normal—most of these experiences are.

Early Discoveries of Orgasm

Virtually all of us have impulses in infancy and early childhood to stimulate our own genitals. How we perceive adult reactions when we act on these impulses at this stage of life appears to be critical. If we learn privacy, but are not too inhibited by our interpretations of what adults want, we continue to self-pleasure and, sooner rather than later, we may discover orgasm.

If we take apparent parental disapproval to mean "just don't let them catch you" and then continue our explorations, a bit of individuation will have occurred. With a clear sense of identity—of self separate from parents—we may feel somewhat guilty, but we just won't get caught next time. Sometimes, a girl reacts to parental prohibitions by taking self-pleasuring undercover, or, more accurately, under the covers. **Josephine (1913)** said: "I masturbated when I was four or five but my mother said I should keep my hands on the outside of the covers, so I knew it was forbidden. Still, I did it. Masturbation went on my whole life here and there. I had orgasms with masturbation very early, when I was about seven or eight." (Notice how often in these examples women give an early age as one of several, e.g., "seven or eight." This pattern is strong evidence that our memories are not precise as to exactly when these kinds of experiences took place.)

Even though the experience of orgasm is discovered at an early age, it may remain private well into young adulthood, as it did for **Susan (1958).** "I first played with myself when I was pretty young, eight or nine. I remember my mother coming in and catching me. She said that I shouldn't do that, and I said, 'Well if I shouldn't do it, why is it there?' It didn't make a lot of sense, because it was so accessible. Later, orgasm just kind of happened, *because the more you rub, the better it feels, and the better it feels, the more you do it, and then it just happens.* Still, my orgasms were private. I didn't let myself have an orgasm with a partner, a man, until I was twenty."

Each of us is unique in our sexual self-development. There is wisdom in Susan's acquired understanding that *the more you rub, the better it feels, and the better it feels, the more you do it, and then it just happens.* This discovery can be made in early childhood or not until much later.

Learning from Others: Explorations with Friends

Learning about genital pleasure and orgasm isn't just a solo activity. It also takes place in the company of friends. From childhood to late in life, information and permission from peers can be powerful facilitators of sexual exploration and experimentation. For example, **Cecile (1952)** said that her first sexual education occurred in first grade: ". . . through a girl who told me that if I climbed the tether ball pole in the school yard and squeezed, that it would feel really good. So I was climbing every pole I could find. I was climbing the clothesline. I was climbing the Stop signs, just going crazy with little mini-orgasms. And then I graduated to wrapping my legs around each other and elevating myself between two places—the kitchen sink, between two chairs—so that my legs were free and hanging. I would do this in school when there were other children around. I would be making these little mini-orgasms at home when there were other people around but they didn't know what I was doing and I knew that they didn't know what I was doing. It was my little secret."

When **Maggie (1965)** was five or six she had a "windmill lamp you could unscrew, and it had a little metal thing on the end. And I remember my best friend and me playing doctor and inserting it in each other. It was definitely pleasurable."

Pam (1968) remembered that "In first and second grade, I used to play sexual games with my best girlfriend. We'd sit in the hot tub and play Truth or Dare. She'd say, 'Run over on the deck and pose like a *Playboy* model.' We never touched each other sexually, but it would be like, 'Touch your right breast and put your finger on your vagina.' And we would look at ourselves with mirrors. I remember her having a very different looking vagina than I did and being very curious about that. We never talked about any of this later when we were older, but when we were young we did it a lot."

At some time or another in our growing up, many of us have some kind of exploratory experience—impelled by our curiosity—with one or several others. If we are fortunate, we are not harmed and what we learn is essentially beneficial to our developing sexual selves.

Shame and Guilt in Exploring with Others

As with solo activity, even when we aren't discovered, our already internalized parental values may lead us to imagine what will happen if our parents do find out. Or an inner voice may say, *You shouldn't do that.* For example, **Peg (1948)** remembered "a tremendous amount of guilt and shame for sexual experimentation—touching each other—with my brother and a neighbor girl when I was six and they were seven. I felt a tremendous amount of shame, not because my mother found out about it, but just because if she *did* find out about it, I would probably be sent to Antarctica or burned at the stake."

When **Angela (1971)** was four or five, all of her playmates were boys. She said, "I wished this one neighbor boy could be my brother. He was kind of my little boyfriend. We would play doctor and other stuff. We liked to take off our clothes and lock ourselves in the bathroom and just hang out there and then put our clothes back on. We kind of had the feeling that *you shouldn't do that.*"

But there are mysteries to solve. *How are boys different from girls?* is a major source of fascination. We see how, as a girl moves through childhood, she must confront and resolve the tensions between her own wish to do and social prohibitions against doing over and over again. In testing the limits of the boundaries her parents and others establish, she must invoke her will to cross the edge marked by feelings of doubt, shame, and guilt.

Some women I interviewed related memories of their mothers' actual reactions to their childhood expressions of curiosity with friends and siblings. For example, **Monica (1940)** said, "I remember having sexual feelings, genital feelings, by age four. When I was four or five, the little boy next door wanted to play doctor, and his idea of this was that we showed each other our genitals. Then he would dig a hole and he would pee in it and I watched. My mother was very upset. She was angry and talked to his mother about it."

If Monica and her playmate were equally curious, about the same age, and neither was coercing the other to participate, their play was probably a useful exchange of information and more helpful than harmful. I can imagine circumstances under which I might be concerned, however. These would include, for example, if either Monica or her playmate was physically hurting the other or if they were engaging in this kind of play obsessively day after day.

Victoria (1946) provides another example of a girl whose mother intervened when she was playing exploratory games. "I became sexual at a very early age, around six, with a little neighbor boy. I didn't know the word 'sex.' I was raised Irish Catholic and sex wasn't part of the scene. We got nude and played with each other. My mother found out and handled it very gently and sweetly, sitting down and talking to me, looking at me, being really quiet. And not yelling. The message was that it wasn't right, it wasn't good, it was sinful."

It wasn't right, it wasn't good, it was sinful. This is one aspect of a theme deeply embedded in traditional religious teachings of our culture—a very strong social prohibition against doing. In finding our way to sexual selfhood, we move toward exploration and self-development, including sexual self-development. At the same time we continue to be influenced by the external values and limits imposed by the society in which we live, our families, our peer subculture, and the other important people in our lives.

First Experiences of Self-Stimulation and Orgasm

There is tremendous variability in the age when women first experience purposeful self-stimulation for pleasure. Some Survey respondents remembered engaging in intentional self-stimulation long before they ever heard the word "masturbation." Others either didn't remember childhood self-pleasuring or did not wish to give information about it.

Of the 2,284 women who gave the age at which they first intentionally stimulated their genitals while alone, 9 percent had done so by age five, 32 percent by age ten, 56 percent by age fourteen, 81 percent by age twenty, and 95 percent by age thirty. Nine percent of *all* Survey respondents indicated that they had never masturbated, and 4 percent didn't answer the question.

Of the 2,448 women who gave an age of first orgasm, 4 percent had experienced orgasm by age five, 16 percent by age ten, 33 percent by age fourteen, 76 percent by age twenty, and 98 percent by age thirty. Thirty-eight respondents said they had never experienced orgasm, and ninety-five others weren't sure.

It fascinates me to compare our findings with those of Katharine Davis and her colleagues (1929) who asked 1,000 unmarried women about orgasms in 1921-1923. They found that "the experience of the orgasm in nearly 62 percent of the cases does not occur until eighteen years or over" (p. 113). In the Ellison/Zilbergeld Survey, the findings were virtually the same: 61.32 percent of the respondents were eighteen or over when they had their first orgasm!

My First Orgasm Occurred Spontaneously

An event that occurs spontaneously is actually the outcome of one thing leading to another. When we are going through the little steps of experience that get us there, we may not even be aware that such an outcome is possible. Nearly half (44 percent) of the women who had experienced orgasm said that their first orgasm occurred spontaneously. Some explained how it happened:

♀ While rubbing with my clothing on; ♀ Moving against my P.J.'s; ♀ By masturbation, but at age seven I didn't know what that was; ♀ I was touching myself and it just happened; ♀ I was twelve, rubbing or rocking against my pillow in my bed on a Saturday morning; ♀ While toweling myself; ♀ On the playground, shimmying up the swing set; ♀ Riding a horse; ♀ From a dream.

I continue to be amazed at the tremendous variety in how we learn about the various aspects of our sexuality.

My First Orgasm Occurred When I Was Trying to Have One

First orgasms for 29 percent of the respondents occurred when they were trying to have one: ♀ I didn't know to call it an orgasm, however, it just felt good! ♀ I had read *For Yourself* (Barbach 1975) and was using a vibrator for the purpose of discovering orgasm; ♀ I was trying to achieve "something," I didn't know what; I'm not sure I knew what to call it; I was ten.

Later in this chapter, you will find more about *For Yourself* and other books that influenced our consciousness about women's pleasure, masturbation, and orgasms.

My First Orgasm Surprised Me

Nearly two out of three of the respondents, 62 percent, were surprised by their first orgasm. Some explained: ♀ My first orgasm *with a man* surprised me; ♀ I hadn't known what to expect; I was moved; ♀ I didn't know what it was; ♀ I realized this was "it;" ♀ My first orgasm that I identified as an orgasm surprised me.

Pam (1968) in her interview, when questioned about her first orgasm, said, "I didn't have an orgasm 'til my first year in college. It was the first time anyone had oral sex with me. And all of a sudden, *Holy shit, what is going on in my body?* And I thought, *This is what they mean.* I had touched myself before, but I thought I would maybe mature into orgasm. I guess I just thought the self-affirming rush I experienced with all the many, many boys in high school was it. After I learned what an orgasm was with this boyfriend, I learned to bring myself to orgasm."

More Survey respondents reported that their first orgasm occurred during sexual activity with a partner than said their first orgasm occurred by themselves. Some mentioned manual stimulation by her partner, cunnilingus, petting, and foreplay; one noted that her first orgasm occurred spontaneously during sexual intercourse. Among the written-in notes were the following comments:

♀ My first orgasm was during a dream about my husband; ♀ My first orgasm was by myself, my first *intense* orgasm was with a partner; ♀ My first orgasms were in my sleep in my late teens. I didn't' know what they were but I felt guilty; ♀ My first orgasm was with a woman; ♀ My first *fun* orgasm was with a partner; I was seventeen and totally in love with my beau.

My First Orgasm Frightened Me

Something happening in one's body that is totally unexpected and never experienced before can be scary. The sensations of their first orgasm frightened 11 percent of the respondents. Some added the following comments:

♀ More guilty than frightened, I was nine; ♀ I was perplexed; ♀ I thought something "broke" inside me; ♀ I thought I was peeing at the time, so I was a bit embarrassed and anxious about that, not exactly frightened.

For some women the feelings were too foreign or too frightening to enjoy. For example, **Donna (1949)** said, "I had my first orgasm as a result of petting in junior high school, but I didn't know it and it was such a strange feeling that I rebelled against it. *Oh, I don't like that feeling. Let's stop. Forget it.* And that went on for the longest time through my first real boyfriend. He had to tell me, *'This is an orgasm, this is what you're supposed to be feeling.'* But to me it was a tingly feeling that just didn't feel good . . . like when your leg falls asleep. The other part was just the unknown. I think my subconscious had set up a *'No'* to it . . . to saying I was sexual. Until Jon, the man I've been with the last few years, I didn't achieve orgasms very easily. It got easier as I got older, into my thirties, and now that I'm forty-three, I enjoy them."

In a different context, **Teresa (1946)** experienced genital stirrings and her first orgasm in response to the sexual energy of her parents; she found the feelings overwhelming. Her family was poor and lived in a very small house. She said, "I was very young, not even in high school, but I had started my period, and one time I heard my mother and father having sex, and I had what I know now is an orgasm. I got sexual feelings hearing them, but I didn't identify them as such, and it was too much for me to handle because I didn't know what it was. I wasn't touching myself; I was actually trying not to hear them and had my hands over my ears."

Teresa's parents were both alcoholics and often had violent fights. It is not unusual for a child in such chaotic circumstances to be hyperalert and to attune herself to her parents' energies in order to monitor that she and they are safe. As Teresa's narrative demonstrates, sometimes children will resonate not only with violence, but with their parents' sexual energies as well.

You will find more about how women create and experience orgasm, as well as more about spontaneous orgasms without physical stimulation, in chapters 10 and 11. If you have not yet experienced orgasm, or are not sure, and this is an experience you wish to have, you will find useful information in those chapters.

Critical Periods for Orgasmic Responsiveness

In human maturation and development, a "critical period" is a limited time during which some aspect of the developing individual is particularly open to influences that can bring about specific and permanent changes. It could be called "the window of opportunity." There is, for example, a critical period during which we can learn language with relative ease. In analyzing the interviews and questionnaire data, I have concluded that there also is a critical period—or actually there are two critical periods—with respect to developing orgasmic responsiveness. One of these is early childhood, the other occurs during adolescence.

Early life self-pleasuring is one of the ways we prepare for adult sexual responsiveness. In childhood, some of us become comfortable with our early impulses for genital self-pleasuring and continue to act on them; others are influenced to postpone acting on them until later in life. Like other developmental impulses, these reemerge at various times to be explored again. New opportunities to experience orgasm are particularly likely to occur during important life transitions—the hormonal shift into puberty, for example, and at the time of first sexual experimentation with a partner. Impulses to experiment also may be reawakened by new information or upon receiving permission from a book or friend.

We have opportunities over and over throughout our lives to replay and work out dynamic developmental issues—*to find our way*. However, that which seems spontaneous and natural in childhood or when we are entering puberty may require conscious effort and present some difficulty when we are older. Yet, as long as we remain able to move and continue to feel sensation, we can learn more about our bodies and genital pleasure if we wish—even into our eighties, as you will see before this chapter ends.

Middle Childhood and Early Teens

The physical transition from girlhood to adulthood is not an abrupt one. Typically, a girl's ovaries begin producing the hormone estrogen before she is ten, several years before her first menstrual period. Under the influence of estrogen, a girl's body gradually changes from that of a child to that of a young woman. Curves appear where there were none before, breasts bud and develop, pubic and underarm hair begin to grow. By the time the girl has her first menstruation—which may occur as early as age eight or nine or, for some, not until ages sixteen or seventeen—irregular hormonal cycling has already been influencing her body, moods, and biorhythms for a year or more. Hormones have begun to trigger sexual thoughts and images.

For **Kathy (1949)** it began when she was around eleven. "I was watching *Gunsmoke* and I found myself feeling really warm between the legs. I felt like I needed something inside of me. I found my stepmother's douche in the bathroom and experimented with that. That was the first time I had this wave of 'I need something.' It was probably the first time I actually ovulated, because I started having periods around that time."

Beth (1961) remembers getting her first bra in sixth grade. "I thought that was really big, like *Wow, I am becoming a woman!* I can remember always running in my room and lifting my shirt up and looking at myself. I remember feeling different and special." **Marcy (1967)** carefully watched the growth of her body. "I was becoming a woman and sometimes I would like what I saw and sometimes I wouldn't like what I saw." **Pam (1968)** noted: "In adolescence my body changed completely, so that seventh grade was really difficult—braces, frizzy hair, acne, the message from my gymnastics coach was, 'You've got to go on a diet.'"

Pam was not overweight according to any accepted health standards. Essentially, her gymnastics coach wanted her to diet and keep her body immature so that it would be closer to an ideal shape for gymnastics. The message from her coach was: *It's not okay to fill out and add the body fat that signifies you are physically becoming a sexually mature woman.* And, indeed, if a maturing young woman can keep herself thin enough, she won't have the body fat to support estrogen production and cycles of fertility. At some sacrifice to her health and emotional well-being, she will keep herself sexually immature.

What do you recall of your physical metamorphosis at puberty? Puberty is one of the most dramatic of life's transitions. It is a time in which we must make all kinds of adjustments to having a new body. Later we will acquire a new body at other times, for example, during pregnancy, at menopause, and after major surgeries.

Self-Stimulation and Orgasm in the Teen Years

Of the women in our Survey, about half who had ever masturbated and 60 percent who had ever experienced orgasm did so for the first time in the decade between the ages of ten and twenty. These are the years I consider to be the second critical period for girls' development of orgasmic responsiveness. Surely this emergence of sexuality in the teen years is related to the hormones that change a girl into a woman and arouse in her sexual interest, desire, and the readiness for sexual activity.

In addition to these biological changes an adolescent girl has access to more sources of information and more variety in value systems than a younger child does. The adolescent is in the process of separating as an individual from her family. She may experience more social or peer acceptance for self-stimulation than she did when she was younger. She may even experience parental acceptance if her parents are among those who provide books that promote self-pleasuring.

Even in the era when masturbation was said to grow hair on your palms or cause you to go blind, there were proponents of sexuality-affirming sex education. In 1929, Mary Ware Dennett wrote:

> In the new education, the scientific truth about masturbation will be told. The fact that there is no sound evidence that any physiological harm results from ordinary masturbation, but only psychological harm—and that due solely to the person's own feelings of wrongdoing—has already reached the knowledge of many young people, but nothing like the majority.

Some of the oldest women I interviewed reported discovering masturbation and orgasm in the years they were growing up. **Hilda (1915)** said, "I discovered masturbation—and orgasm—sometime in high school when I was fourteen or fifteen." And **Ann (1934)** said, "I discovered masturbation in high school. That's when I discovered orgasm and also that orgasm could relieve menstrual cramps. I could reach orgasm whenever I wanted to. I don't know how I learned about it but I'm sure my mother didn't tell me."

Probably, almost none of us can imagine when we are young that the women who preceded us were as open and knowledgeable about sex as we are. I suspect that each new generation thinks that they have made discoveries about sex and sexuality that their parents' generation did not know. In the 1970s, when I first began teaching human sexuality courses, the idea that masturbation might relieve menstrual cramps was presented as a new idea, but Ann already knew this in the late 1940s.

Solving Some Mysteries

Sexual decision making is an ongoing aspect of our development. The narratives that follow dramatically portray certain aspects in the formation of one's sexual self-image. Two developmental questions stand out:

1. *How do you do this?* which also includes *Am I doing this right?* and

2. *Should I be doing this at all?*

I Don't Think I'm Doing This Right!

While we are growing up there is a lot about the doing of sex that is hidden. Even how to stimulate oneself for pleasure may seem like a mystery to be solved. *There must be some right way, but what is it?* **Jessica (1970)** first tried masturbating when she was sixteen, in high school: "It was my first time to try ... so I didn't really know what my feelings were. I kept wondering, *Am I doing it right? What's going to happen?* I touched my breasts mainly. That was pretty much it for the first time." **Kirsten (1970)** first masturbated during her junior year in college, when she was twenty, ". . . after I found out from other people that people did that. I was just exploring to see what it was like. I took off all my clothes in my little dorm room and just started rubbing my breasts and my clitoris. The first time, I didn't know if I was doing it right. I didn't achieve orgasm or anything. I'm pretty confident that I wasn't doing it right. I felt kind of inept that I hadn't been doing that and other people had. I had to experience it for myself."

As girls seek answers to their questions about technique, they also wonder about the values that surround these behaviors.

Should I Be Doing This?

As we experience again and again the tension between the urge to do and explore and the urge to conform and keep the approval of those who are important to us, we are likely to wonder *Should I be doing this?* Because our parents may have one set of values, our peers another, our religion a third, and the books and magazines we read still more, we may have to consider conflicting views as we try to determine our own.

For **Deanna (1971)**, "It was just one time—about the same time that I got my period. I was fourteen. I just kind of rubbed my vaginal area, outside of my clothes. I didn't put my hands in. I guess I felt kind of bad about doing it. It was late at night. My feelings were, *Should I be doing this? I'm not sure.* I was kind of questioning myself why I was doing this: *Is this right or wrong?*"

The emerging urge to masturbate can in itself be confusing because it's so new, so unlike "the *me* I've known up to now." **Andrea (1972)** related in her interview that she first masturbated during her senior year of high school ". . . when I started reading a lot of adult romance novels, fictions that just sort of just happen to have very explicit sex scenes in them. It was largely an imagination thing. Just reading along, you'd sort of feel things and touch yourself while you're reading, sort of for two or three minutes as you go through that part. And then you'd just keep reading from there. At first I was little bit nervous, like, *This is a little weird.* The first time after it happened I was kind of like, *Now why did I do that?* I didn't really feel like it was wrong, just from everything I'd learned before, so it wasn't a shameful feeling. It was more that I just hadn't really thought I'd needed that before."

Finding Our Way in the Teen Years

There are many parallels during the junior high and high school years to sexual self-discovery in early childhood. Suppression of sexual exploration can occur in adolescence, just as it can for young children. For example, Penny's urges to explore her new adolescent feelings were squelched in her early teens by the presence of her mother, described in her interview as "very intrusive and inside my boundaries." Later, away from her mother, she got another chance to find her way to self-pleasuring and orgasm. **Penny (1946)** put it this way:

> I discovered masturbation my second year in high school. I was always curious about sex and I was a horny little thing even though I'd never had sex. Masturbation just sort of happened in bed one night. I was moving my hips around, having sexual feelings. I'm not even sure I was touching myself with my hands. After I'd only done this a couple of times, my mother almost caught me. She came in the room and said, "What are you doing in here?" And I went, "Ah-hh-hh [sharply draws in and holds breath, and then says, very tightly:] Nothing." Mom had antennae—ears and eyes in the back of her head. And I didn't do it again until I left home. When I was eighteen, a freshman in college, my roommate told me how good it felt to roll a pair of socks into a ball and use that on her genital area. Of course I tried it right away.

Can I act from my own will and still be loved and accepted? is a dilemma of the young child that follows us into adulthood. Penny perceived her mother's reactions as so negative that her impulses to self-stimulate for pleasure were completely squelched until she left her mother's home.

Considering variety in experience, we see how different sexual-self development was for **Mary Jo (1947)** whose adolescent urge to explore not only was not blocked, but was encouraged in her home environment. A home where adults are comfortable with their own sexuality and are clear about sexual boundaries may safely contain a young girl's—or a teen's—experimentation and discoveries. Mary Jo said, "For some reason I figured out the vibrator thing. My parents had a vibrator around the house—not the ones that look like dildoes, those other ones—and so, from the time I was thirteen or fourteen on, I was having orgasms, which meant I was used to pretty regular orgasms before I was with any man. And it wasn't much to translate that into intercourse when I was eighteen."

If you sought to solve the mysteries of sexuality by looking for what your parents (or parent) might have hidden—or perhaps not hidden—you are not alone. If within the boundaries of home we feel more or less safe to explore, most of us will do that at some time or another. **Bonnie (1966),** nearly twenty years younger than Mary Jo, also discovered her parents' vibrator. She started "masturbating and having orgasms with the vibrator Mom and Dad had" when she was "around ten, eleven, or twelve."

Acquiring Language

Another important aspect of our sexual development is learning the words to name and label our experiences. Here we consider some of the consequences of naming our experiences.

Erotic Experiences Without Words

We have already heard from some women who, as girls, had erotic experiences before they had the language to define or name them. There were many others. Comments like **Marsha's (1940)** were not uncommon: "I was seven or eight when I began touching myself by rubbing myself against the bedsheets and I must have had some orgasmic experiences. But I didn't put two and two together. I didn't learn to touch myself to masturbate or that I could create orgasms deliberately with my hands until I was fifteen, after I'd had my first petting experiences early on in high school."

Mary Jo (1947) got a horse when she was about eleven years old: "I remember riding around on him. And the difference between sexuality and feeling good physically, you know, like feeling like an animal with your body, it's a strange, a funny shift. I remember mostly when I was with that horse it was not sexual, but later it became the rhythm and all that. At the beginning you don't exactly know what all this is."

One Survey respondent **(1964)** was thirteen, fantasizing, when she had her first orgasm, but only "... discovered later that these good feelings I was making myself have were orgasms. I think I was in my twenties when I finally understood what had happened."

As children, we solve the mysteries of our sexual responsiveness one step at a time. Marsha's rubbing against her sheets, for example, laid down a foundation of understanding before she had adult language or concepts to explain to herself what she was experiencing; petting with a high school partner added new experiences and understanding; further self-pleasuring then added more.

Naming Experiences

When we have an experience without the words to name it, we have body sensations together with the feelings and images that accompany those sensations, but we don't have to deal much with society's values and prohibitions. But attach a label—like the word *masturbation*—or *bad*, or *naughty*, or *disgusting*—and suddenly all the values, judgments, myths, and other bits of information that we connect to this word become attached to the experience. In a sense, there is an end of innocence. Verbal language is another vehicle—in addition to the nonverbal responses of adults—through which naive curiosity and interest come face to face with embarrassment, shame, and guilt.

Emily (1919) exemplifies the tension we experience over and over throughout our lives between how much we enjoy doing something and what we have been told about the dangers or the wrongness of doing it:

Around age eight I accidentally discovered that touching my clitoris—I didn't know the name at the time—could be fun. One night my nightie crept up and somehow my hand just touched my genitals and I wanted to explore further. Soon I had discovered orgasms. Although my parents had never mentioned masturbation, I somehow knew it was a no-no. I was careful that they didn't find out about it. I had a very strong drive to masturbate, but when it was over I would swear off it like an alcoholic swears off drink after a binge. I began to hear things as I got older like I would go blind or crazy, all of those negative myths. I didn't really think I'd go crazy but I had such strong guilt that I would swear off. But then the urge would return because it was such a pleasure.

Chris (1970) shows us that a label also may bring naive curiosity and interest face to face with positive recognition and acceptance:

When I was probably six or seven—it was always in my bed, usually in the mornings—I had a teddy bear that I would hold really tightly between my legs and squeeze and kick my legs—like putting pressure specifically on your vulva area. I didn't usually use my hands, although sometimes I would feel my breasts. It didn't feel wrong or bad or anything like that, especially because I don't think that I knew what to label it until much later. As I got older, there was a little bit of embarrassment around it and I sort of had this feeling that I didn't want anyone to walk in. But it never felt like something wrong. It wasn't until later that I really knew, *Oh, so that's what I was doing.* And then there was much feeling like it was normal and natural and all that.

Without a label, the response is not to the idea, but to the direct experience: *This is interesting; it feels good; touching there is fun.* But, as Emily said, "I began to hear things as I got older, like I would go blind or crazy, all of these negative myths." Chris, on the other hand, had learned that "it was normal and natural and all that."

A label also may elicit an *Oh, my God!* reaction that squelches excitement and leads, at least temporarily, to not accepting some aspect of one's sexual self. **Allison (1971)** demonstrates that sometimes years can pass between having an experience and naming it: "When I was in first or second grade, my best girlfriend and I would go in the van parked in the front driveway and touch ourselves. Not each other, but at the same time. And then we would come out. And that was it. We didn't even take our pants off. I just rubbed my hand on my clitoris. I didn't understand what I was doing, and I didn't know why I was doing it. I don't even think an orgasm came of it. It was just something that felt good. I guess it would be called masturbation. I never even realized until about a year ago even what it was, and that I had actually done it. And then I thought back and, *Oh my God!*"

Oh my God! Even though nearly fifteen years had passed before Allison linked her experience with the word "masturbation," the moment of realization zapped her with a wave of shocked shame and judgment.

Was it really masturbation? Some might say yes, some would say no. Not all of us use words that we apply to aspects of sex and sexuality in the same ways. In this instance, however, it's not important that we refine our definition. It is important to notice the consequences of translating "we went in the van and touched ourselves" —a phrase that describes action or process—into the label that calls it a name: "It was masturbation." For Allison, the word "masturbation" was loaded with meanings and associations.

For **Maggie (1965)**, this word was so loaded that for years she resisted applying it to what she was doing: "After I had my first orgasm with my female partner when I was nineteen, I started masturbating with a vibrator, which I still do. I never brought myself to orgasm with my hands. And I never called it *masturbating*. I would say, *I used my vibrator*. Only in the last year would I even say I *masturbated*."

Labels Are Links to Information

Labels are not only links to the judgments and values of our peers, parents, and society, they are also links to their acquired wisdom and knowledge. Knowing what to call experience is useful. We can look a word up in the dictionary, look for books that satisfy our curiosity, ask others what a word means, and exchange information about experiences. If the word isn't in the dictionary, that, too, teaches us something.

Deborah (1949) described what happened after she met and danced with a "really nice young man" while at Disneyland with her family when she was twelve years old: "I was very, very shy and not really into boys much yet. Once I was home again, I was thinking about him, and I must have been touching myself, because it felt so good and I had this really spontaneous, wonderful feeling. Looking back, I know that was an orgasm and that I was masturbating. But it kind of caught me by surprise. I didn't know how to recreate that wonderful feeling. I thought it was thinking about him that had caused it, not my hand. After that, I didn't get into masturbating until I was twenty and happened to read *The Sensuous Woman* ["J" 1969], which a roommate had lying around."

When we are young, the learning process is often one of finding our way *from the experience to the words* linked to it. When we are older, we know more concepts and words and may, quite literally, want *to flesh out their meanings through body experiences*, as Deborah did after she read *The Sensuous Woman*. **Madeline (1915)** also was much further into adulthood when she did this: "I don't know if I even knew there was such a word as 'masturbation' as a child . . . maybe I heard about it by other names, like 'playing with yourself.' But as an ongoing sexual practice that adults were involved in—it was like homosexuality—it never occurred to me that there was such a thing. In a college psych course I began to hear about homosexuality and masturbation as something that adults did. And it was news to me! I thought masturbation was just something little kids did that they weren't supposed to. But it had nothing to do with me, until I finally decided way long and far down the line, when I was fifty, sixty years old, that maybe I should try it, and I did just to see what it was about. I thought, *People talk about this all the time and I should figure that out.* My work at that time was counseling students at the university, and they talked about it. So I did it, and it was okay. It was all right."

Lori (1969) was much younger. "I was seventeen, housesitting for some people, and I was just by myself. And I thought that I would give it a shot. I was in the living room, and I was kind of sitting upright, and I just used my hands—just as if you would have sex, kind of doing the old rhythmic insertion into the vagina. It was fine, it was pleasant. It was something that nobody discussed before, so afterwards I didn't know what to think about it. I wasn't positive that real people actually did this."

Of course, real people do actually do this. Almost everyone, at some time or another, in the quest to understand their own potential for sexual arousal and pleasure, will do personal exploration.

Deliberate Exploration of Self-Pleasuring

The deliberate exploration of self-pleasuring is another parallel in the teen years to sexual self-discovery in early childhood. Just as some girls do at a younger age, adolescent girl-women embark on a quest to understand the sensations and pleasure potential of masturbation. By the time they are teens, girls are more likely to know concepts and words and be seeking to *flesh out* their meanings, while at the same time their rapidly changing bodies are presenting them with new sensations and the readiness to experience sexual feelings. **Mindy (1965)** was fourteen, new to high school, when, she said, "I consciously knew that that's what I was doing, and for what purpose. I'd read some book that my mom had about masturbation and how to touch yourself, and this was my own personal experimentation. That I could potentially make myself feel this way—Oh, wow! I don't think I was orgasmic then. I remember saying, *Oh this feels really good.*"

Melanie's (1970) first masturbation experience was just before she began her freshman year of high school. She said:

> When you're young, you hear talk about masturbation and sex and all this, but you don't really understand what it means. I had just finished going to the bathroom, and there were just these feelings that I was having, sort of urges, and I went to get a mirror. I was sitting on the toilet, my legs were open, and I put the mirror down there, just kind of looking around. I'd never really looked at it before, and I just started touching the clitoris area, just a soft rubbing motion. And it felt really good. I didn't orgasm, but my heart was just pounding. I was just like, *Oh my God, this is really weird.* After a couple of minutes, I put the mirror away, and went back into my room, thinking only about that: *Just exactly what was that? What was I doing?* It was kind of confusing. . . . I wasn't sure why I was having all these strange feelings I'd never had before. After that first experience, it took me about six months to figure out exactly what I was doing and to know what to do to make it work good. I'd guess I was first orgasmic with masturbation when I was fourteen or fifteen. But it was very secretive. I didn't really feel guilty about it, but it seemed really powerful to me. There would be certain times that I would have to do this, and I would carry around a little compact mirror. It was like I wanted to watch. I still do this every so often, but I know what it is now, and it's normal; it's not quite as secretive and weird.

Personal explorations of pleasure in adolescence are typically private and secret, although friends do exchange information. Frequently, feelings of pleasure are accompanied by at least a twinge of confusion, shame, embarrassment, or guilt.

Self-Acceptance

An aspect of finding our way to sexual pleasure free of shame and embarrassment is gathering information and various bits of experience and, one step at a time, putting them all together. These become integrated into our sexual self-image. The more informed we are, the clearer our values become and the easier it is to make sexual decisions. There are many paths to self-acceptance. Cynthia reveals to us some of the steps she went through as she grew into understanding and acceptance of her capacity for sexual pleasure. For **Cynthia (1954)**, who started to masturbate when she was sixteen, it was acceptance from another that freed her to accept herself and her own experiences: "I felt embarrassed and ashamed about masturbation even though it felt so good and I loved the orgasms. But when I was eighteen I became close to a girl in school and she told me that she masturbated, too. I was so relieved. No more shame or embarrassment. I'm not the kind of person who'll go out and get a book or somehow else find out what's okay or normal. I needed to hear from this other person that masturbation was okay."

Changing Sexual Mores

There have always been some people with positive attitudes about sex and sexuality who have been accepting of masturbation for pleasure and the relief of sexual tension. Katharine Davis wrote about the prevalence of masturbation at length in her 1929 book; so did Alfred Kinsey, et al. in *Sexual Behavior in the Human Female* (1953). The number of thinkers and writers who openly accepted this practice—particularly for women—progressively increased throughout the twentieth century until the 1970s. Then, in the mid-1970s three important books irreversibly shifted the national consciousness. Betty Dodson's *Liberating Masturbation: A Meditation on Self-Love* (1974), Lonnie Barbach's *For Yourself* (1975) (dedicated to "all women who want to develop their sexual and nonsexual potential"), and *The Hite Report* (1976) *encouraged* women to use masturbation to teach themselves about pleasure and orgasm. Betty Dodson, Lonnie Barbach and Shere Hite didn't just give women permission to masturbate; they *advocated* the practice.

It was clear from our Survey, however, that not all women who had ever been orgasmic learned through masturbation. Forty-seven percent said their first orgasms were by themselves, but 53 percent said their first orgasms were during sexual activity with a partner. In addition, there were 164 more women who said they had experienced orgasm than there where who said that they had ever masturbated.

Women Who First Masturbated After the Age of Seventy

Although virtually all of the participants in our research who had ever been orgasmic had reached their first orgasm by age fifty, sixteen Survey respondents and several women I interviewed did not intentionally masturbate until they were older than fifty. **Lillian (1905)** was seventy-six the first time she tried it. When I interviewed her, she told me: "There were a few years before my husband died when he wasn't able to have sex anymore; that's when I first masturbated a couple of times. One of my girl friends (a woman about my age, widowed) said do that if you get too lonely. I can talk to her about anything. But then I said, *This is silly*. So I said, *Just cut it out*. So I didn't do that anymore. I didn't like it. I just felt guilty. You know, I think it's the upbringing, it's so strict on morals and things like that. A bit of it still lingers."

It seemed to reassure Lillian a little, and to give her permission, when I told her that another woman I had interviewed, **Ellen (1910)**, first masturbated at eighty-one, after her husband became quite ill:

> I don't think I ever did any of that [masturbation] until after my husband had prostate cancer and we quit having intercourse. I think the idea of doing it then came to me through reading about it in books. I grew up with the idea that masturbation was evil, it was wicked, it would drive you crazy. But then you read about what a release it is and so on, and so I just decided, *Well, I might as well try it*. So, I did. Sort of like saying: *Well, if John can't give me what I need, maybe I can give myself what I need*. It's kind of a conscious decision. I don't do it very much anymore. For one thing, I've been battling bladder infections for the last thirty years or so. So I finally decided that maybe it wasn't such a good thing to be doing. Actually, I don't think I would have quit masturbating if it hadn't been for this bladder because there are still times when I very much would like to do it but I don't because of that. I think some of the best orgasms I've ever had were the ones that I gave myself in the last few years.

Sexuality: A Lifelong Work in Progress

The sexual self doesn't have to retire. As these older women demonstrate, your sexual self can be a lifelong work-in-progress. Lillian experienced, in her seventies and eighties, a reprise of that dichotomy we all first experience in early childhood. She finds herself, even in her mature years, continuing to confront and resolve the tension between the *wish to do* and *prohibitions against doing.* Ellen experiences a parallel theme: the tension between *the wish to do* and the *problems caused by doing.* Sex and sexuality are with us all our lives. Lillian had received information about sex and sexuality from her girlfriends when she was a teenager and she found that she continued to receive sexual information from a friend when she was in her seventies and eighties.

These interviews demonstrate that no matter how old we are, new life situations can pose new questions about sexuality. As women get older, some continue to talk together about sexual matters and advise each other about the adjustments they need to make when their circumstances, their health, and the health of their partners change. Little girls and women of all ages advise each other on matters of sex and sexuality and pass along gems of information they have discovered in this sometimes mysterious and hidden realm. Sex and our sexualities are with us all of our lives.

What Does This Mean to You?

Now, if you wish, pick up your notebook and express the thoughts and feelings you're having about your early sexual impulses and experiences. Here are some questions you might want to consider after you've done that.

- What do you recall of your early impulses and experiences? Some themes you might consider are secret moments of pleasure; your earliest memories or images of a sense of privacy; the messages you received from adults about your sexual curiosity; and your emerging awareness of the pleasures of your body.

- What kinds of pleasurably aroused sensual experiences did you have as a child—either specifically sexual or more generally sensual like Mary Jo's experience with her horse—before you had language to describe the experience?

- What do you recall of learning language? You might consider, for example, the word "masturbation," which for many of us is a taboo word. How did you first learn it? How comfortably do you use it? What other interesting words did you learn? What has been the impact of applying these words to your experience?

- What is your judgment, right now, about the okayness or not-okayness of creating and experiencing body pleasure? How did you arrive at that value?

- If you are recalling experiences that you now regret, consider the circumstances, the roles of others, and how you saw your options at the time. Then, sit quietly with your eyes closed and imagine what you could now gently and lovingly tell your younger self that would be healing and lead to greater self-acceptance.

3

Thinking About Sex: Attitudes and Values

Many of us find it easier to imagine just about anyone else in the world having sex but our own parents—or our own children. Educator-humorist Sam Levenson once put it this way: "To think that my mother and father would do such a thing! My father—maybe, but my mother—*never!*" (Berezin 1972). Yet, for most of us a significant part of our sexual heritage evolves from how our parents, or those who were like parents to us, felt about their sexuality and conveyed that to us. Our sexual heritage includes not only the verbal messages our parents gave us, but the ways they touched us and the behavior they modeled for us. And our parents were affected by their parents who were affected by their parents, and on and on back through the generations. There are many subtle incidents—solo, with friends, and within the context of family life—that give us sexual lessons without anyone saying, *This is about sex.* This chapter continues to demonstrate that much of what we learn about sex and sexuality in childhood is indirectly taught to us.

Your Sexual Heritage

What do you know of the influences on your parents' sexual beliefs, attitudes, and knowledge as they were growing up? What did they learn about sex and relationships, and where did they get that information? What was their courtship like? You may be surprised at how much you know of your parents' sexuality through clues in family anecdotes, pictures, souvenirs, or traditions. You may be able to trace your sexual heritage back even further—to your grandparents or even earlier generations. As you consider it now, how much of what your parents and grandparents believed about sex and sexuality do you think has affected you? Even more important: how much has affected your children, if you have them?

Ronni (1955) talked about her mother's values and how they had been shaped by her grandparents' values. "My mother was raised in a very Catholic house and she actually rebelled very strongly when she was growing up. She didn't want to instill in us any sense of guilt or shame about sex, so when I was a kid she talked quite openly to me and my brothers about sex. My mother called a *penis* a *penis*, a *vagina* a *vagina*. She made sure my brothers knew the difference between clitoral stimulation and vaginal orgasm before they had sex when they were teenagers. She described birth control. She made it clear that you didn't have to be married to have sex, but she didn't want a free love sort of thing. She did want me to be sensible, monogamous, and in relationships. I learned about oral sex from my mom. That's one of the things I thank her for. But there was also a real contradiction . . . mixed messages. On the one hand she was very open about things, but when I started to experiment sexually as a teen, she was clearly unhappy about it." (See chapter 5 for more about how Ronni's mother felt and reacted when Ronni became sexually active.)

Earlier, I described the *finding our way* process in which words, images, ideas, and experiences lead each of us, step by step, to clearer understanding of how our sexuality fits into who we are and to fuller acceptance of our sexual selves. **Alicia (1967)**—like most of us—has had to find her way through values and influences on her sexuality that go back to an earlier generation: "Even though I don't like to admit it, I'm still affected by what my parents think. I think it was the values they grew up with from their parents; they're very conservative. Living with your boyfriend is just not something you do; an engagement ring would probably make a big difference. I was brought up in a Unitarian environment which is pretty free thinking, so it's not religion, it's culture and human nature. We had sex education in high school when I was fifteen and, other than that, I started to release myself from a lot of guilt just by talking to people when I went away to college."

Donna's (1949) experiences were quite different. She, too, has had to *find her way*: "I learned almost nothing from my parents about sex. My parents, being Chinese, were fairly traditional and my mother literally was a prude. I never saw them being affectionate, and they'd go into the bedroom separately to change into their night-clothes or else sit on opposite sides of the bed facing out. My mother was the nicest lady but she never learned to accept her own sensuality, her sexualness. My mother's parents had a fixed marriage, and my parents almost did. They got married right out of high school; they were dating, and my father was going to be sent back to China for school; also his parents had arranged a marriage for him to a woman there. My father didn't want to move back to China, so he picked the first available woman who would say, '*Yes*.'"

While we are growing up, we are solving a mystery and constructing an inner mind/body picture of sex and sexuality. What we learn from our parents is only one piece of this puzzle that we put together. We get other pieces from our siblings, our classmates, and our teachers. We also learn from religious teachings, the books we read, magazines on the newsstands, television, movies, our own experiences, and many other sources. In this construction we gather information not only about what people do when they have sex, but about attracting partners, having babies, and the roles of women and men in relationships.

As you think about it now, how are you still affected by what your parents, or those who were like parents to you, think or thought about sexual matters? Which of your own values are thought-out agreements or disagreements with theirs? Which are in reaction to their values or behaviors? How much do you think your parents are or were affected by their parents' views and behaviors?

The Primary Roles of Parents

Very few Survey respondents (about one in eight) selected their parents as among their most significant sources of helpful or useful sex information. Sexual partner(s), sex education book(s), and same-age friends(s) were the significant sources of sex information selected as most helpful by more than a third of the respondents. It is interesting that parents were more likely to be regarded as significant sources of misleading or harmful sex information, although only a relatively small number of respondents (one in five of those answering the question) put their parents in the *misleading or harmful* category. Media (TV, movies, magazines, etc.) and religious teachings were the sources most often selected as misleading or harmful.

Based on my research, one important conclusion I have reached is that, with respect to sex education, parents are not the primary sources of directly taught information. Most typically, the primary role of parents—at least in our contemporary United States—is to convey their values to their children and to model what a relationship can be.

Everyone Except Our Own Parents and Children

I often jokingly say, as I did earlier in this chapter, that many of us can imagine just about anyone else in the world having sex but our own parents and our own children. I think there's some kind of built-in barrier between us and our kids when it comes to talking about the specifics of sex, some kind of inherent psychological boundary. Perhaps it is a built-in incest taboo that keeps parents and children from seeing each other as sexual and therefore as potential partners. This boundary is not absolute and is sometimes crossed, but I think it does exist.

Lisa (1970) described how sex was something private for her: "I've learned a lot of good things from my family. All the people in my family have stayed married. So I remember learning that *monogamous sex is wonderful.* Growing up, I heard jokes on my mother's side of the family that implied that the women are very sexual ... that they liked to have sex, and that sex was okay. It was something that they were kind of proud of almost. So I always had good feelings about sex. But there was a lot of my mother and my aunt, trying to be very liberal, always wanting to talk about things. And I didn't want to talk to them about sex. That's private stuff to me."

I know only a few people who have *comfortably* talked to their own kids about sex; I know many more who have not, although some of them wanted to. Either they, their kids, or they and their kids, just felt too uncomfortable. The impulse to talk and directly teach never broke through what were often mutual inhibitions. I do know many parents, though, who very comfortably advise their children's friends about sex and sexual matters while their own kids are taking their questions elsewhere—to teachers, their friends' parents, older relatives, or to peers.

One teacher told me in her interview: "It's nice being a teacher of fifth graders because I get to find out what kids are really thinking about at this age, and what they really know and what they think they know. For example, they have myths about how you can and can't get pregnant, like the sperm can all of a sudden come alive and can swim through bathwater and get into your vagina. They know that AIDS is out there and that there are all these other diseases, but they are not sure how you get them, or how you get infected and how to prevent infection. Also, kids have a hard time talking with their parents about the questions they have. I did this thing where you had to write your questions on a piece of paper without your name and I would pull them out and answer them. A lot of students said, *I'm really glad that I can talk to you because I can't talk to my parents.*"

Families That Provide Information

In spite of the likelihood of awkwardness or discomfort, there are some families in which providing information about sexuality is a conscious part of the family agenda, especially when it comes to conveying the particulars of the "sexual plumbing" or the mechanics of "the sex act." Parents are, however, unlikely to tell their children much about creating pleasure, although some do talk about that subject as well. **Emily (1919)** first heard of sexual intercourse from a girl cousin when she was about nine. She said, "I told a friend of mine who told her mother who told my mother. So my mother then took charge of my sexual education. She apparently had been waiting for me to ask questions and I never had. But now she started telling me about sex. My parents made it clear I should feel free to ask them any questions I had about the subject. I did and they were very good about answering."

By the time she was eight, **Helena's (1943)** mother had told her "... about the reproductive system, how erection occurs, how the man puts his penis in the vagina and so on. It was very cut and dried and specific and cool and kind of unemotional. But I knew there was more to it." Helena continued, "I felt kind of impish after my mother delivered her lecture, and I said, *So sex is for making children,* and she said, *Yes. So you never have sexual intercourse unless you want to make a baby?* and she began to waffle. I knew that I had her and she knew I had her. Then I took it further. I said, *I'd like you and Daddy to demonstrate how this sexual intercourse works.* I thought it would be great if I could see this. I didn't think she would comply, and, of course, she didn't."

Karen (1957) remembers her mother telling her about sexual activity and then asking her mother whether she enjoyed it. Karen told me, "That really threw her off. That was not open for discussion. She wanted to feel like she had told me about the mechanics. It was years after other kids had already told me about it. It was very uncomfortable for both of us, but I sort of felt respect for her and positive about the fact that she had talked to me about it. My father didn't talk about it at all." I wonder how typical it is that when parents do get around to talking about sex, their daughters have already acquired the information elsewhere. Was that your experience?

Infancy—The Language of Touch

When you were an infant, did your mother breast-feed you? Were you held while you were bottle-fed? If so, your parents, or those who were like parents to you, gave you some preparation for wholesome adult sexuality that you previously may not have recognized.

The first language we learn is not the language of words but the language of touch. This is the language that we richly develop—or do not—in those most formative and most developmentally open months inside our mother's uterus and in "the in-arms phase" (Leidloff 1977) between our birth and when we begin to crawl. Learning the language of reciprocal touch through touching and being touched in the first months of our lives seems to be a prerequisite to the fullest realization of healthy adult sexuality. This language between mother and infant is so finely attuned that most mothers of newborns can identify their own babies when they are blindfolded so that they can neither see nor smell the babies. If they spend five to ten seconds lightly stroking only the backs of the hands—not even the fingers or the edges of the hands—of their own and others' infants, they can identify their babies (Kaitz, Lapidot, Bronner, et al. 1992).

For babies fortunate enough to be breast-fed, it is in the breast-feeding relationship that much of the foundation of this language of touch is laid down. Breast-feeding is the newborn's first experience of a reciprocal relationship. A baby's hungry cry stirs the release of milk and a multitude of other changes in her (or his) mother's body; her mother's nipple touching her cheek stimulates a baby's suckling reflex. The suckling relationship is mutually beneficial—physically, emotionally, developmentally, and more. The baby gets nourishment. She also gets sensory stimulation that leads to important neurological development. Through the feedback loop formed with her mother, her nervous system, incomplete at birth, forms a multitude of connections.

Suckling at her mother's breasts activates all of an infant's senses. The baby smells, tastes, and touches her mother; her little hand feels and strokes her mother's breast as she suckles; she hears her mother's voice, gazes at her face, eyes, and smile; she smells and tastes the sweetness of the milk. She is learning feelings she will later call warmth, love, and being wanted. As she receives nourishment, her suckling induces beneficial changes within her mother's body and releases endorphins that give her mother a sense of well-being. Ideally, both mother and baby experience pleasure. With a sense of wonder we can recognize, in the words of Ashley Montagu (1986):

> ... how beautifully designed the suckling of the baby at the mother's breast is, especially in the immediate postpartum period, to serve the most immediate needs of both. ... What is established in the breast-feeding relationship constitutes the foundation for the development of all human social relationships, and the communications the infant receives through the warmth of the mother's skin constitute the first of the socializing experiences of [her] life (pp. 92-93).

Being fed and held as an infant in the breast-feeding or bottle-feeding relationship is a distinct phase in the development of our sexuality.

Breast-feeding their babies is a life experience unique to women. It is a distinct phase of the reproductive dimension of a woman's sexuality. Breast-feeding is part of the reproductive process that is comprised of attraction, lovemaking, sexual intercourse, pregnancy, giving birth, and the nurturing and feeding of the infant born of that union. The nursing experience at her mother's breast (or with a bottle) while being held in loving arms, lays the foundation for the eroticism of the sexual woman this baby girl will become.

Unfortunately, some people feel confused and threatened when they contemplate the pleasure that babies have in physical contact with their parents and parents have in touching and caressing their babies. They confuse satisfying those most basic needs that babies and their parents have for skin contact and for loving, affirmative touch with being perverse. They confuse the pleasures of touching that establish a sense of being loved and wanted with foreplay and sex. They confuse nakedness and skin-to-skin nurturing with abuse.

Some are shocked, too, that nursing a baby can feel wonderful and that nursing may stimulate waves of pleasure for both the baby and her or his mother. Breast-feeding can be a deeply sensual experience that stimulates perfectly normal physical and emotional stirrings much like those that a woman experiences in sex. When **Marsha (1940)** had an orgasm as a result of nursing her first child she didn't then know that many women have such experiences; she now regrets the outcome: "Around eleven weeks after my first daughter was born, I was breast-feeding her and I had an orgasm and scared myself. I weaned her at twelve weeks because I had no idea that I was supposed to enjoy breast-feeding. I felt weird. It makes me cry to realize how ignorant I was. I didn't breast-feed my second child because I was still scared and had no understanding."

With her baby's suckling, the mother's uterus rhythmically contracts, facilitating its return to only slightly larger than its pre-pregnant size. Sometimes spontaneous orgasms do occur during these contractions. We should not think of nursing our babies as separate from the fullness of the reproductive dimension of a woman's sexuality. This very important pleasurable aspect of women's lives is of utmost importance for both a woman and her infant.

Mutual pleasure of mother and infant is not abuse. It is not sex. Instead, it is one of a girl's first learning opportunities about sensation, safety—and, yes—eroticism and pleasure.

Positive Modeling

It seems that families or orgin in which strong positive modeling occurs are not the majority, at least among the Survey respondents. Only about one in three said that their mother and father openly demonstrated physical affection for each other, while even fewer, about one in four, agreed that their mother's or father's attitude toward sex was generally positive. Even taking into account the incidence of single-parent families, these are low numbers. A higher percentage, not quite half, agreed that their mothers had affectionately touched (for example, hugged) them, while about one in three agreed that their fathers had done so.

Even though families of origin in which strong positive modeling occurs are not the majority, some of the women I interviewed did recount positive memories of the relationships their parents modeled for them. Women whose parents did express affection are represented in the narratives that follow. **Ruth (1943)**, whose parents have been married fifty-four years, said that she got wonderful messages from her mother. "They have a great marriage. My mother's very sexual, but she was always quite vague about it without being very specific. I can't say anything she ever said to me, but just being around her, I know that they have a very healthy sex life. They don't like to be apart from one another at night, have always slept in a double bed together so that they could be close, have never wanted a bigger bed. So I got affirmation of sexuality in growing up, but without the details."

Beth (1961) described growing up in her Catholic family: ". . . my parents, my four brothers, and me. Just watching who my mother was, and our family and how she related to my dad made me think, *Oh, this is what I will do.* As if sexuality was a thing where you grow up and find a mate and have children. They were somewhat affectionate, they would hold hands and kiss now and then, but more of what their life was about was this family." **Diana's (1968)** parents, too, are affectionate with each other. She described them as "always hugging and kissing" in front of her. She concluded that seeing her parents "very free and open with each other" is one reason she feels "free to be affectionate and express what I want with my body."

Janet (1955) received a mixture of positive and not-so-positive nonverbal and verbal messages. Her mother's discomfort with nudity shows us how, as parents, our own histories can be reflected when we are making an effort to model something for our daughters that we have not comfortably experienced ourselves: "My parents made a point of always having an open-door policy on the bathroom so that we would see them nude. My father was comfortable with it and my mother was uncomfortable but did it anyway. When I was young, my parents would kiss and my mom would sit on my dad's lap and occasionally he would grab my mom's breast or her behind." Janet went on to talk about her father's dirty jokes: "As I got older I realized how much these jokes perpetuated the double standard that it was okay for the guys to sow their wild oats but girls had better keep their legs crossed or they weren't respectable."

There were others who also reported that their parents' relationship had a mixture of qualities that they both did and did not want for themselves. Although **Alicia's (1967)** parents are "very much in love" and have "a great relationship," it's not the kind of relationship she would want for herself. She said, "My mother's a little too dependent, doesn't stand up for herself as much as I think she should, and my father is a bit overbearing and does pretty much what he wants. But then that's what makes her happy, so they fit together just perfectly. They give me hope in this day and age of so many divorces that marriage can last a long time."

The Parents' Dilemma

Parents want the best for their daughters, but parents are also shaped by their own values and experiences. Before they convey their values to their daughters they must confront the dilemmas within their own value systems. For example, is experiencing and responding to pleasure something that we want to teach our children to enjoy and do well at, or is it something we want to keep them from learning at all costs? Is sex for reproduction only or is reproduction only one of the reasons we engage in sex? Is it okay if our children freely explore their capacity for sensual pleasure and use it for self-comforting, or is this capacity for pleasure sinful and to be controlled and eradicated? Will self-pleasuring lead to a healthier child or to warts, hair on the palms, and a need for glasses?

Today, most of us would say that reproduction is just one of the many possible reasons to engage in sex. Nowadays, most adults don't give a second thought to having sex for relaxation, relationship enhancement and the pleasures of making love, or for play and, sometimes, just plain "getting off."

Earlier in the twentieth century, however, the mainstream view was that reproduction was the primary function of sex. The morality or immorality of birth control was a hot political issue and a strong stigma was placed on sex before marriage. Even worse was living proof of doing it, a child born "out of wedlock." Society required state- or church-sanctioned marriage to create a social structure and continuity for children. Before a woman had sex she was supposed to have wed a trusted partner with whom she could raise a family. Marriage was required to "legitimize" sex and having children.

Among the values that the parents of the older women I interviewed had conveyed to their daughters were several themes. Parents then—and now—want to protect their daughters from the dangers of sex that they perceive or imagine. These themes can be summarized as follows: Sex is pleasurable, but it is dangerous. Be careful. I don't want you to get hurt. I don't want you to ruin your chances for marriage, a good life, and the best future possible. Specifically, the older women heard from their parents that:

- **All boys and men want is one thing; they're not to be trusted.**

Lillian's (1905) parents were "... very stiff. My mother was a southern belle and they thought sex was dirty. When my sister and I got to the age where we wanted to date, my mother told us, *When you go out with a boy, all he wants is one thing.* We didn't know what the one thing was. To find out what that was, we had to ask our friends." **Emily's (1919)** father wanted her to know "that men will push you as far as they can but when it comes to marriage they're looking for virgins. That was the idea he grew up with and he assumed it was still that way when I was a child."

When she was twelve, **Judith (1940)** got an inappropriate and insensitive sex lecture from her stepfather that left her terrified. "I liked the feeling of being horny, but I didn't know what it was; no one ever talked about sex. But one night when my mother and brother were out, my stepfather said, *How much do you know about sex?* I was terrified and yelled *Enough!* Consciously, I really didn't know anything about sex. He said that he didn't think I knew enough and he was going to tell me. He said, *All men ever want from you is to put their thing in yours. And don't you forget it.* I didn't know what a 'thing' was. I had seen my brother's little penis but never a man's that I remember. I didn't say anything, just sat there at the piano frozen. And he said, *Old men will rape you.* The next day downtown with my girlfriend I was terrified, scared out of my wits at every man I saw. That feeling lasted for a long, long time."

- **Be a good girl or no man will want you; don't get pregnant; save sex for marriage.**

Essentially, the logic went like this: Be a good girl—be "chaste" and "pure," don't have sex. Having sex will ruin your reputation, you will be "soiled goods," no decent man will want you, you won't be marriageable. Don't get pregnant. If you do, the world will know you aren't a "good girl." Save "it" for marriage; marriage to a "good man" is the prize; then you can have sex. (None of the older women and only one or two among the younger women interviewed mentioned their parents saying anything to them about the possibility of being with a woman.)

When "living together" wasn't a socially acceptable option and effective woman-controlled contraceptives weren't as available as they are today, parents had genuine concerns about their daughters' marriageability. They wanted their daughters to be able to maintain or improve their social status and to have the best lives possible. Parents feared, often realistically, that if a daughter became pregnant she would lose status. Parents, strongly influenced by religious teachings, addressed these concerns by holding up the age-old madonna/whore dichotomy (there are *good* women and *bad* women, with *good* and *bad* defined by how they express their sexuality) and by defining sex outside of marriage as sin, i.e., as violating not only the rules of society but of God. Imposing guilt rather than teaching informed decision making was at the forefront of parents' efforts to control and protect their daughters' sexuality.

Did guilt prevent women from engaging in sex or just interfere with them enjoying it fully? In chapter 5, where women talk about their first experiences of sexual intercourse, we will see the interplay between the urge of young women to "do it" and the powerful social prohibitions against "going all the way" before marriage. In her interview, **Emily (1919)** talked about the effect that guilt had on her:

Compared to many, many people from my era, my upbringing was quite liberal. But still, I had to break away from certain of the values my parents had and find my own path. Like this thing of being a *good woman*, and if you didn't behave in a certain way you were a *bad woman*. Whenever a girl we knew, a relative or someone in the neighborhood, got pregnant outside of marriage, this was a big topic of conversation in our house. It was pointed out that she didn't say *No* and she should have said *No*; it's not a smart thing to do and it's going to affect the rest of her life. My father always said that, *When there's no money coming in the door, love flies out the window.* He made it clear that unless a man had a way of making money, there would be trouble and instability in marriage. My parents had very, very definite ideas about what was right and what was wrong. There was no middle ground. So when I strayed from that path, I felt very guilty. There was one guy I dated who tried his best to get into my pants and he almost succeeded, but I always heard my father in the background saying I shouldn't be doing this, and I always stopped.

Gloria (1944) heard similar values espoused in her African-American family: "When I was around ten, eleven, twelve, I was told there were good girls and there were loose, bad girls, and you wanted to be a good girl. The loose girls were the ones who were fooling around with boys and those girls were going to *get into trouble*. The word *pregnant* was never used, just *get into trouble*, until my period began, when I was twelve. Then I got the talk: *Stay away from boys because now you can get pregnant.* Nothing about how you 'get pregnant,' but I knew already because all the girls were talking about it."

Katherine (1938), whose parents were born in Europe, specifically got the "preserve your marriageability" message: "My parents' message was not to do it: *Nobody worthwhile is going to want you if you have sex before you get married.*"

Although less practiced, the message of waiting for marriage is still with us. College student **Allison (1971)** received this value from her parents, too. She first had sexual intercourse as a senior in high school after dating her boyfriend for two years, but she felt guilty about it for a long time. At the time of her interview, she and her boyfriend were still partners. She said: "The message I've always had from my parents was, basically, *Don't do it; don't do anything until you're married.* That value has restricted me and held me back in a lot of ways. Sex is bad, something to feel guilty about. Although it's better now, for a long time I felt negative about doing it."

Books and Magazines

Emily, who first heard of sexual intercourse from a girl cousin when she was about nine, demonstrates that if parents wait for their kids to ask about sex, that may never happen. One way some parents get around their own reticence to talk about sex, and their children's reticence to ask or listen, is to provide books on the subject. **Josephine (1913)** reported, "I had read books when very young. I knew the most important things when I was ten. My mother didn't tell me much about sex and when she did, I could tell how hard it was for her."

A number of women mentioned *Growing Up and Liking It*, a booklet about having periods that could be sent away for from a company that manufactured sanitary napkins. **Barb (1955)** said that, when she was thirteen, her mother "literally threw it down on the bed and said *Read this and tell me if you have any questions*. That was the sum total of my sexual education. I read it, but it didn't tell me anything I didn't already know from the streets."

When **Lisa (1970)** was eleven or so, her mother gave her "a book with all these passages of different experiences of like, going through puberty, dating, and sex, and it went through all sorts of things, like birth control, and it also talked about developing. I read that a lot." However, Lisa's emerging sexuality seemed so private to her that, like many of us, she couldn't acknowledge her sexual curiosity to her mother, even after her mother had introduced the subject. Lisa's inhibition is a good example of what I'm calling the "psychological barrier" between children and their parents. Lisa said, "When she gave it to me, she was like, *Oh, I want you to read it.* And I always brushed it aside and did not want her to know that I had it under my bed and I read it all the time. I had it memorized. So I learned a lot from reading. From pretty young, from nine to now, I tried to get my hands on books where there were sexual passages."

Nearly 40 percent of the questionnaire respondents said sex education books had been among their most significant helpful sources of sex information. Fiction was much less likely than sex education books were to be considered helpful or useful, and nearly one in four of the *Survey* respondents listed fiction as among their "most significant misleading or harmful" sources of sex information. However, women born in the 1960s and 1970s mentioned Norma Klein and Judy Blume's novels for teens as beneficial. For example, **Alicia**

(1967) said, "My first awareness of my sexuality was probably at fifteen, reading a book by Norma Klein, an author who has written a lot of books about young people, young girls. It was about a girl who was fifteen, too, and she was talking about masturbating and things like that in language that was not spelled out. And for the first time I started to understand the language the characters were using that had been confusing to me in books before. She was talking about feeling close to this guy and feeling that she was one person with him, and for the first time I started to identify with her. I started to think of a guy I liked and I felt the same about him."

One woman who found books both helpful and misleading noted: "Women's novels were useful; romances, harmful." Another who found both books and the media harmful said: "They promoted idealized couplings and body confusion!"

If Their Parents Only Knew!

Much about sexuality is hidden, so there may come a time when we go in search of, or perhaps just discover, something our parents think they have hidden from us; or we may see something while away from home. Numerous women mentioned discovering *Playboy* or similar magazines while they were growing up. Looking at such magazines when young is likely to give a girl distorted images of sex and her sexuality. Some interviewees thought the images they saw in *Playboy* had influenced their sexual fantasies; a few who were aroused by the images of women's bodies in these magazines became confused, at least for a time, about their sexual orientation.

That is what happened to **Marybeth (1972)**, who said, "When I was eight or ten, I found my father's *Playboy* magazines. I was shocked that my father would have these in the house, but I was interested in reading them, too. I found it kind of disgusting the way they portrayed the women with all their clothes off. *Where did they get such big breasts?* was my question. I didn't see them as particularly beautiful. Even when I was as old as eighteen, if no one else was home, I sometimes would see if they were still where he kept them and I'd look at them." Marybeth's parents would have been shocked that this was going on when Marybeth was eight or ten, because at that time they were monitoring the movies she was allowed to see. She added: "The *Playboys* were my first experience with visual erotica. I wasn't allowed to watch any R-rated films until I convinced my mom when I was about fifteen or sixteen. Then I saw things like girls kissing guys and heavy kissing and sex. Watching that kind of behavior still makes me uncomfortable."

When interviewed, Marybeth was still confused about being aroused by images of naked women—not in *Playboy*, but in *Cosmopolitan*: "I really don't like the women on the covers of *Playboy*. I like it when I see beautiful photos of naked women, like some of the photos in *Cosmo*. It is slightly erotic for me. It makes me worry. Homosexuality is not discussed in my family at all. And I don't consider myself to be a homosexual person, but I don't know how you can decide that you know you are a homosexual person. So, initially, I'd be kind of interested because they would be so beautiful, and I would think, *I must be gay.* But then I consider, *it's not strong enough for me to be gay.* I find myself way more interested in men than women. It's just that naked women are something that I don't see a lot, and it's kind of shocking and it's kind of interesting."

It's true that at times most of us are aroused by images of our own gender. As Marybeth is realizing, this in itself doesn't mean that we are gay. That we can enjoy and appreciate the beauty of other women's bodies doesn't necessarily mean that we want to act on our arousal and have sex with other women, although some of us will want to—and do so. Probably more of us would explore our attraction to other women if society in general were more accepting of women exploring sexual pleasure with each other. This is another situation in which trying to fit a label to a person (*gay, lesbian*, or a derogatory word) instead of describing behavior (*exploring sexual pleasure with each other*) can be confusing or problematic.

Some of Marybeth's earliest sexual fantasies perhaps were influenced by images she had seen in her father's magazines: "My sexual fantasies used to be sort of S and M kind of thoughts, only the guy was the one being chained and bound. When I was thirteen or a little older, I would work out these elaborate light S and M movies in my head, and that would excite me. And then I'd think *I'm a really evil person for thinking these things; this is the wrong way to think about sex.* So they don't interest me anymore. I think I've developed. Now that I'm twenty, it's your standard guy meets girl and the act, sort of." As Marybeth demonstrates, seeing magazines like *Playboy* when we're young and impressionable can be problematic. Her fantasies did not make her an evil person, but she thought that they did. The pictures and advertising in magazines like these present women as sex objects and often misrepresent how most people relate in sex. These magazines present a girl with sexual themes that are outside mainstream sexual comfort zones and could be better understood and integrated when she is older and her sexual self is more developed.

Cecile (1952), whose orientation is bisexual, realized that *Playboy* images distorted her view of women: "My first boyfriend and his brother had a stack of *Playboys* in their bedroom. As I started to get more curious about women, that's where I started looking at women. My sexual focus on women in the beginning was sexual and graphic. So I didn't approach bisexuality from the same love place that I approached my heterosexuality. I saw women as sexual objects. Which I am not totally proud of at this point."

Responses to *Playboy*-type magazines weren't all negative. There were others for whom the images were not problematic. I do find it interesting, however, that this college student **(1971)** equates being desirable with being sexy, which is exactly the value these magazines promote. "I don't recall my parents ever teaching or talking about sex: Instead, I remember learning about body parts and sensuality/ sexuality from the *Playboy*-esque magazines we kids discovered in the bathroom at my father's workplace. I thought the women were beautiful and sexy, and now, after imitating them to the best of my abilities in my late teens, I realize I have easily accepted myself as sexy and desirable."

Consider for a moment: What other qualities, in addition to sexy, might we—and this young woman—associate with being desirable? What other qualities do we want to encourage teens to develop within themselves?

The books we find in pursuit of sex "education" may be relatively benign, like the novel **Cheryl (1937)** found on her parents' sunroom bookshelf: ". . . a biographical novel about Robert Burns. There was this little passage where he finally embraces a young woman—kisses her, I guess—on a rug in front of the fireplace. I read those two pages over and over and over again from when I was about nine or ten until maybe twelve. It certainly wasn't explicit or genital, but it sort of got me glowing. Later, as a teen, I used to read *True Confessions*, obviously a turn-on."

The books we find also may be potentially more harmful, like those on the crammed bookshelf in **Penny's (1946)** home: "My dad was hooked on Mickey Spillane mysteries which always had all sorts of hot little things in them. When I was in junior high I used to regularly take *Peyton Place* [Metalious, 1956] from the bookshelf and read it. And the other one was Henry Miller's *Tropic of Cancer* [1961]. Those were real risqué books in those days. I only had the vaguest idea of what I was reading." The pornography **Sara (1949)** found in her neighbor's garbage was substantially misleading: "When I was twelve or thirteen, the nurse who lived downstairs from us in this apartment building threw out an incredible collection of pornography, and I found it in the garbage. All kinds of stuff. She read good porn! I liked the gay male stuff; I found that very sexy; I found they all turned me on. She also threw away an unexpurgated version of *A Thousand and One Nights*, which was beautiful poetry. It didn't really get me hot, but it was just lovely to read. I read all this stuff. And of course it was written by men, so the women were multi-orgasmic . . . always swallowed *cum* . . . took it up the ass. They did everything. And so this is what I thought you were supposed to do." (See chapter 5 to read about how these images and the assumptions they created for Sara about what you do when having sex were played out in her first intercourse experience.)

Siblings

Although relatives, in general, weren't high on the list of the most helpful sources for sex information, siblings were frequently mentioned as sources of support and sex information. For example, a Survey respondent (1955) wrote: "My parents' attitude about *their* sex was definitely positive. They had seven kids, and growing up I knew they still 'did it' and 'liked it.' But my parents *never* discussed sex with me, which I wish they had. My older sister gave me the most guidance about morals and values and outcomes of relationships and having sex." **Beth (1961)** said that "As far as just learning about sex, I have a brother close to my age so the two of us would do a lot of talking. He was an important influence on my sexual development." Not all siblings have a positive influence on their sister's sexual development. See chapter 4 for a discussion of the negative impact siblings can have, and a description by Beth of a period of time when she and her brother—whom she still values highly—engaged in mutual physical exploration that became problematic for her.

Changing Mores

The advent and increasing acceptance of readily available contraceptives, particularly of the birth control pill introduced in 1960, brought dramatic changes in customs and cultural mores. In the 1929 Davis survey, only about 20 percent of 958 unmarried women, all college graduates, believed that premarital intercourse was ever justified, either for women or men (Davis 1929). In national surveys of women and men in 1937 and 1959, more than half of the respondents felt it was *not* right for either the woman or the man to have had previous sexual intercourse at the time they married (Hunt 1974). During the "sexual revolution" of the 1960s and '70s this changed considerably. A 1974 survey found 90 percent of young women approved of premarital intercourse for a woman in a love relationship (Hunt 1974).

Alicia's (1967) comments illustrate both the changes in mores and a shift in emphasis from guilt to informed decision making. "My mother was a big influence in my growing up because she is the one who taught me, or tried to teach me, everything. When I was fourteen or fifteen, she gave me a very liberal book—*The Facts of Life and Love* by Alex and Jane Comfort [1979]. I liked it a lot and that got me thinking. It wasn't didactic and preachy like the Ann Landers' books from thirty years ago that she had also given me. Those were very preachy: *You shouldn't do this, and you shouldn't do that.* The Comfort book was very nonjudgmental, saying that when you want to have sex, if you feel you're ready, take the proper precautions and that's okay."

Themes for the 21st Century

Beginning a new millennium reminds us to be thoughtful about where we've been, where we're going, and the values that guide us. We want the best for our daughters, their daughters, and the women of future generations. What follows are guidelines we can offer them garnered from our collective acquired wisdom.

What Would You Want Your Daughter to Know About Sex?

The narratives thus far have been from the point of view of a daughter. But many daughters grow up and become mothers and fill other roles as well—aunt, teacher, therapist, friend, to name but a few—in which they will influence the sexual values of their children and others younger than themselves.

The women who were interviewed wanted the best they could imagine for their daughters. Each one, even if she didn't have children, was asked, *What would you want a daughter to know about sex?* Consider for a moment how you might answer this question. How might your mother have answered this question when she was the age you are now? What about her mother?

Six interrelated themes emerged from their responses. When we educate our daughters about sex and sexuality in the twenty-first century, we want to convey the following ideas:

1. Value yourself.

2. Value that aspect of self that is your body.

3. Be aware that sex can be dangerous.

4. Sex is pleasurable.

5. Don't be pressured into sex that isn't right for you or that you don't want.

6. Balance pleasure and responsibility.

Value Yourself

To create satisfying relationships, you need a developed sense of self. This includes a sense of what you want, of your right to be treated well, and of your entitlement to pleasure. Getting to know and understand what you think, feel, and want will provide you with a foundation for satisfying relationships and informed sexual decision making. Here is what several women had to say in their interviews:

Penny (1946) would "bring a daughter up in such a way that she felt that she had a lot of self-worth and a good self-image and good strong personal boundaries, and then that would spill over into sex." **Katie (1955)** would want her daughter "to know everything about sex" and "to have a very healthy respect for herself, that's the most important thing." And **Jennifer (1965)** said: "What I want for her is *not* what I tell her to do and *not* what I say is right, but what she believes in her heart is right."

Value That Aspect of Self That Is Your Body

It is through your body that you experience and express your sexuality. Value, protect, and honor it. And enjoy it. Beware of society's messages about women's bodies. The media and advertisers will try to tell you your body is not okay unless it looks a certain way, but ultimately, you have to be happy with yourself.

In her interview, **Fran (1965)** said, "I would want a daughter to know that sensuality and eroticism are okay—conveyed as she grows up through a lot of physical affection . . . and nudity is great. Being totally accepting of her body and her physicality and sensuality would help her sexually." **Chris (1970)** would tell her daughter "everything about the basics of pregnancy and disease, but, also, physical facts about her body and how it develops so that I could tell her, *This is your clitoris. And this is your . . .* And I'd want her to know that her body is absolutely fabulous the way it is, no matter what it is; that there's no perfect body."

Be Aware That Sex Can Be Dangerous

Sex can harm you both physically and emotionally, particularly when sexual activity is outside the safety net of a committed relationship. Sex can lead to unwanted pregnancy and to diseases, some of which are merely annoying, some of which compromise fertility, some of which are fatal. A partner who does not treat you well, respect you, or honor what you thought were mutual agreements can bring you emotional pain and leave you emotionally wounded.

Cecile (1952) put it this way: "It's a complicated subject, honey! Try and take care of your emotional feelings first. And be careful that you don't place yourself in dangerous situations. And try and find a loving, caring partner to learn with. And be very careful about birth control; use condoms all the time." And **Michele (1972)** mentioned diseases and added that "although people say they love you, be committed, be sure. Don't do it because everyone else is doing it. I'd tell her that I'd rather have her pregnant than have her catch a disease. I definitely want my daughters to be safe. I want them to be healthy."

Don't Be Pressured into Sex That Isn't Right for You or That You Don't Want

With a partner and circumstances that fulfill your personal conditions, sex can be absolutely wonderful. Think about what your conditions are for wonderful sex, because there may be times when you will experience pressure to participate in sex with partners or under circumstances that do not fulfill the conditions that you need. In all sexual situations, pay attention to your inner sense of what is right for you.

For women who reached sexual maturity during and after the sexual revolution of the late 1960s and the '70s, there was a much weaker social imperative to wait for sex until marriage than there had been for women of earlier generations. But there was also no longer the strong—and protective—societally imposed "No." When these younger women said they would tell their daughters that sex could be fun or pleasurable they were also likely to add a few sentences about not being pressured into sex you don't want. Many added, too, that sex is even better within an established friendship or relationship.

"I would want my daughter to know," **Anna (1949)** said, "how to recognize her own needs and to take pleasure in sex, but also to know enough to protect herself against unwanted sex." **Susan (1958)** said, ". . . that she doesn't have to do anything that she doesn't want to. That sex is this really great thing and it's even greater when you really love someone and when you are committed to someone."

What **Alicia (1967)** thought most important for her daughter was "that she not be pushed into anything she didn't want to do. I would probably stress that most of all. And I would hope that she would go slowly, wait until she had had many relationships, or at least knew what she wanted from a man . . . that she would wait until she felt mature enough to have sex (intercourse) and would build up to it slowly, learning what she liked. And, of course, birth control. I wouldn't stress marriage so much." And **Leslie (1971)** would "want my daughter to wait to have sex when she was ready, and not at a young age, and just to know that it can be something that's positive. Always use protection, practice abstinence until you're in a relationship. No casual sex. It's about pleasure. It's also about responsibility."

Balance Pleasure and Responsibility

Ultimately, it is up to each of us individually to learn how to fulfill our potential for pleasure and how to protect ourselves from unwanted physical and emotional consequences of sex. The challenge is to achieve balance.

Karen (1957) said, "What I value in sex is connectiveness in pleasure. I would want her to know about pleasure, and that she needs to at least share responsibility for having that happen; someone else can't fully give you pleasure. Knowing about her potential for pleasure is part of empowerment for a woman."

Luci (1959) would want her daughter to know "about orgasm and how to have them and that it's okay to enjoy them. That she has the right to be as sexy as she wants. I'd tell her about sex when she was about thirteen or fourteen. I'd warn her about sixteen- and seventeen-year-old boys. I'd say that all they want is to get laid and they'll do anything to get that. And she has to watch out about getting pregnant. I'd definitely tell her about birth control." Luci's message is familiar. It's the same one the women of her mother's generation heard: *All boys and men want is one thing—they're not to be trusted.*

Some women talked about how they would want to spare their daughters from repeating some aspect of their own sexual lives that they now regret. **Carole (1930)** said, "If I was raising a daughter now, I would teach her really to respect herself and to say *No* when she felt *No*. Because that was something I didn't learn for a long time." **Doris (1930)** "would not want her to be uptight like I am. I would want her to be knowledgeable about not only the physical aspects, but the mental."

Don't Repeat My Mistakes

Connie (1956) would tell her daughter about what she went through in *finding her way*: "I would tell her everything I went through, all my stories. I would say, *Just don't be stupid.* Don't go off with a man and do things with him if you're not prepared to have sex with him. Don't put yourself in a situation that you might be trapped into doing something you don't want to do. Think about it before you act. Be smart. Don't dress provocatively unless you want a response. I was stupid. But I guess you have to learn through your stupidity. I would say, sex is a very wonderful thing, it can be very enjoyable, but I didn't enjoy it for a long time. I tried to, but I didn't. It's something you share with somebody because you care about them. It's a physical enjoyment but it's also an emotional enjoyment. So make sure you really care about whoever you're with."

I wouldn't call Connie *stupid*, as she called herself. I would translate "learn through your stupidity" into *find your way in spite of, your inexperience, emotional needs, and lack of knowledge.* **Amanda (1970)** also would like to spare her daughters from repeating an aspect of her sexual life she now regrets. "I'd try to talk to a daughter a lot about sex, especially about guarding her sexuality. Just to really make sure that she's going to feel comfortable with it. I would tell her that there are certain people that are going to try and take advantage of her and to be strong and to say *No* like, *You're not going to do this to me.* Just to have respect for her body, and really I hope that I can raise my child, especially a female child, to demand respect and have a sense of who she is; and that she can assert that sense through a relationship, or, in general, in her life. And that she doesn't have to play second fiddle to all the men who will be around her. 'Cause I just feel a lot of times I've got really caught up in that."

What Would You Want Your Son to Know About Sex?

A parallel interview question was *What would you want a son to know about sex?* How would you answer this? Women want their children to be safe and many said they generally would give sons and daughters similar information about the risks of disease and pregnancy and the importance of being responsible. But, in addition, women wanted their sons to develop their capacity for respect and some other qualities that I suspect these women would find ideal in their own partners. **Carole (1930)** said she would tell a son to "wear condoms and keep his dick out of places where it shouldn't be. To have great respect for the women he has sex with. And to understand that *No* really means *No*." **Gloria (1944)** told her sons "that responsibility goes with privileges. If they're going to be sexually active they have to be responsible and take care of themselves and their partners—use protection and do safe sex. I told them about being gentle and loving and kind and sharing. I told them that sex was wonderful."

Maggie (1965) thinks that "we don't raise boys to respect girls enough." She would "talk about sexual desire as a healthy motivating force [and] about the sacredness of sex; I don't think people should be with other people until they can have that perspective. And I would encourage them to masturbate. I would teach a girl about getting her own needs met and a boy about pleasing his partner. I would let them know that if they end up gay or straight, either is fine." **Bonnie (1966)** would treat sons and daughters alike. Both "would probably get condoms for their twelfth birthday. *These are what they are, play with them. I'd rather you wait, but if you don't, here's the necessary stuff you'll need.*"

We also want our sons to be sensitive and to understand women's feelings. **Sharon (1962)** would tell a son to "be really conscious of your partner. Try to find out what her needs are, what it takes to turn her on. What it takes for a woman to really appreciate sex is someone who is tender and makes her feel like she's wanted and cared for not just before but even after the experience. Kiss and hug her and make her feel wanted." **Marie (1965)** would want her son to know "that women are more than just objects for a release, that they are people and that they are sensitive, that they have this whole body and a mind to go with it; you better beware!" **Marcy (1967)** would say, "Don't always play the stud or Mr. Macho. You're not the same gender, but you both want the same thing, pleasure. Be honest and open." Similarly, of course, we want our daughters to be sensitive, open, honest, and to try to understand men's feelings.

Parents Really Can't Win

No matter how well we instruct our children, they won't always follow our advice. The fortunate ones are those whose parents are able to let them *find their own way* without abandoning them. **Diana's (1968)** children will be among the lucky ones who know their parents will always be there for them:

> I think the more informed our sons and daughters are, the
> more they will make intelligent choices for their lives. They

probably won't listen to me, but I hope they'll know that I'm supportive of them, no matter what choices they make—that *even if you get yourself into situations you can't handle, you can come to your parents. That maybe I'll get mad at first, but then I'll understand, and I'm always there for you, because I love you.* I think about all the stupid choices I made because I was afraid to tell anyone, or afraid to ask somebody, when the information was there. Like when I was having unprotected sex with my first boyfriend. Wow! I could have really made a big mistake. My mom had warned me. She sat down and said, *You be careful,* and she told me that she wanted me to be protected. Later, when I was in college she asked me to be on birth control. And I just didn't listen.

Here's that psychological barrier again. Diana notes that she *just didn't listen* to her mother and suggests that her sons and daughters *probably won't listen* to her, either. It fascinates me that so many of us think we got so little from our parents while at the same time, over the years, I have talked with so many parents who were concerned about doing a good job of educating their children about sexuality.

It is obvious in these narratives that, as parents, we want the best for our daughters and sons, whatever we perceive that best to be. Yet when we were growing up (and also in retrospect), we did not perceive that our parents acted on these intentions. It may be that most parents really can't win. That is, from their children's point of view, they aren't going to get it right, no matter how concerned they are and how supportively they behave.

If parents aren't perceived as sufficiently open, they will be faulted for that later; on the other hand, they also may be perceived as too open. For example, in the following narratives, the women all had well-intentioned parents, but they were presented with information they didn't feel ready for or that they felt was invasive of their personal boundaries:

When **Doris (1930)** and her brother were little, their mother got them a book about reproduction: "She sat us down and read that to us very seriously, and then off we went to bed. I don't think we were ready at that time, because I didn't know what it was all about, and I think she was uncomfortable with it."

When **Ronni (1955)** was in her late teens, before she went to college, her mother took her to a seminar in which "We actually saw a film of a woman masturbating, one of these instructional feel-good-about-your-body sort of things. I was distressed by it. It was funny that I would feel that way, but it was a little bit too much for me. I wasn't quite ready."

Pam (1968), whose dad is a doctor, reported: "Talking about sex and anatomy in my family was always very open. But when my older sister got her period for the first time, my parents went into this elaborate ceremony of getting out a mirror and showing her cervix to her and teaching her how to use tampons. It was like no way in hell was I going to go through that. I taught myself how to use tampons. It was always just really private for me. I remember my mother and sister having talks and never wanting to talk about any of that myself. When the time came for birth control talks, I just did it on my own. My boyfriend and I went together and bought condoms and spermicide."

Having Different Values Than Your Parents

We also may go off in an entirely different direction with our sexuality than our parents ever imagined for us. **Liz (1951)**, whose partner is a woman, is a good example of this. "I grew up in a typical Catholic family and went to all-girls' parochial schools. There was no doubt I was going to find a husband and have kids and fulfill the American dream. I had a hard time with my sexuality. I did know at a young age that something was kind of different. I went out with men quite a bit until I got my current job. I had an interest in women then but it wasn't until I felt more secure with myself that I explored my own side as far as being with women."

Finding Our Own Way

No matter what our parents tell us, each of us, as an individual, has to *find her or his own way.* **Melanie (1970)** described her process: "They had a sex education excerpt in my ninth-grade health classes in high school. I certainly had heard about it before, but I still didn't get what it was supposed to be. But it was like a development thing through high school, because I think you sort of learn—you hear all the names, the fancy names, and all these long words, but you just kind of grow into them. And when you have the experiences and it kind of becomes part of you, then you put the whole picture together. And you kind of understand what it's supposed to be about. But for a long time it was just confusing to me."

Most Parents Really Do Care

Parents always have been concerned about the sexuality of their children. We were the daughters. Now we are the parents. Perhaps our parents really did try to teach us about sex and sexuality. Perhaps some of us had parents who did not care, but it is clear that many more of our parents really did care. If you are a parent, you may find it helpful to keep in mind the psychological barrier that exists between a child and her or his parents. In most families, even when we want to talk openly and honestly to our children, there will be some intergenerational discomfort or embarrassment. That's just a fact of life.

We probably best convey sexual information to our children by teaching them to value themselves and how to make effective decisions, by letting them know we value having sex within a context of physical and emotional safety, by giving them books and providing them with opportunities to attend classes that convey our values, and by being sure there are relatives or other supportive adults in their lives to whom they can go for advice.

What Does This Mean to You?

Now, if you wish, pick up your notebook and express the thoughts and feelings you're having about your sexual heritage. Here are some questions you might want to consider after you've done that.

- What kinds of messages did you get from your parents about sex?

- What do you think their adolescent ideas were about virginity and intercourse? Where did they meet? Do you think they followed the values of their parents or worked out their own values?

- If you have a sibling or siblings, think for a moment about the role they played in your sexual development and you played in theirs. What values did you get from your sibling(s)?

- If you have children, what kinds of messages did they get—or will they get—from you?

- If you are recalling experiences that you now regret, consider the circumstances, the roles of others, and how you saw your options at the time. Then, sit quietly with your eyes closed and imagine what you could now gently and lovingly tell your younger self that would be healing and lead to greater self-acceptance.

4

Love, Sexuality, and Sexual Boundaries

As children anticipate adult roles in their fantasies and play, they actively seek out the rules of adulthood. In early childhood—particularly between the ages of three and six—a child explores the belief that she has the right to love and to be sexual. A girl may experience love and sexuality within the context of her family in a number of different ways.

As Bodynamics researcher Lisbeth Marcher (1991) explains it, if a girl experiences "that she is valued and respected through both her sexuality and her love," she is likely to grow up able to "identify with both love and sexuality and [to] adopt the sexual-self image *I can sense my love and sexuality at the same time and I decide how I act with it.*" If "her parents *negate* the sexual components of her love," she may then identify with her love but repress her sexuality; "she may adopt the sexual-self image *My love is pure, unspoiled by sexual desire; someday I'll find the one to whom I can give my heart.*" Alternatively, if "her parents *over-focus* on the sexual components of her love," she may "identify with her sexuality and repress her love and adopt the sexual-self image *Love is in reality sexual need; life is sexuality; sex makes the world go round*" (Marcher 1991).

These descriptions are not absolute statements. Aspects of love and sexuality may be experienced differently at different times during childhood, and we also learn about love and sexuality outside of our families. Love and sexuality themes and issues are played out over and over again throughout our lives, particularly within our intimate friendships and relationships.

Caution: Some of the sexual experiences described in this chapter—and in the chapter that follows—were abusive. You may find that the narratives in these chapters will evoke images of your own childhood very powerfully. If you have ever been sexually violated, and you think that reading about other women's nonconsenting experiences may be a problem for you, I recommend that you read these chapters when there is someone available with whom you can discuss the material contained in them.

Nurturing Fathers

The relationship with her father is a major contributor to a girl's image of her sexual self. If he is absent, her image of him influences her. When a girl's father—or a man in a fatherlike role—has clearly defined sexual boundaries, she can learn a lot that is positive about love, sexuality, and sexual relating through play and discussions with him.

A father can appreciate and allow his daughter to experience in his presence the energy of her excitement—of general nonspecific arousal—without sexualizing it. Fathers do, of course, sometimes have sexual feelings in the presence of their daughters, but a man with clear sexual boundaries recognizes these feelings as his own and reins them in and contains them when he is with his daughter. This means that he does not act out his sexual feelings and needs with her, even when she is playing at flirtation. He does not make her his sexual partner either physically or energetically. When she is being flirtatious in her play, there may be some sexualized energy because she is practicing the dance of courtship and sexual initiation. He keeps this energy within the game they are playing and limits how far it is allowed to go. And he doesn't continue—or allow her to continue—the *dance* outside the limits of their playtimes.

In the narrative that follows, **Emily (1919)**, an only child, recalls some of the ways she indirectly learned about sex and sexuality in play with her father. She also speaks of the values her father directly imparted to her through discussions. Emily was ages two to twelve in the years from 1921 to 1931. She was first married in 1940. Clearly, with respect to the roles of women and men, family values were in some ways quite different then from what they are today.

I played in bed with my father every Sunday from the time I was two until just before I began to have my period. I would crawl in bed with my parents on Sunday morning, my mother on one side and I on the other, and we would cuddle up to my dad. And he would tell us fun stories. And then it was time for us to have our time together, and we would push my mother out of bed with much fighting and laughing and playing, and she'd finally fall out of bed and go in the kitchen and make brunch. She always left me with my dad to have this time with him. When I was quite young he taught me to massage his back and shoulders with my feet. It was great fun and lots of body contact, but he never tried anything sexual with me and he always had his genitals covered. In return for the massaging, he would tell me stories and play games like Elevator, where he would lie on his back and put his hands flat and lift me up so I could sit on the crossbar of the bed. Then I would say "Elevator," and he would put his hands up and lower me. One of my most favorite games was Bronco Riding. He would be on his hands and knees, and I would climb on his back and hang on around his neck. I loved all of this. Without any of us being aware of it, I was getting strong encouragement that it was pleasurable to be in bed with a man. It was over when I started to get breasts. It just sort of gradually was over—my father would say, *No, I don't think we'd better do that anymore.* And I was ready. A year or so after that I was dating.

The appropriate age for that kind of play had come to an end. In games like Elevator Emily learned as a child how to ask for—and get—what she wanted; she also learned how to stop an activity when she had had enough. Emily's mother, supportive and available in the kitchen, also played an important role in safely containing Emily's experiences. In no way were the games hidden or secret. Emily's father continued to offer his values and define sexual boundaries for her as she became a sexual adult. In fact, when it was time for her to marry, he, as she describes it, "set her free" to enjoy sex.

I come out of an era when virginity was an important state to maintain. In my own home, it was strongly encouraged. My father wanted me to know that men will push you as far as they can but when it comes to marriage they're looking for virgins. But about a week before I was to be married, my father said to me, *Have you taken care of yourself in regards to not getting pregnant right away? I said, I've taken care of it, Dad. I went to a women's center and got a diaphragm. He said, Well that's fine. Because, honey, after marriage, anything goes.* I never forgot what he said. It really set me free.

What were your reactions to reading about Emily's childhood experiences? Some parents of young children have told me that they enjoyed reading Emily's narrative and felt affirmed in its validation of how they are raising their own children. Yet, a woman who had experienced the violation of her own sexual boundaries in childhood had a difficult time reading it. She was disturbed that Emily's play-times with her father took place on the bed, and she saw no reason for Emily to be in bed with her father for any reason whatsoever. Our histories clearly affect what we consider appropriate behavior.

Emily herself assesses these girlhood experiences of hers as a positive influence in *her* sexual development. I agree and respectfully accept her interpretations. As I see it, Emily's family contained a young girl's developing sexuality in a positive way. Her mother was clearly her father's *sexual* partner; in fact, as she got older, Emily realized that her parents' Saturday naps when she was sent out to play were their playtime; she was able to be aware that her parents had a sexual relationship without being included in it. But Emily, an only child, also was able to have her own times with her father without his crossing generational boundaries inappropriately. This family separated sex and love and had no trouble expressing both. Emily's description of her discovery of self-pleasuring (see chapter 2) is further evidence of this. Emily learned that she was valued and respected for both her ability to love and her sexuality, and that these were separate aspects of her developing self.

Violative Fathers

Father/daughter incest is a very serious psychological violation of a girl's sexual-self image. Contrast Emily's experiences with those of Sara, whose "games" with her father had a different quality altogether. They were injurious rather than beneficial. Sara's father was inappropriately sexual with her in those very important childhood years when a little girl begins to learn the rules of love and sexuality. The crucial boundary between sex and love was not observed in this family—it was inappropriately crossed. When asked about her first experience of feeling sexual **Sara (1949)** replied:

I can't really tell you when I discovered my own sexuality, because it was introduced to me. Because my father was sexual with me starting when I was about two-and-a-half years old. My father was a night worker. So he would come into my bedroom after his shift and, from what I can remember, touch my genitals very lightly and rub his penis on me. And then, when I was about four and a half I approached him in front of my mother. I think I touched his penis, and it was clear that I wanted to play. Because it was a game. My father was hardly ever around, so this was my context with him. And, at that point, I was beaten, by the two of them. I was grabbed by the neck, and my father would shake me, my mother was hitting me: *How dare you do that? It's disgusting! What's wrong with you?* And then my father left . . . just disappeared. I didn't see him again until I was twelve years old, when he returned for a time and was again sexually inappropriate with me. There's a place inside where I blamed myself for all of this.

Sara was introduced to sexual feelings and behaviors long before they were appropriate in her development. Her father's abuse and her mother's reactions to her prematurely sexualized behavior created significant trauma for Sara's emerging sexual self. Notice, too, that Sara was a passive recipient in her father's "game"; in fact, she was punished when she attempted to become more active. Emily, on the other hand, was an active, mutual participant in her Sunday morning play with her father.

A child has an amazing ability to perceive and respond intuitively to the needs of her parents and to take on roles that are unconsciously assigned to her (Miller 1990). When a young child's parents are overly focused on her sexuality, she learns that love is, in reality, sexual need. This belief becomes a part of her sexual self-image.

Some girls who are prematurely sexualized seem to draw the sexual attention of older males, and this happened to Sara. She noted: "I did seem to draw a share of sexual attention. Like from an older kid down the block. We had these weird vibes, and I knew it made me feel funny all over. I was eight years old, he was seventeen. So I knew that there was something funny, but I didn't know what it was." It is not that girls like Sara are deliberately seeking sexual attention; their premature sexualization has taught them to seek attention through behaviors that are steps in the dance of sexual initiation. They may want attention, but what they get is sexual attention.

Sexual exploitation by an adult robs a girl of her childhood innocence—that sense of curious wonder that impels children to experiment, explore, and seek to understand their world in age-appropriate ways—wonder unfettered by the values, judgments, myths, and other bits of information that later become attached to experience. Sexual exploitation also has physiological effects; research indicates that some kinds of sexual abuse result in girls becoming physically mature earlier, on average, than their nonabused peers (DeAngelis 1995).

An Unprotective Mother

It is not only fathers and stepfathers who may prematurely sexualize their daughters. Susan's mother was unclear about her own sexuality, and she had problems with alcohol. One aspect of parenting is to offer a view of what is right or wrong; even when a child pushes or rebels against the guidelines, the standards are there. Instead of giving Susan guidelines for making appropriate sexual decisions, Susan's mother unconsciously and inappropriately facilitated Susan's precocious sexual development. She failed to provide a healthy, protective environment of concern and restrictions for her daughter's emerging sexuality. **Susan (1958)** provides another example of how significant the sexual heritage we receive from our parents can be.

> I don't know what it was about me, but I think my mother promoted a lot of it, because she didn't have an active sex life. When I was ten, she let me have a fourteen-year-old boyfriend who I would make out with a lot. As a mother, I would never let my child get involved like that; that was just really neglectful. When I was fifteen, a man who was thirty-six asked my mother if he could take me out; she said *Sure*, and gave him my phone number. I didn't go out with him; I just didn't want to. My mom was really loose and didn't keep an eye on me, and I didn't know what was right or wrong. But I wish she had been protective of me. When I was ten, she put me in a beauty contest. She was very promoting in those ways. At the same time, if I wore things that were too provocative, because that's the message I was getting from her, she would call me a slut. I've worked very hard for many years on all this stuff in therapy.

When Susan was ten, her eighteen-year-old baby-sitters, two women, molested her; this was another circumstance in which Susan was not protected. Susan experienced the confusing combination of pleasure, fear, and shame that those who are being sexually abused often feel.

They took me into their mother's really dark, smelly bedroom. I remember being on the bed with my pants off and liking how I was feeling. It got into a pattern and went on for several months. My mother was working and was also an alcoholic and neglected me quite a bit. I think I got into what these baby-sitters were doing because someone was paying attention to me. They were masturbating me, inserting their fingers and kissing me and like that. At first I was scared, but it just felt good. That was really hard for me, that what they were doing felt good. For years after that, I would avoid them and I felt really ashamed when I saw them and I thought something was wrong with me. It's really awful I had to think so badly of myself. It wasn't my fault at all. Even as a little girl I went to the library and read things about lesbians because I was worried that I had magically become one because of what these women had done to me.

Now in her second marriage, Susan describes herself as bisexual: "For a good period of time I was involved with women. I find myself attracted to women and I have a lot of fantasies, that if my husband were to die or I was ever divorced, that I would probably end up with a woman. I am with a man because I really wanted children. I also see myself as very much a man's woman; I don't see myself as either-or."

I can't help but wonder: If I could interview Susan's mother, what life story would she have to tell me? What were the factors that shaped her sexual-self image and, consequently, influenced the sexuality of Susan, her daughter? Susan's sexual heritage may well go back many generations.

Sexual Abuse

What is it that constitutes sexual abuse? We know that Sara was abused; I believe that Emily was not. How do we determine that? Sometimes the answer is obvious; sometimes it is not.

As discussed in chapter 2, the naming of experiences has consequences. When we just have experience without words to label it, we have body sensations and the feelings and images that go with those sensations. Without a label, the response is not to the *idea*, but to the *direct experience*: "This is scary; the way he's touching me feels good; he smells awful; I want this to stop; I don't want to be here."

There are consequences of attaching labels to experience—for example, sexual abuse, incest, or rape. Sometimes these are helpful.

We can use these labels for intervention, prevention, and forming social policies. But sometimes the labels get in the way. In the context of considering many of the narratives in this chapter and those that follow, I think it might serve us better to say: "This is what she experienced. That's how it is." We can then go on to consider: *How has that affected the woman she has become?* In what ways has it damaged her? Are there ways in which she was empowered? Experiment with thinking this way as you read this chapter and see how that affects your perception of what you read.

In other chapters you will find additional narratives from women quoted in this one. These will let you consider further how their childhood experiences may have influenced them.

Stop for a moment now to reflect on the experiences of Emily, Sara, and Susan in the previous examples, perhaps comparing their childhood experiences of their sexuality with your own. If doing that causes you distress, move on to the next paragraph; otherwise, consider: What was healthy and affirming in their experiences? What was harmful and even traumatizing? How do you imagine these experiences have affected the sexuality of the women they became?

With respect to a history of some kind of trauma, a stance of self-acceptance begins with "That's what I experienced. That's how it is. Where I am right now is my starting place as I go on to create the kind of life and experiences I want to have."

Brothers and Cousins: From Curiosity to Coercion

Brothers, sisters, and cousins are often childhood partners of opportunity when it comes to satisfying sexual curiosity. About 3 percent of the respondents who had had a childhood or adolescent experience with a male said their first sexual activity with a male was with a brother, another 3 percent that theirs was with a cousin. These experiences ranged from fully to not-at-all consensual. The Survey respondents, of course, had many other consensual and nonconsensual experiences with brothers and cousins that were not their *first* sexual activity.

Many of the incidents that involve brothers and provide information useful to a girl's developing sexual self are subtle. **Katherine (1938)** and her father and brother (two years older) took baths together until she was seven "and never thought anything of it. That's the way we did it. There was nothing sexual about it. It was just we didn't have clothes on. And then we would get dressed and go to bed, in our separate beds." **Diana (1968)** was about four when she noticed the differences between boys and girls: "That's when I asked Mom how come my brother had a penis and I didn't."

The women I interviewed reported interactions with their brothers that ranged from clearly positive to terribly abusive.

Sometimes with an older brother, explorations that were benign when younger became less so as the boy began to mature sexually. When **Carole (1930)** was eight or nine, her older half-brother crawled into bed with her. She said, "We were playing around and my mother caught us and yelled at us. There was never any explanation of what was bad or why, but my mother was really mad and that was the end of us sleeping in the same room. Later, when he was a teenager he would come to where I was living and push me up against the wall and rub on me. He had an erection and I could feel it. It was a mixture of feelings. I didn't like him doing it, but it was a turn-on."

When **Vickie (1957)** was three or four, she and her four-years-older brother would play in the bathtub and, she said, "identify our private parts, our genitals. A lot of it was very playful."

But their relationship gradually gravitated toward "some kind of sadistic abusive stuff."

She continued: "We would play with sort of the edge. I think I went along with it at the time. There was something exciting about it. But when I was around five or six, there was an overstep. We were playing in our basement and he kind of threatened me—told me—asked me—to strip. I ended up stripping and he tied me up some way. There may have been some kind of anal or vaginal penetration. Mostly it was just very scary. Up to then it had been our exploration and play. It went over the edge at this point and it became too scary for me. It was no longer fun. I think after that we no longer played the games. My guess is that we knew we had gone too far and that was that. I don't know if it ever occurred to me to tell on him. I didn't really have a sense of what had happened at the time."

The Edge

When Vickie described her experience, she said, "We would play with sort of the edge. . . . There was something exciting about it." Here we see the tension, the excitement of testing the limits, the *edge*—that edge of experience where curiosity, a little danger, excitement, and the slightly forbidden meet. And one way we learn is to go just a little over the edge, seeing what the consequences are.

As we are finding our way to sexual selfhood, we confront and resolve over and over again the tensions between *curiosity and the wish to do* on one hand and *prohibitions against doing*—and sometimes the *dangers* of doing—on the other. Within many families, there is enough safety for children to confront and resolve these tensions. But even in protective families, it may be fairly common for mutual exploration between a girl and an older brother to go awry at some point. Older brothers are bigger, stronger, and may mature before their younger sisters. Both a girl and her brother are finding their way—seeking information, seeking to understand the mysteries of sex and sexuality. Both are pushing limits and boundaries. But there is an age and power difference. There are other family constellations, too: a sister may also be older; or two sisters or two brothers may explore together. By the time Vickie's basement incident with her brother occurred, he would have been nine or ten, moving into pre-pubescence.

These days, if Vickie and her brother—or Carole and her teen-aged half-brother—were discovered, it would be called sexual abuse or even rape by some, and the brothers would be punished accordingly. But is this the most life-affirming response? Was Vickie's brother, for example, deliberately harming her or had mutual experimentation gone too far? If we call him a rapist or juvenile sex offender instead of, for example, a curious pre-pubescent boy with an equally curious and more-or-less-willing sister, we could do them both serious harm. We could create a situation much more severe and traumatizing than the sexual exploration gone awry that Vickie and Carole described. Whatever labels we applied would affect the rest of their lives.

If a wise adult had been aware of what Carole and Vickie and their brothers were doing at the time, she or he might have counseled them and created a safer context for their time together, as Carole's mother attempted to do. I see, though, no benefit in punishing Carole, Vickie, or their brothers. If Vickie's brother's one-time over-the-edge behavior had continued or if he had been intimidating other children as well, then I would have advised professional assessment and perhaps professional counseling.

Just when does play at the *edge* become sexual abuse? Where do we draw the line between sexual abuse and experiences that prepare us to be sexually healthy adults? These are not easy questions to answer. We might even say, It *depends* . . . Beth and Amanda provide other examples of the edge where mutual, curious exploration becomes problematic. These examples may help to clarify our answers.

When **Beth (1961)** and her brother were in junior high, they would, she said, "touch and stimulate each other but there wasn't any kind of intercourse or kissing or those kinds of things. It just seemed like we were experimenting. At the time, I would just do anything for him. I was curious at first. I had changed my other younger brothers' diapers so it wasn't like the male body was foreign to me. I was familiar with how it looked. I was just curious about what it did, how the penis would get hard. Then that curiosity was gone, but he would continue to have ideas like *Let's try this.* There was a mixture of feelings. Because of my connection with him, I would do that for him, and at the same time feel like I didn't want to be doing this anymore."

I asked Beth what—if she'd known the words and felt powerful enough to say it—she would have liked to have said to her brother. She replied, "If I could have, back then, I would have said, after the second or third time, *What are we doing? What is really going on here? I really don't want to do this anymore.* We never talked about ending it, but we moved to a new home in the ninth grade and we didn't do it after that. It wasn't like there was much dialogue. Even now, as adults, I've only talked about it with him once and he is fuzzy about it. No one else in the family knew about it."

What began as mutual exploration became a predicament. Once her curiosity had been satisfied, Beth did not know how to stop it. Because at the time, as she said, "I would just do anything for him," perhaps she didn't feel it was okay to let her brother know she'd had enough. Some other women who, like Beth, talked as adults to their brothers about similar incidents, reported that their brothers, too, are fuzzy about their recollections.

Amanda (1970) was another who explored sexuality with her brother:

> My first awareness of my sexuality would probably be an incestuous relationship—more an exploration—with my brother, off and on when I was nine, ten, eleven. He is two years older. In the beginning it was just something that was happening, playing in the house. I didn't feel like I was being violated really. It was just an exploration, doing the acts, but not actually doing everything involved in it: feeling each other, maybe him being on top of me, but never really intercourse. He never penetrated me. I touched his genitals, penis, probably his chest and everything. And the same with him, touching my breasts, touching my vagina. Sometimes he would have erections. Maybe later I began to realize that this really wasn't something that was supposed to go on. But I wouldn't say that I saw it as a violence against me, but more of an awareness that this wasn't

supposed to occur. I'm not really ashamed of it anymore, because I look at it as more innocent. We didn't really understand what was happening. I don't see my brother very much now, but we continue to have a caring relationship and encourage each other.

Amanda's narrative is very interesting to me, because she seems to be arguing with those who gave her the value-laden phrase—the label—"incestuous relationship." *It was more an exploration*, she says. *I didn't feel like I was being violated. I didn't see it as a violence against me.* It seems to me that she is saying strongly that how she remembers what happened with her brother does not fit the victimization interpretation she has heard from others. When asked how this relationship affected her sexuality, she replied: "That and other experiences have made me a lot more skeptical of what is occurring in a relationship and what somebody wants. When you actually engage in sexual intercourse, what does that mean? What are you giving and what are they receiving? And in terms of how they feel about me: Do they care about me? Do they love me? Do they respect me? That kind of stuff. If I'm engaging in this act, then what is coming out of it?"

Pause for a moment and consider: This is what Amanda experienced. How did those experiences, through which she was finding her way and decoding some of the mysteries of sex and sexuality, affect the woman she became? It seems to me that, although there were indeed some negative aspects to those early experiences, her ability to choose a sexual partner who values her was enhanced, as was her awareness of how important it is to her that the sex she engages in be meaningful.

Brother Abuse

There is no question in my mind that this next narrative is an example of sexual abuse. **Doris (1930)** describes experiences with her brothers that were not mutual curiosity and exploration gone over the edge, but experiences to which she clearly did not consent. These victimized her and deeply wounded her sexual self, two criteria I use to describe sexual abuse. Doris, the youngest of twelve children, had six brothers. She said:

A lot of my feelings about my sexual self are not good, and I think are directly related to my brother who is a year older than me. He molested me a lot, starting when I was five, six, seven. He'd take me out in the field and put his arm around me, and lay me down, and do a lot of touching and rubbing around my vagina. It left me distressed. From a very young age I felt that sex is dirty. I watched my older brothers laugh a lot about inside jokes . . . it was funny, but it was dirty, and I wasn't supposed to know what it was about. And two of my brothers set me up a couple of times with other boys. One time we were all upstairs just playing around and having fun and my brother shot downstairs and left me with this other fella, and, again, he grabbed me and was feeling my breasts and feeling my vagina. It was just touching, but I was the victim . . . over and over again . . . the quiet little girl who never said anything.

As I had asked Beth, I asked Doris what—if she'd known the words to use and felt powerful enough to say them—she would have liked to have said to her brother. She replied, "I wish I'd said, *Goddamn it, get your hands off of me!* My mother and older sisters weren't aware of this at all. I didn't tell anybody. I think that's really affected my sex life. The only time that I really enjoyed sex was when I was married, and that was just sometimes. Because then it was legal, and right . . . okay. My husband gave me the feeling that I had a nice body and that I was loved for more than just my body even though I always thought I was fat."

Judith (1940), too, was identified by her older brother and his friends as an object for the satisfaction of their sexual curiosity and exploration. She, too, was abused.

When I was four, my brother—three years older—and two of his even older friends—I remember them as very big—called me into the bedroom and told me to take off my clothes. I recall lying there with my legs apart, and I think I was raped. That still isn't totally worked through. I had a strange childhood. My parents were divorced when I was one and my mother, brother, and I lived with my grandfather and there was no supervision.

For Judith, there was another abuser besides her brother and his friends, a man who used to visit:

I can still smell him and it makes me nauseous. I can see him and the image makes me disgusted and angry. The sexual feeling was very pleasurable—scary. It does feel good, and it's—it was—very scary. There's still some residue of the feeling good and the shame that goes with it. And it's secret. There was nobody to tell, nobody to listen to me. He'd put me on his lap and pull me against him . . . fondle me . . . put his hands down in my crotch . . . rub what I now know was his hard penis against me. This happened many times from when I was six until about eight or nine. I don't know if he ever actually penetrated me. He smelled horrible. I would dread it when he came over. I would go into my room and hide. I was so relieved when he stopped coming around.

Emotional Reactions

Judith experienced *terror*, one form of which is *anticipatory dread*, ongoing anticipation of abusive events. Abuse that involves fearfully waiting for the abuser to show up again and again is going to have enduring trauma effects (Hindman 1989). Judith also experienced other confusing and conflicting emotions—moments of pleasure mixed with feelings of shame, strong fear, and disgust. Such mixed emotions are frequently described as linked to situations like hers.

Another who experienced this confusing combination of pleasure and shame was the woman (1966) who appended the following note to her questionnaire. Her experiences started out as abusive and completely nonconsensual but ended up feeling good and filling some of her needs for affection. She wrote: "I was raised by two very cold parents. My mother never hugged me or told me she loved me. My father never showed much love to us either. I was fondled by my older male cousin from age nine to ten or eleven years old. At first I hated it—but then it felt good to have orgasms. We never had intercourse. When I was fifteen years old, I let a married man fondle me. I felt ashamed but again it felt good to be touched and to be brought to orgasm. We didn't have intercourse either. I had boyfriends who fondled me. I guess I always loved being touched that way. I met my husband, who is sixteen years older than me, when I was nineteen years old and I was a virgin and he introduced me to intercourse."

Sexual responsiveness is an appropriate physical reaction to sexual stimulation, but in a circumstance of misuse by another, the context is unhealthy and the stimulation is inappropriate. Consequently the girl or woman may feel pleasure, but it is mixed with other feelings such as disgust, anger, fear, and confusion. When she physically responds, it is because her body has a healthy capacity to do so. In the right context for her and with a partner of her choice, sexual response and pleasure are desirable. One of the consequences of sexual violation is that pleasure responses are sometimes blocked from occurring freely. They may stay blocked until the confusing overlapping feelings are untangled or neutralized through a combination of therapy and a loving relationship or some other means of healing the wounded sexual self.

When sexual boundaries are violated, there are some conditions that can help make the outcome less traumatic. A girl or woman usually will experience fewer continuing emotional consequences and can begin to heal and neutralize the experience almost at once if she is able to tell someone about what happened immediately after the abuse takes place; if she is believed; and if the person she tells is supportive and affirms that she did not cause the abuse—it was the person who violated her who was responsible and wrong (Hindman 1989).

Unfortunately, for both Judith and Doris none of these conditions was met. Even now, years later, Judith is still addressing her early childhood experiences in therapy, through which, over time, she has been able to develop the perspective: *That's what I experienced. That's how it is.*

Dirty Old Men

Outside of the family, another source of sexual boundary violations is what women of my generation called "dirty old men." Sometimes a girl observed male behavior that validated what she heard from her parents—*All boys and men want only one thing; they're not to be trusted.* **Nan (1917)** said, "An older man tried to have a relationship with my sister when she was only eight and I was six. Nothing really happened, but he tried. I was told about it, and it was impressed on me that there were men who wanted younger women, children even. That's stayed with me all these years . . . the feeling that some men aren't really nice."

Other girls, such as **Lorraine (1957)**, were actually groped or touched. She said, "At least four or five different times during my childhood, men—neighbors or people at my mother's church—tried to put their hands in my pants."

Self-Efficacy

A girl is likely to feel confused and powerless in such situations. But some girls are able to avoid men who treat them this way, or to fight back. They recognize, although probably not in these specific terms, that these men are obnoxious, that they have unclear boundaries, that they are not respectful, and that they treat girls as objects who have no feelings and sensitivities of their own. These girls are empowered by that recognition to exercise self-awareness, sidestep what is distasteful, and take measures to protect themselves.

Through their own efficacy the girls in these following examples rescued themselves from men who were behaving inappropriately with them. Ann and Bonnie were able to transform feelings of victimization into empowered confidence and a sense of *I can take care of myself.* **Ann (1934)** spoke of an experience when she was ten or eleven. "I wasn't sexually abused but I was fondled by an adult male one time. My father was overseas in the Navy and this man was like a surrogate father to me and we went to his house a lot. I was sitting in his living room and he was massaging my back and then he started massaging my breasts. And suddenly something clicked and I was aware this was not what I was accustomed to. So I just avoided him from then on." **Bonnie (1966)** said, "I had an incident when I was around twelve, maybe older, when one of the kids around the corner who was about sixteen basically sexually attacked me. But I was very strong and threw him off me. I got hold of a wine bottle and threatened him with it and told him to leave and he did."

When a girl clearly identifies herself as being victimized and clearly identifies the other person as wronging her, she will experience a sense of personal power that can help to diminish traumatic effects and make them less enduring, particularly if she is able to take defensive measures. Not every girl is able to do this, however. We do the best we can at the time.

Cynthia (1954) was sexually violated by her father and was definitely traumatized by this emotionally complex experience. But once she became aware of her father's potential to violate her, she was able to keep it from happening again. Cynthia's parents separated when she was eight. She adored her father until he molested her when she was twelve, while she and her younger brother were visiting him. From the emotion in Cynthia's voice as she relayed the details of her molestation, it was clear that recalling the shattering of those positive childhood images is still painful.

> He was drunk; it was late at night and I was in bed but not quite asleep. He just started fondling me. Not intercourse, but he undressed me and licked and touched me. He penetrated me with his hands, but he stayed dressed. This was my first experience with sexual touching. I was so incredibly shocked and confused. I kept crying the whole time, saying *Daddy, please don't, please stop, please stop.* I couldn't believe he was doing this. Up to then, I had him on a pedestal. I thought he was the most handsome, wonderful man in the world. My mother hadn't shared with me how he had

treated her. I knew he always had a can of beer in his hand but I had no idea of alcoholism. When he molested me, it was like the statue had fallen off the pedestal and had busted. Earlier that day I had watched him beat my step-mother, the first time I had seen that. So it was more than him molesting me, it was everything that happened that day. I didn't know what to think. I didn't understand his interest in my body. I hadn't begun to think about sex yet. It really hurt a lot emotionally. I didn't have anybody to turn to. Mom wasn't there and I couldn't tell my grandparents. I was stuck in my own head. When I got home, my mother sat me down and said there was something she wanted to tell me before I visited my dad and she hadn't been able to stop thinking about it . . . that he had a drinking problem and when he gets drunk he might look at me as just another girl and forget that I was his daughter and might try to do things to me. I was sitting there thinking, *It already happened, Mom.* I wanted to tell her, but I couldn't. I don't know why. I only visited my father once more and that was because I didn't know how to tell my mother why I didn't want to go. But I protected myself that time. I stayed out of his way the whole time I was there and managed not to get stuck with him.

Cynthia's experience was incredibly complex psychologically. It has continued to affect her into adulthood. But included in her sexual self-image is the empowered and healthy statement: *I protected myself that time.*

The Wounded Sexual Self

Child abuse researchers have determined a number of factors in abuse experiences that are likely to make the trauma more severe. These include, for example, sexual responsiveness to the stimulation; terror; not clearly identifying the molester as wrong and herself as victim; being under age twelve at the time of the abuse; not telling anyone about it; disastrous responses from others when the abuse is revealed; and ongoing contacts with people and situations that continue to elicit feelings and thoughts connected to the experience. Someone who has been abused is likely to deny, rationalize, minimize, and rearrange the facts in order to avoid looking at what happened. This may involve such powerful forms of denial as amnesia and dissociation or behaving *badly* so that she herself becomes apparently *deserving* of blame or guilt (Hindman 1989).

Effects of Childhood Abuse on Adult Sexuality

What are the effects of childhood sexual abuse on adult sexuality? **Maggie (1965)** spoke of the enduring effects abuse had for her. She described her family of origin as one with a multigenerational history of sexual abuse; she herself had had numerous abusers. Maggie began engaging in adult-like sexual behavior with peers by the age of ten, and she had so many male partners in her last year of high school that she lost count. That same year she also had substance abuse problems and was taking drugs to try not to eat. Her brother who was four years older and his friends molested her. She said: "When I describe my childhood, a lot of it is about sex—positive, negative, who I was being sexual with, who was being sexual with me, what I was doing. It was very hard for me to be assertive about what I didn't want. I never had a clear sense in sex with men that it was about my pleasure at all. It was about what they could get out of it."

As an adult, Maggie has undergone individual therapy and been in a therapy group for women who have experienced incest. Since she was seventeen, most of her partners have been women. She talked about the problems her early sexual abuse created for her in relationships:

> It's more of a problem in ongoing relationships because I've let someone in emotionally and I start to feel pressured by having someone around me who wants to be sexual. I was with a woman for five years. We had incredibly wonderful creative passionate sex—but getting to the point of having sex was the problem. I would usually shut down in the kissing stage. There were times when I was completely nonsexual. I wasn't clear about what I wanted just for myself ... how to set boundaries ... so I set too many. As soon as I learned to say *No*, I couldn't say *Yes* again. I fought against accepting myself as a sexual person ... that I had desires. I was completely unclear where my own desire came in ... what I wanted ... and how to integrate someone else's desires with my own without feeling responsible, guilty, or angry. I always experienced her desire as threatening to me, as something I either had to capitulate to or push against. I still wrestle with giving myself permission to want to be sexual with someone. Physically I'm aroused but mentally I come up with all sorts of excuses.

Maggie was sexually abused and had a highly sexualized childhood and adolescence. Her experiences went far beyond the typical curious exploration and experimentation of most children who have not experienced sexual abuse. Being sexually misused by others had many consequences for her developing sexual self. Her experiences taught her that sex with men was about what they could get out of it, not her pleasure. She was robbed of her ability to enjoy certain kinds of sexual stimulation such as tickling on the outside of her vulva, because, as she told me, that had been done to her by a live-in maid when she was young.

After a lot of therapy and other healing experiences she is finally beginning to accept that she is a sexual person with desires of her own. She is beginning to accept that a sexual invitation from another doesn't require a rigid *No* or an unqualified *Yes*. There are many options in between. She is still working on understanding a realm of human activity that poses problems for many of us, whether we have a history of sexual abuse or not: she doesn't have to be guilty or angry to say *No* to another's sexual desires. And she doesn't have to feel totally responsible for her partner's feelings and reactions, although it is important that she be sensitive to how her partner may respond to what she says and does.

Each of us is responsible for how we treat our partner and entitled to and responsible for our own reactions, feelings, and desires. When we don't get our way, we may experience anger or disappointment. That's how it is. What we do with these feelings is our personal responsibility, just as a partner's feelings and actions toward us are hers or his.

Healing the Wounds of Sexual Trauma

There are lessons about sex and sexuality that, ideally, we all would learn as we grow up. Among these are the following:

- To appreciate that we can engage in sex for our own pleasure

- To understand that partnered sex can be a process of creating mutual pleasure

- To recognize and accept our own sexual desires

- To recognize that we have choices about how to express these desires—or not

- To set boundaries that allow us to integrate someone else's desires with our own without giving up what we need and want for ourselves.

- To negotiate sexual invitations—how to say *No* and when and how to say *Yes*

These are difficult lessons to learn under the best of circumstances. In childhood and adolescence, during mutually curious play and exploration with age peers, we may begin to understand some of them experientially. Throughout our lives we continue to refine our understanding of these lessons and ideals.

A sexual abuser honors none of these ideals. An abuser robs us of the opportunities to experience ourselves in these sexually healthy ways. An abuser acts out of his—or sometimes her—own desires. A girl or woman who is being sexually misused is not learning to negotiate her own desires. In fact, she may experience that she is powerless to do so.

Now, here are some accounts by other women describing what they did to heal their sexual wounds. **Victoria (1946)** recounted how she worked through the impact of early abusive experiences with her older brother on her own. When she was six or seven and he was thirteen or fourteen, he twice came into her bed at night and played with her genitals while having her play with his. There was "no penetration." These experiences really scared her. After the second time, however, she told him to go away, and he did. She said: "I didn't remember the abuse until early on in my first marriage, when flashbacks would cause me to feel like I was sinful; I felt bad and would draw back during sex. But I worked it out. I just thought about it and realized it wasn't my fault. I didn't need to feel guilty or bad, there was nothing I could do about it then; it was an unfortunate thing to happen to both of us. I knew he was sorry about it. Life goes on." Victoria's conclusions demonstrated that she had arrived at sexual self-acceptance. She went on to say that she now enjoys sex. Although Victoria was able to reach these conclusions on her own, many people in similar circumstances will need therapy or other help to arrive at self-acceptance.

Another Survey respondent's (1947) report of abuse by her brother provides us with both a sense of the impact molestation can have later in life and the knowledge that healing can take place when a couple can confront their histories together. She wrote:

I met my husband in college. We were both virgins. We touched and kissed and reached orgasm but didn't actually have intercourse until our wedding night. It was wonderful. We enjoyed each other sexually and in every other way. We were, and still are, twenty-two years later, best friends. But in our third year of marriage, I seemed to lose interest. I still felt sexual desires but something was "in the way." I remembered the molestation by my brother, when I was ten and he was fourteen, and I kind of figured that was the problem. My husband wanted sex much more than I did but I turned away. I couldn't tell him—I couldn't tell *anybody*! I felt so ashamed of what had happened with my brother. My husband was so frustrated with me. I cried a lot and kept saying, *It's not you, it's me.*

Unfortunately, many years went by. It wasn't until our early forties, when I was in counseling, that I realized that my counselor was the one I could tell about my brother. About the same time my husband realized that he had been abused by his parents when he was young. When his abuse came out, that's when I told him about my brother. He was furious that I hadn't told him many years ago. He still doesn't really understand why I couldn't. All those years he thought there was some way *he* was lacking sexually because I turned away. But—I am happy to report that we are getting help. Our counselor is terrific, I thank God that she came into our lives. Now my husband and I are like two newlyweds. There are times we can't wait to get into bed! And in the last year we have engaged in oral sex (both of us) which I was too inhibited for before.

Not only does this narrative demonstrate that healing can occur when a couple address their histories together, it also shows us how, in some instances, when we think we are sexually lacking because a partner keeps turning away, our partner may be sexually blocked by her or his own life experiences. Furthermore, it demonstrates powerfully how important it is to seek help as soon as possible, so that potential opportunities for pleasure and intimacy can be fulfilled.

We all have some sexual wounds. The consequences of having one's sexual boundaries violated can range from annoying, as they were for some of the women who were pawed by older men, to seriously traumatic. For almost everyone who experiences violation of her or his sexual boundaries, it is helpful to talk about what happened to a supportive, accepting other, whether friend, therapist, or intimate partner. It is best if you are able to talk about what happened very soon afterwards, but even if years have gone by, it is not too late. If you have experienced sexual violation, some of the ways you might approach healing your wounded sexual self include the following:

- Individual therapy

- Group therapy with others who have had experiences similar to yours

- Sharing your history with your partner and learning about your partner's history

- Writing about your history and feelings in, for example, a journal, short stories, or poetry

- Drawing or expressing your history through other art forms

- Engaging in movement forms such as belly dancing and other kinds of dance, tai chi, or martial arts, etc.

- Creating sexual experiences—solo or partnered—that give you pleasure

A Narrative for Your Consideration

I end this chapter with a narrative that takes the question of *What constitutes sexual abuse?* even further. It contains a situation that goes against acceptable social mores and pushes a lot of our judgmental buttons—he's a teacher in his twenties and married; she's a teenager. As you read this narrative, notice your thoughts and feelings about the experiences **Ruth (1943)** describes. These experiences took place in 1959 and 1960.

> I had my first very nearly sexual experience when I was a junior in high school. It was with a guy who was married; he was twenty-four and I was jail bait—sixteen, seventeen. We worked at a summer camp together. God, I loved him! I thought he was wonderful. His wife taught school with my mother. Isn't that scary? And he taught junior high school. We would meet in his classroom and make out. I didn't touch him under his clothing; he would touch under mine; he would touch me genitally. He would be very erect; I would walk in the room and he would have an erection, and that would really turn me on. But even then, I had very little knowledge of women's sexuality. I did not masturbate at all; I didn't know you could. But I would come home and sort of daydream about what it would be like to have sex with him—up to a point—and then go to sleep. I never had orgasms with him, but I did have a lot of experience with sexual feelings and sexual arousal.
>
> I would have had sex (intercourse) with him in a flash. He had the sense not to; I had the ignorance to do it.

To me, it's a miracle that we didn't get in trouble in some way. But, again, when I look back on my life, I really have taken risks in several areas; I consider that was a big risk, when I was a teenager. That lasted two summers; during the winter nothing happened; I went to school and did all my stuff. But in those two summers we worked at this day camp, we had a great thing going except that it just never went to intercourse. But it was still very real to me; I really have no idea what it was like for him. In retrospect, I wonder: *What was his angle in that?* Because we never discussed him divorcing. It was all very casual and yet it was deep to me. I was in love with him.

I recognize that in the context of our society there are distinct rules and laws that apply to this situation. Since Ruth was not yet eighteen, this would be labeled as statutory rape under the laws in most states today. A teacher discovered behaving with a student in this manner would be seen as violating the ethics of his profession and would probably lose his credential to teach. He was married, so his church or synagogue, if he had one, also would be likely to label his behavior as sinful or immoral.

But this is a book about how women experience and express their sexuality. I am asking you to consider what Ruth actually experienced, not how society might judge her. In that spirit I ask: In your opinion, is this situation in some way sexual abuse? If so—or if not— why do you think that? How do you think Ruth may have been harmed? What may have been positive or empowering for her in these experiences? If the man involved were to be interviewed, what do you think he might tell us of his experiences with Ruth?

The fortunate young girl grows up in a situation that provides a protective environment of acceptance, concern, and reasonable restrictions for her impulses to explore her emerging sexuality, but such circumstances may be the exception not the norm. We have seen that consent and age-appropriateness are important factors. We have seen, too, that sexual feelings and exploration are appropriate for a girl in childhood, when the exploration is impelled by her own curiosity. Furthermore, experiences involving mutual curiosity and exploration with siblings, cousins, and other playmates are often positive although—even in protective families—they may sometimes go over the *edge* and become unpleasant or harmful. And we have seen that positive experiences are quite different from experiences with age-peers or adults in which a nonconsenting girl is regarded as an object for the satisfaction of others' curiosity.

What Does This Mean to You?

Now, if you wish, pick up your notebook and express the thoughts and feelings you're having about your family and your experiences with sexual boundaries. Here are some questions you might want to consider after you've done that.

- How was love expressed in your family when you were growing up?

- What was the major impact of your father—or the man who was like a father to you—on your learning about sexual boundaries? (Consider the behavior and values he modeled for you as well as his words.)

- What was the major impact of your mother—or the woman who was like a mother to you—on your learning about sexual boundaries? (Consider the behavior and values she modeled for you as well as her words.)

- Is there a sexual incident you recall from your childhood or adolescence in which—if you had known the words and felt powerful enough to say them—you would have made a situation stop or change course? Do you know the words now that you have a broader perspective, more life experience and more awareness of your power? Imagine the situation with a new ending in which you effectively stop or change it.

- Most girls are at some time the recipients of unwanted touches and attention. If you've ever had an experience in which someone was inappropriate with you, imagine now—even if it really didn't happen this way—what it would have been like to overpower that person and run him or her off or totally erase him or her off the face of the earth. (You realize, of course, that this is a healing fantasy image, not something you would do now in reality.)

- If you are recalling experiences that you now regret, consider the circumstances, the roles of others, and how you saw your options at the time. Then, sit quietly with your eyes closed and imagine what you could now gently and lovingly tell your younger self that would be healing and lead to greater self-acceptance.

5

The First Time

Almost every woman who has "done it" clearly remembers her first time. If she has chosen for herself when, where, and with whom it will be, a woman's first intercourse can be a momentous event. It can be the culmination of years of curiosity, erotic imaginings, romantic or lustful crushes, and physical experimentation that began when she was very young and evolved through increasingly complex solo and partnered sexual exploration.

Getting Ready

Few women have consensual intercourse for the first time without having first wondered and fantasized about it. Who will he be? How do you do it? What will it feel like? Will it hurt? A young woman who has not yet had intercourse may imagine being swept away by the man of her dreams, feel frequent arousal, and regard giving up her virginity as a significant rite of passage into the sisterhood of adult women. As she gets ready she is also experimenting and talking about it with friends. If a woman has been sexually violated, she may not consider the instances of violation to be "sexual" experience. For her, giving up her virginity may come later, through her own choice and with her consent.

The Preteen Years—Figuring It Out

As preteens approach puberty, they have a range of questions and concerns about sexuality and close relationships on their minds that many adults find astonishing. They want to understand all they can about sex and relationships *before* physical metamorphosis and powerful hormone-driven urges transform them into adolescents. Once they become adolescents their attention will be focused on new matters in new ways. They need as much information as they can get before that happens.

In a 1985 survey of fourth- to sixth-graders who ranged in age from nine to eleven years old, sex educator Eric W. Johnson found that they thought and worried about questions of difference, belonging, relating, love, and how people treat each other. The students were given open-ended anonymous questionnaires that consisted entirely of blank pages except for the following headings: "1. *Facts* You Want to Know About People, Love, Sex, and Families" and 2. "*Questions* You Want to Ask." The most frequently asked questions sought information about how people have babies and how men's and women's bodies work to have children.

The second most frequent category had to do with the feelings associated with having sex. These girls and boys were curious about what having sex feels like: "Does it feel good?" "Does sex hurt?" "Is sex dirty?" "Is it the best thing in the world?" Some wanted to know "What do you mean by having sex?" Most seemed to assume that actually having sex was something they would not do now but would do later in their lives. They wanted to find out now about what would happen later. They were curious about dating rules and when, where, and how they would have sex.

By about age eleven, some girls are already having strong sexual feelings. In general, boys' feelings become very strong two or three years later than girls' do. Many girls and some boys wondered whether it is wrong to feel that you'd like to have sex. "Is it wrong to want to have sex at this age—not have, but want?" asked a sixth-grade girl, and a fifth-grade girl put it this way: "Is feeling a sexual attraction for a boy wrong? Or is it just a part of life?" (Johnson 1985).

How Do You "Do It"?

As girls approach puberty, questions they were addressing earlier with respect to self-pleasuring are now addressed to partner sex.

One of these questions is, "How do you 'do it'?" Misinformation and vague explanations can cause great distress for girls in their ongoing attempts to decode the mysteries of sex. For example, During **Penny's (1946)** sixth-grade sex education class she learned that the way to get pregnant was "... to be *in love*. They could not say *by making love*. I thought since I had a crush on one of the boys that I was going to get pregnant, even though he didn't even know I existed. I was terrified."

When **Kathy (1949)** was about ten, her year-older sister told her: *They put the place where they pee into where you pee, and that's what sex is.* Kathy said, "I knew I had two holes and ... that the man put his cock inside of me, but I didn't know which hole and I didn't have anybody to ask." From jokes, snatches of conversation, and TV she would try to figure out how you had sex. "But," she said, "in those days TV was fairly tame; usually they would kiss and then, when they would go to lay down on the bed, the scene would be cut; I couldn't even tell if they were facing each other or not or which one was on top. It was so frustrating!" When **Melanie (1970)** was young, she thought "the way you got a baby was that you could just say, *I want a baby* and you would get one." She was terrified of saying those words. So when she first heard about sex, her reaction was, "That's a big lie. That's not how you do it."

Decoding the Dance of Courtship

Do you remember learning to tie your shoelaces or to ride a bicycle? You were probably awkward at first, but then you practiced the basic movements until they became a part of your unconscious memory and thereafter they seemed spontaneous and automatic, as if you had always known how to do them. Similarly, the processes of courtship and adult lovemaking are learned one step at a time.

Although we don't realize it when it is happening, throughout our childhood and teen years we are learning the basic steps of adult romance, courtship, and sex. We learn, for example, that there are courting and sexual scripts, and that in these scripts girls have certain roles and boys have different ones. **Michele (1972)** described an experience she had in third grade: "When I was nine it didn't dawn on me that guys and girls were supposed to like each other. I always played a lot more with boys than girls. I had a best friend, and he was a boy. And all of the sudden, he started calling me up. It was fine; it was like talking to a girlfriend. And then one night, he called me and asked, *Do you like me?* And that was the first time it dawned on me like, *Oh no! He thinks I'm a girl.* I was crushed. He was my best friend. Friends don't do that. *Oh, no!*"

Learning "Sexual" Skills Through Play

One important way we learn is by rehearsing adult behaviors. As girls we may wrestle and experience excitement and the tensions and resistances of physical contact. We feel *in love*. We may kiss or hold hands. Each of these mini-experiences allows us to rehearse a step in the sequence of adult courtship and lovemaking. **Joan (1944)** kissed one of her brother's friends when she was seven. "I had him down, and I was sitting on top of him. And I thought he was so cute. I wanted to kiss him, desperately, and I just sat there for the longest time; it was kind of like standing on the high diving board, trying to get the nerve up to jump off. Finally I kissed him on the cheek, and my face turned bright red and I went running off."

Some girls attempt to figure out how you do it by going through the motions with each other, actively rehearsing the basic skills of adult sexual expression. That this is done with another girl usually has more to do with opportunity than with sexual orientation. **Jessica (1970)** said, "My first experience of myself as sexual was probably in sixth grade, just kissing and exploring, with my cousin. She was on top of me, and that was it. We didn't know anything."

Although some girls are quite active in exercising their curiosity, others, like **Pat (1945)**, learn more passively. They are observers of the scene, more aware than active: "Around twelve or thirteen I became very aware of sexual needs, but because I was Catholic that was a verboten area. I didn't become sexually active as a teenager, but I was very sexual, very aware of my sexuality."

Curiosity About Penises

Girls of all ages are fascinated by penises. Some seek through their own agency and curiosity to know more about this mysterious *something* boys and men have that girls don't. At the swimming pool when she was about ten, **Katherine (1938)** observed "those guys in their little bathing suits," and, she said: "I thought, *Those guys are so weird looking!* Their bathing suits were so tight you could see everything." **Harriet (1938)**, who had no brothers and so didn't know much about males, said, "I didn't know what a penis looked like. I remember my father sleeping out in the yard one day in his boxer shorts. They were a little bit open and I walked by and tried to see what was in there."

Sometimes a girl's curiosity takes her to the edge of greater excitement and also greater risk, as it did for **Connie (1956)**, who was a "tomboy" and "liked boys." "We were always playing with each other. I remember playing doctor with the little neighbor kids and we would inspect each other's little parts. I was fascinated by penises. I remember one time one of the neighbor boys peed on me. I thought that was very weird. It was sort of exciting, but I was angry and then we fought. I was maybe eight and he was six. But it was exciting at the same time."

Most children engage in some kind of curiosity-impelled experimentation. Occasionally, experiences like the one Connie described are labeled as "abuse perpetrated by the boy." However, when I consider the circumstances and the ages of Connie and this boy, I conclude that it was *not* "sexual abuse" when he peed on her. It is through activities like these that we learn about the differences between girls and boys, begin developing skills that become the foundation for our adult lovemaking, and solve the mysteries of adult sex and sexuality. However, some childhood sexual play is less benign. **Janine (1921)** described one such experience. "From the time I was five or six, I would play and experiment with the neighborhood boys. We looked at each other's genitals and touched them; I remember it as pleasurable. I didn't carry any guilt but I knew this was something you didn't tell people about. When I was about seven, there was a boy who was twelve, old enough to ejaculate. He did ejaculate on me and I got very upset and very frightened because I had heard about babies and I remember going home and washing in the bathtub and thinking I'd never do that again. We moved after that and I found a girl playmate in the new neighborhood. We did genital touching, just experimenting; it was pleasurable."

Janine didn't describe being frightened by the boy's penis or his ejaculating; she was frightened because she misunderstood how a woman becomes pregnant. Her statement: [*I thought] I'd never do that again* affirmed her capacity for self-efficacy. This frightening experience "at the edge" was a learning experience for her. She was there because she wanted to be and seems not to have been unduly traumatized. It did not bring her experimentation and discoveries of pleasure to an end. Yet we are not all alike. Although apparently not terribly traumatic for Janine, that kind of experience might have been so for someone else. Because of that, the age differences of the children might be of concern to a wise adult. *Understanding Your Child's Sexual Behavior: What's Natural and Healthy* by Toni Cavanagh Johnson, Ph.D. (1999) is an excellent guide for assessing when children's sexual behaviors are "natural and healthy" and when they may be "indication[s] of some distress or disturbance."

Traumatic Experiences

Some girls are exposed to penises without their consent and in situations that are not entered through their own efforts to satisfy their curiosity. Such experiences tend to be more traumatic, but how much so depends on many factors including whether most of the girl's later experiences empower and enhance her sexual self. **Anna (1949)** had such an experience: "When I was six, my girlfriend's brother locked me in the garage, backed me against a wall, pulled his pants down, and stuck his penis in my face, and asked me to touch it. I remember getting out of the garage, but I don't remember if I touched him first; that's blocked out."

Like Doris and Judith in chapter 4, Anna was a passive recipient not a mutual participant in this activity. The experience was impelled by the boy's curiosity and needs, not her own, and Anna clearly did not want to be there. Her experience was unlike Doris's and Judith's experiences in that, for Anna, this happened only once, and she does remember her own ability to get away; she got out of the garage. Anna told me, *I don't think there was any lasting effect of this event.* Still, the experience was dramatic enough that she remembers it; traumatic enough that she blocks out part of it.

Bonnie (1966) had an experience when she was five in which "the guy next door touched me and wanted me to touch him.... Sometimes I think this still makes me a little insecure around males, but for the most part I think I've overcome that." Again, we see an experience impelled by the male's curiosity and needs that introduces a girl to sexual behaviors long before they are appropriate in her development. Bonnie told us in chapter 4 of the time when she was twelve and used a wine bottle to chase off a sixteen-year-old who sexually attacked her. Even if she is a little insecure around males, she has demonstrated that she also can take care of herself.

Penis Envy

Only one person I interviewed, **Joanna (1957)**, described what might be the penis envy that Freud attributed to all women (see chapter 10). Since her early thirties, Joanna's partners have been women. She told me, "I remember sometime before I was twelve not liking that I didn't have the same parts as a boy and sitting on the toilet backwards trying to pee like they did. I was a little jock and played with the boys. And boys are always playing with themselves. I didn't have anything there to play with and I didn't like it. I remember exploring my body but not with any kind of stirrings. I knew I wasn't supposed to do that because I was this Catholic girl and sex is bad when you're Catholic, so I wouldn't touch down there." It is interesting that Joanna's adult orientation is to be partnered with women, but we should not draw any conclusions connecting childhood "penis envy" with being a lesbian from just one woman's story. That these two characteristics occur together in this person may be entirely coincidental.

Who Will It Be? The Dimension of Romantic Attachment

Among all the other important questions pre-teens and teens are considering are these: *How do I attract a partner?* and *Who will my partner be?* In their active lives and in their fantasies they are addressing the dimension of adult sexuality and adult sexual expression that involves forming a romantic attachment—falling in love and bonding with another.

As girls try to figure out the mysteries and rules of sex and romance, fantasies may be shared and information exchanged. They wonder about the contexts in which sex will occur. In grade school, **Lori (1969)** and her friends were reading books like Judy Blume's *Forever* (1975). When they talked about sex, it was not so much about genital sex as about partner qualities and the rules pertaining to when and with whom you do it. Among the examples Lori gave were these: "We talked about, *Would you want to marry a man who's had sex before?* And we had this continuing fantasy story. The perfect man would be someone who loved me, and who was always nice to me. The sexuality was really confined to the issue of virginity. Because I think all my friends thought that women were not supposed to have sex before marriage, but it was okay for men to."

And one day, for many girls, there is an awareness that *Oh, yes! They're boys!* **Andrea (1972)** described her experience in this way: "Sometime in the middle of junior high you start actually thinking of these boys in your class as somebody other than just other people in your class, that they're actually boys. You start gossiping with your friends about, *He's really cute,* thinking of them in a more personal way." At that age, Andrea was still spending more time in mental and emotional romance than in actual activities with boys.

Crushes

Crushes are another aspect of mental and emotional preparation for real-life romance. Girls of all ages engage in adult-role rehearsal by having crushes. When **Katie (1955)** was in second grade, she had "a big crush on the school bus driver. I and two other girls were in love with him. We bought him Easter candy and did all kinds of crazy things." **Connie (1956)**, who when she was a three-year-old had a crush on Moe of the Three Stooges, added: "Later, other idols came along who I developed crushes on—like the Beatles and Herman's Hermits. I have always loved boys, always, so I was always sexually conscious."

Crushes occur most frequently in adolescence and, for some girls, become a bridge from imagination to actual dating. **Joan (1944)** had her "first real big crush" in the seventh grade: "And then he was my boy friend. He was shorter than me and the extent of what we did was kiss and hold hands. Which was pretty exciting then." **Pam's (1968)** crush on a summer camp counselor in eighth grade was "such a huge thing, it was like we had a love affair going. I wrote to him a lot and he would send me a postcard once in a while. And whenever I got one, it was like the world had shaken."

Not all crushes involve boys. **Liz's (1951)** crushes and early mental rehearsal involved primarily women, and, for her, the orientation toward women carried through into adulthood: "I was seven or eight and there was this older gal up the street I had this mad crush on. I had crushes on women, very few men."

Fran (1965), whose first sexual relationship was with a woman, spoke of a deep childhood friendship with a girl. Now dating men, she describes herself as bisexual. "I was raised in an incredibly repressive Catholic family. I had really intense, good, committed childhood friendships. When I was three or so, through the third grade, I loved my little friend Sara more than anybody. I guess it was a little crush."

Almost Dating

The skills of adult sexual relating and sexual expression are accumulated one step at a time. Among these skills are attracting a partner, flirting, consenting, saying *No*, kissing, necking, petting, orgasm, and *doing it*, all of which themselves are made up of many smaller steps or skills. As more skills are acquired, experiences gradually increase in complexity. As **Katy (1970)** explained, "I think sexuality first meant something to me when I was first sexually attracted to other people, which was probably in eighth grade. I can think of my first kiss, but I don't think that was when I was first sexually motivated. It was kind of a gradual thing rather than an event. I gradually became sexually aware of myself." For many, "going together" may at first involve seeing each other at school, writing notes, calling each other on the phone, perhaps some kissing, and, now, sending e-mail. Having a boyfriend may not, at first, involve much physical contact but instead be a bridge between mental and emotional rehearsal and being with a boy. As **Angela (1971)** explained, her seventh-grade boyfriend "was more of a status thing. I mean you at least had to be able to say that you had a boyfriend."

How Do You Get a Partner?

One dilemma a girl has to resolve is *How do you get a partner?* What are the rules? What is my unique way of being attractive? How do I get a boy—or girl—to like me? In the seventh grade, **Beth (1961)** became sexually aware: "Reading about what the female body is all about and then checking it out for myself, looking at the photographs, touching myself and exploring. That's when I started to feel, *Oh this feels nice.* Also being aware of how I looked. I wanted to look cute or a certain way so that I would be noticed by guys. I was interested in guys back then. So there was that awareness of wanting to attract others." (Beth gradually became aware that her sexual preference is to be with a woman.)

Genital Stirrings

At puberty and beyond, genital stirrings become more and more linked in imagination with having a partner and having sex. These stirrings may be coupled with romantic fantasies and sometimes vicariously with the sexual activity of others. **Ronni (1955)** remembered: "In my early teens I would come home and watch old movies. My first rush of genital arousal was when I was watching Rock Hudson and Doris Day kiss in a 4:30 movie."

The Dance of Courtship: Intermediate Steps

As she begins to have opportunities to kiss, touch, flirt—to practice the actual steps of the dance of courtship—a girl moves to another level in feeling the feelings and acquiring the skills of the dance of sex.

Josephine (1913), one of the oldest women I interviewed, remembers that she was interested in boys early, at age ten or eleven. She described the teen activities when she was young: "youth meetings, trips, camps in the summer, times of exploration, some kissing, like that." When **Penny (1946)** was in seventh grade an older boy from the neighborhood challenged her to a game of strip poker out in the woods: "And I whupped him; I only had to take off my blouse and I had this proper undershirt underneath. He had to take everything off, and he was horribly embarrassed. It was very lucky that I won 'cause I didn't know anything about it."

The exploratory play of early childhood was likely to have involved more looking than touching; now kissing and other physical interactions are added. New steps are learned. When **Cindi (1952)** was ten to twelve, an almost-teen, her family went on camping trips with a family with five boys. She told me, "I was attracted to one of the boys, about my age, a cutie pie, blond, freckles, and blue eyes. We would make out a little bit. I really got the body sensations. When I was twelve we would go off alone and sort of pet and kiss and do all that kind of stuff. It was kind of neat."

Dating

Early dating can involve a lot of confusion and more rules to figure out. A girl may become involved in experiences that go beyond her understanding and the girl-boy scripts she knows. If the context provides safety, dating can give her affirming circumstances in which to practice the steps: necking, petting, and sometimes more. She can continue to find her way.

Jennifer (1965) described her progression and her limits. "When I was around twelve, I wanted to kiss my first boyfriend; by thirteen, it was kissing, petting, things like that. Petting included feeling my breasts and then went into all over; towards the end, a little bit of genital stimulation, but not really. I wouldn't go that far." For **Lori (1969)** at seventeen, "There was a lot of fondling, but never to the point of not having any clothes on. It was exploration without the visual cues."

In the teen years, "sexual" activity for girls is often less about having "sex" than about being accepted by boys and by one's peers; about belonging and being affirmed in one's "okayness" and attractiveness—having a boyfriend. Girls seek the status bestowed by having a boyfriend. Because it is not a predominant cultural message, most girls do not think of sex as the process of creating mutual erotic pleasure with their partners. **Pam (1968)** explained how, in the sixth through eighth grades, she "acted out a lot of my insecurity with boys—kissing and touching with no genital contact. It affirmed something in me, I was okay; I was desirable, although I didn't know what desire meant. I had no idea of what sexual pleasure for me was. I was getting pleasure out of being touched, but I had no idea that I could initiate things or do the touching."

More About Ruth

Remember **Ruth (1943)** from chapter 4, who described her summer experiences as a sixteen- and seventeen-year-old with a married teacher in his twenties? Here, we learn more about her as she talks of dating in the late '50s and early '60s: "I certainly had many dates through high school and college where men—boys—just pawed all over you.

"I never felt threatened, like I was about to be raped or anything. I just thought it was boring that these people I didn't have much interest in were wanting to paw all over me. And have their wet sloppy kisses. Yuck-o! It was usually at a drive-in movie or something when all that stuff was going on. I didn't walk out of the car and go home. But I can remember being repulsed by it. I didn't feel any guilt about any of this, but I think I would have had I had intercourse. In college, there were three categories for girls: those who slept around, those who were in committed relationships, and those who didn't do it. And I was in the *didn't do it* category. I had a lot of friends who were committed; they had a boyfriend that they were pinned to or engaged to. And they slept together. And that was okay. It was the ones who slept around who were *really* not okay."

Coming of Age

Here is a long narrative from **Mary Jo (1947)** that illustrates many elements of the coming-of-age process in which skills for adult sex and relating are acquired one step at a time. Although she is from a wealthier family than most, Mary Jo had coming-of-age experiences and realizations that were similar to those of many other women. When she was eleven and twelve, she "didn't feel so much physically sexual but wanted to be part of the boy/girl scene . . . everybody was dating, doing things in groups, having parties. And I was pretty naive. I remember things like riding my horse and being with the guys, and they would take my boots and tease me. They'd say, *We'll give them back if you sleep with me* and they'd all laugh; obviously it was something wrong or stupid but I didn't know what it was. There was a lot of that kind of thing."

Oh, no, I'm a girl! Mary Jo went on to tell of a realization she had in her teens similar to the childhood realization of Michele (*Oh no! He thinks I'm a girl*), who discovered in grade school that boys treated girls differently than they treated each other. "At the beginning, I could ride out with the guys and do whatever they wanted to do. But then I got a little bit older, and I couldn't spend the night at this cave with the horses because I was a girl. That was the first of many, many, many, many, many, many more resentments that I had about being a girl. It just kept me from doing all of the stuff I wanted to do."

Oh, yes, I'm a girl! Themes of gender change form and play out over and over again as our sexual self-image evolves throughout life. At each phase there are new realizations. Mary Jo continued, "Later I found out that there was some power there, with the sex. Being a girl was useful and interesting and boys were exciting. But before that I was pretty insecure, self-conscious about my looks. And I went through all the romantic wonderful stuff—the excitement and all the agony of teenage years, sighing and looking at the moon, that kind of thing. You know how it is. When I was fourteen, I ended up going steady with one guy of that group. We would kiss, make out, and it was wonderful. The big event was a party at somebody's house during the day with blankets put up to cover the windows and you would kind of kiss and things. That was about it, but we thought we were really bad, very risqué. By high school, I ended up with a few more boyfriends and things went a little further, but I was raised so that you didn't have sex before marriage. It was sort of everything else went."

The Edge in Adolescence

The edge: the outer limit of experience where curiosity, danger, excitement, and the slightly forbidden meet. Adolescence is a time of dramatic changes; adolescence itself is the *edge* between childhood and adulthood. It is a period of great physical and emotional vulnerability. It is a time when sexual contact becomes increasingly complex and, consequently, may become increasingly dangerous.

For centuries societies controlled the sexuality of the young with a protective structure built of rules, limits on opportunity, and social sanctions. There were bundling boards and chaperones, rules that you didn't have sex until you were married, and separate living quarters for adolescent girls and boys who weren't married. Traditionally, it was assumed that the young unmarried needed to be protected by their wiser elders from their turbulent hormones and irrational sexual desires.

That situation held until the sexual revolution of the 1960s. Within one generation dorms became co-ed and sexual experimentation with many partners began to be encouraged. We can get some idea of the tremendous changes in dating patterns by considering the changes with respect to oral sex. We can see, too, in some of the narratives that follow, that the results of sexual liberation have not been entirely beneficial for young women.

Oral-Genital Sex

For women born before 1950, oral-genital sex was not a dating practice. Engaging in oral sex while still in high school was almost unheard of; for those few who did it, oral sex usually meant the woman stimulating her partner. Fewer than one in ten born before 1950 had any experience with oral sex before having sexual intercourse for the first time, and intercourse, for the majority, occurred after marriage or, at least, after becoming engaged. Typically, oral sex came later in a relationship and was often a sign of deepening intimacy and sexual comfort.

But for those born after 1950, who became sexually active between 1965 and 1990, there was an increase in pre-first-intercourse oral sex with each succeeding generation until, by 1990, about half of all college students had engaged in oral sex (Rubin 1990). It is significant, then, that **Barb**, born in **1955**, matter-of-factly mentions oral sex as a part of the game strategy for not losing her virginity in high school. Sexually, she came of age during the sexual revolution, and she represents a new generation. "In high school, there was sexual energy, but I wasn't going to lose my virginity. So you play these games. Basically, the rules were that you could do anything as long as you didn't lose your virginity, so basically anything but penetration was okay—genital touching, oral sex, dry humping, with or without clothes, depending."

Today, oral sex has become a commonplace initiation into genital sexual activity. In a 1994 study with a nationally representative sample, 26 percent of the high school students surveyed had had oral sex. Of those who had had intercourse, two-thirds also had engaged in oral sex (Lewin 1997). Many of today's adolescents see oral sex as safer than intercourse and less a sign of commitment or of an intimate relationship than "going all the way." Adolescent girls see oral sex as a way to remain a virgin and avoid AIDS and pregnancy. A study in 1996 of adolescent sexual behavior reported that boys were as likely to stimulate girls orally as the other way around (Schuster 1996). (Note that some sexually transmitted diseases, gonorrhea, for example, can be transmitted through oral-genital contact; also it is unlikely, but possible, to contract the AIDS virus in this way.)

Leslie (1971), who graduated from a boarding high school in 1987, talked about how she discovered "blow jobs." "I never had a boyfriend in high school. We'd just fool around . . . usually in the dorms, a drunken encounter . . . most of the time it was not positive. Whoever I was fooling around with wasn't my boyfriend. I was sneaking around, usually heavy petting, never fully naked, not really knowing, very unsure of myself. I was always fearful of touching men's penises. As I got older, a boy asked me to give him a blow job, and he seemed to enjoy it so much that then I started giving other men blow jobs. It seemed like such a quick easy way to satisfy them without having to go through the other motions, them fondling my breasts or my vagina, which it never seemed that they really knew what they were doing and never really gave me that much pleasure. It was nice to have human contact and skin against you and all that, but it wasn't satisfying sexually."

For Leslie there were no bundling boards and chaperones, no rules that you didn't have sex until you're married, and no separate living quarters for the girls and boys who weren't married. There were no wise elders in evidence who were "protecting" her sexuality and that of her peers.

Leslie was not provided with a safe context in which she could satisfy her needs for touch and human contact and engage in sexual experimentation. You will read later in this chapter about Leslie's first sexual intercourse and in chapter 6 about her experiences with casual sex. At the time of her interview, Leslie had not yet found her way to much personal fulfillment through her sexuality. She demonstrates some of the consequences a girl-woman can experience when there is no wise adult to guide and protect her.

Out at the Edge

One consequence of the decrease in social protection of young women's sexuality has been an increase in what is called "date rape." Often the male partner is to blame, but, as Karen's narrative demonstrates, sometimes there is a dangerous ambivalence on the woman's part as well. A girl-woman's excitement, curiosity, and desire for new experiences, together with environmental factors such as alcohol and a place to "do it," can put her and her partner at a dangerous edge. In this narrative from **Karen (1957)** we again see the confusion that can arise when we try to label our experiences:

Did I have any sexual trauma or misuse? Not to my memory. I have wondered about an experience I had when I was seventeen and I was drunk at a party and I flirted with a guy and we went out to a truck. It was my first experience with oral sex; he was on top of me and wouldn't get off of me. I was having a hard time breathing. A friend later said, *That was rape.* I said, *I don't think so; it didn't feel like rape.* I would say it was somewhat uncomfortable, but I don't label that as being a bad sexual experience in particular. I wasn't satisfied, but I write a lot of that off to it being my first time. I solicited that experience. I was very curious about oral sex. I wanted him to be doing that. Retrospectively, I wish now I would have known at that time some way to say, *No. This isn't good for me.* But I didn't at the time. I think he suggested the oral sex, but I said, *Yeah.*

This is an excellent illustration that there is a climate of confusion about what is considered rape and what is not. But whether or not we give this experience the label "rape," Karen's ambivalence is obvious. Yes: *I wanted him to be doing that.* No: *This isn't good for me.* Yet she does take responsibility for her involvement in the experience. She consented—and even sought—to do at the time what later—in retrospect—she might not have chosen to do, under those conditions. This is what happens in *finding our way.* We are limited by what we want and what we know *at the time.* Later, we evaluate. Then, we may decide to do things differently—or not at all—another time.

Alcohol and the Edge

Alcohol makes the edge even riskier. Under conditions of safety, a small amount may enhance pleasure; without such conditions, alcohol greatly increases physical and emotional risks.

At age thirteen, **Lorraine (1957)** visited her sister, who was away at college; during that visit she got drunk for the first time. Perhaps her parents were expecting her older sister to chaperone her, but this is what happened: "My sister, her boyfriend, and this nineteen-year-old guy were at her apartment. And I woke up in the sofa bed in her living room with this guy's face and hands where they shouldn't be. He was touching me inside; I'd never been touched like that before. I said *Get out,* and he left. My sister later told me that that night I had stripped and was dancing naked. I have absolutely no memory of that. I do have a very clear memory of that person in the bed. I never told anyone. Because what goes through a young girl's mind—what I said to myself was—*It's my fault. I was wrong.*"

A girl or woman who has an experience like this may have to find her way back to loving herself and valuing her sexuality. It helps if she is able to tell someone about it right away who is both supportive and nonblaming. It helps, too, if she can attribute responsibility to the person who violated her and doesn't blame herself. If she did put herself in danger, she recognizes how she can be more protective of herself in the future, but, ideally, she does that in a gentle, self-loving, and nonblaming way. One aspect of resolving problems resulting from a traumatic experience is to understand the larger picture, particularly the role and responsibility of the one who harmed her.

But it is typical that a young girl does not tell. When she was thirteen, Lorraine did not tell anyone, and she blamed herself. From her adult perspective, she describes how her experiences continued to affect her: "Those early experiences affected my sexuality and my sex life with my husband. Early on I pushed him away. I wanted to be cared for and held and loved and all that, but I didn't want sex to the degree that he did. I kind of felt obligated then, which is *not* how I feel now, because I'm more educated and my self-esteem is very different. I didn't know that I had sexual power and that I had the power to choose what I do or how I do it. Or that it wasn't just what I call *getting fucked*. What I knew about sex is you get fucked. I think in my sexual experimentation as a young adult, that because all I knew how to do was to get fucked, that that's all I got."

Women in every generation have to find their own way. Still, I hope that young women reading this book will learn from the experiences of women like Lorraine and the others who found their way before them, and will therefore have a more informed starting place for solving the mysteries of sex and sexuality for themselves.

Danger Zone: High School Girl-Women and Older Boy-Men

It is clear from the interviews and the questionnaire Survey that it can be uncomfortable and even dangerous for teenage girls to date older boys or men. High school girl-women who date college boy-men are particularly at risk for nonconsensual experiences. A young woman's high school peer group will have its own rules about sexual limits and acceptable behaviors. A college event or a date with a college man can throw her into a situation where the rules, limits, and expectations are different in ways she neither expects nor is prepared for. This happened to **Judith (1940)** when she went out with a "guy from the Air Force Academy" while she was still in high school: "I remember necking with him in the car and when he put his hands under my blouse I said *No*, pushed him away, and got out of the car. I was really panicky. He got angry and called me a *prick teaser*. And I didn't understand what that was about. I was naive on the one hand and overcome with sexual energy on the other. So I can see how he got the impression that I would be willing. But I was unable to do anything about it. I didn't know exactly what I was feeling or what I wanted and I also didn't know what the rules were."

Pam (1968) spoke of an experience that went beyond groping, to rape. She began by describing the social milieu in her high school and her role in that context: "There was a time in high school when I was pretty promiscuous, just needing affirmation of myself from men—boys. Having no idea that I had some stake in sexual encounters. A lot of it was out-of-body stuff, kind of *Here I am, just do what you need to do*. And then I will have had this experience. I was stupid in kind of a safe way. I definitely lived the notion that there's a lot you could do without having intercourse. I would only go so far, only do so many drugs (mainly alcohol, pot, and some cocaine) and would never do intercourse with any of these guys. I led a double life in high school. I was a straight-A student and hung out with a groovy group of friends who did community work. And then there was this side of me that would go to these parties with other friends and do a lot of drugs and drinking and have these one-night escapades."

From the shelter of this contained social group of high school friends, with its shared code of *everything but intercourse*, Pam traveled, during her junior year, across country to visit colleges she might attend. In New England she stayed with one of her sister's male friends, a college student who apparently was playing by different rules with different sexual limits and different interpretations of her behavior than those followed by her high school peers. He raped her. She said, "My first intercourse was with a close friend of my sister's from high school. I didn't have a choice. I was staying in his room, and he forced me. This occurred at four o'clock in the morning, and I was running out of this dorm room in New England in February and ended up spending the rest of the night walking the streets in the snow. And no one was around. Not knowing what to tell anyone. This was my sister's friend. I had chosen to go there. We had gotten stoned together. All of these things. *Like how responsible am I?* And *doesn't he know what he's done?* I was a virgin.

Trauma, trauma, trauma. Pam didn't tell anyone; she didn't clearly identify this man as responsible in her own mind. The trauma manifested, she said, "at unexpected moments in my life, a real fear of just losing control—of where I was—and who was going to help me if I needed help. I repressed the rape for a while and didn't deal with it. Then, in my freshman year in college there was a 'speakout' about this kind of thing and I sat there pretty composed, and then when I went home I got totally paranoid and was afraid to leave my house. I called my therapist and we talked for hours that night. It was that night of the rape coming back, a lot of my anger, my fears, my frustrations, shame about not telling my sister, shame for not being strong enough to deal with it. But I couldn't tell my sister. I was afraid she wouldn't believe me. He was one of her best friends."

Pam's experiences, and many others like them, provide strong evidence about how uninformed high school and college students are about sexual decision making, male sexual scripts, and establishing conditions of safety for themselves. And perhaps Pam was being asked to do a lot on her own that reflected the enormous changes in cultural mores that had occurred in the thirty years that preceded her rape. As I have noted, in general, society was more protective of young women's sexuality in the earlier decades of the century. In the mid-fifties, for example, campus rules of colleges and universities were shaped by a policy called *in loco parentis*—literally, *taking the place of parents*. Then, she would have been unlikely to have made that trip without a mature traveling companion, a chaperone. Girls had curfews and had to sign in and out of their dorms and sorority houses; campus rules would not have allowed a woman to be in a man's dorm room at four in the morning, let alone to sleep there.

There has always been sexual trauma. It seems, however, that in the final third of the twentieth century, with the dismantling of older social structures and the increase in sexual freedoms, the prevalence of sexual trauma also increased. This will be even more evident in the next section where we consider the changes in circumstances under which women choose to have their first experiences of sexual intercourse.

What Does This Mean to You?

Now, if you wish, take a break, pick up your notebook and express the thoughts and feelings you're having. Here are some questions you might want to consider after you've done that.

- What kinds of *at the edge* or *danger zone* experiences have you had? Is there any way you could have been better protected?

- What were your questions about sex and relationships when you were a preteen?

- What mistaken assumptions did you have?

- Was there a distinct moment when you recognized that you were a girl in some kind of dance with boys—or that you weren't attracted to boys in the way other girls were?

- If you are recalling experiences that you now regret, consider the circumstances, the roles of others, and how you saw your options at the time. Then, sit quietly with your eyes closed and imagine what you could now gently and lovingly tell your younger self that would be healing and lead to greater self-acceptance.

When, Where, and with Whom?

This section is about the values and circumstances that guide women's decisions about when, where, and with whom they first have sexual intercourse. This topic elicited what are perhaps the most dramatic differences I have seen between the generations. With her "first time," a woman at last fills in some of the details that were missing from her childhood experimentation and her adolescent fantasies about sex. Finally, she has answers to her questions: Who will he be? How do you do it? What will it feel like? Will it hurt? With this rite of passage she may feel that she has been initiated into the sisterhood of adult women.

For most of us reading this, these decisions are a part of our personal histories. Our experiences were shaped by the times we lived in. In finding our way to these decisions, we did the best we could with what we knew and understood then. It is only in retrospect that we are able to consider whether we might have done things differently or would do exactly the same if we could have the experience to live over again. We may, however, still have opportunities to influence our daughters, granddaughters, great-granddaughters, and other young women we know.

Our collective acquired wisdom makes this a valuable intergenerational dialogue. The experiences women share can lead us to individual healing and self-acceptance. They can inform those readers who are still contemplating when, where, and with whom it will be. They can inform readers who are contemplating sex with a new partner. And they can inform us all so we can wisely provide guidelines for other women who have yet to make these decisions.

First Times in the Early Twentieth Century

Lillian (1905) provides a striking example of the social customs and strong religious prohibitions that once served to constrain the sexuality of unmarried girls and young women. Eighty-nine-years old and widowed when I interviewed her, she had been married to her only sex partner for fifty-six years. Her first sexual intercourse had been on their wedding night, when she was twenty. On that occasion her husband, described by her as "a gentle and sensitive lover," brought her to her first orgasm; she told me that she had never faked orgasm. She also said, "If we'd had intercourse before marriage, we would have been run out of town, and my Catholic mother would have been the first one running us out."

"Someday my prince will come—and I'll come, too—and he'll make it wonderful" is what I call this sexual script in which the woman is innocent and the man is her teacher. How he is supposed to have learned what to do is left to one's imagination. While Lillian's sex with her "prince" was immediately satisfying, that wasn't true for **Hilda (1915)**, who in high school was part of "a sort of a gang of boys and girls that used to hang out together"; her husband-to-be was "one of the boys." She said: "Nobody had any money to date . . . we all went out together . . . and the girls in my group didn't have intercourse outside of marriage. It was when we decided we were going to get married shortly that I finally had sex with him—in the back seat of a car. It was a relief, although not a great experience; I never really enjoyed sex with my husband; I don't think I ever had an orgasm with him. The marriage ended after nineteen years, when I was around forty, and suddenly I sprouted wings. I had a very active and enjoyable sexual life from then on."

Technical Virgins— Everything-but-Intercourse Sex

For many women born in the first half of the twentieth century their pre-marital sexual expression included genital activity and even orgasm. It wasn't always *all* sexual activity that was postponed for marriage or a formal engagement, it was *sexual intercourse*. This custom of deferring intercourse but not sexual activity until a committed relationship was firmly established protected women from unwanted pregnancies and sexually transmitted diseases. At the same time, it allowed relatively uninhibited sexual expression for many couples. Women often came to marriage as *technical virgins*; they already had done almost everything but intercourse and oral-genital sex. In a sexually active engagement that included everything but *doing it*, a couple might develop skill in the dance of erotic pleasure. With intercourse prohibited, they weren't skipping over delightful basic erotic steps and immediately rushing to intercourse as a goal.

Janine (1921), whose "first time" took place in the late 1930s, was only technically still a virgin; she already had been sexually active with several boyfriends and had engaged as well in the exploratory play she described earlier in this chapter She explained what had kept her from "going all the way." "We had a tremendous fear of pregnancy in those days. There were no contraceptives except for condoms, and boys didn't like to wear them and they didn't always work. Abortion was a fearful experience then and in many ways unavailable; in middle class families it was such a scandal. All this protected me although I had boyfriends and we did necking and genital touching and the boys would have orgasms; sometimes I would, too." **Carole (1930)**, nearly ten years younger than Janine, also was a technical virgin; her first time took place at age twenty, when she married. She admitted, "The only reason I didn't have sex a lot earlier was fear, fear of getting pregnant. 'Cause I had some other boyfriends who I really wanted to have sex with. In those days you didn't go to a doctor to get a diaphragm unless you were married, and as far as I knew there was nothing else available."

Trust, Feeling Safe, and Fear of Pregnancy

Today, readily available contraceptives are so much taken for granted that we find it hard to imagine that Margaret Sanger was put in jail for informing women about birth control early in the twentieth century. Or that there was a time when, to get a diaphragm, a woman had to be married and her husband had to grant his permission in writing. Or that in the early 1960s practitioners at many medical centers, particularly government-funded or church-sponsored ones, were prohibited from dispensing contraceptives or even talking about ways to prevent pregnancy.

Still, even today we must be watchful of the right to birth control we take so much for granted. There continue to be factions that would undermine the ease with which we can protect ourselves against undesired pregnancies. It was announced recently, for example, that the only hospital in a community about ninety miles from where I live is being taken over by a Catholic health care organization. Up to now a woman could have her tubes tied (a sterilization operation) at the same time she gave birth in that hospital; after the takeover, that procedure will no longer be available. A woman who wants her tubes tied will have to travel to another city to have her baby.

In the interviews of older women, trust, feeling safe, and fear of pregnancy were recurrent themes. In the years these women were becoming sexually active, *safe* usually referred to the consequences of becoming pregnant. Through the 1950s, the cultural rules about dating, sexual exploration, and when, where, and with whom a woman's first intercourse *should* occur were much more clearly spelled out than they have been ever since. Of course, not everyone abided by the rules, but many women did save intercourse for marriage.

Marriage: the Next Step

Marriage often was seen as "the next step" in a life script. **Ann (1934)** captures the essence of the "rules" of the 1950s: "I first dated in high school and didn't have anything but kissing games until I was dating a fellow fairly seriously my senior year. My values about sex then were that you never went below the waist. You didn't have intercourse until after you were married no matter how you felt. The girl had to set the limits and had to be very up front about it. I remember saying to a guy I dated that *if we had sex I couldn't marry him because I wouldn't think he respected me.* It all had to do with respect and being good. So I didn't have intercourse until I was married which, looking back on it, brought me very naively into marriage, when I was twenty-two. My husband wasn't very pushy, and I wasn't passionately in love with him. I think I got married because it was simply the next step."

In those days, wanting to legitimize sex was often a stronger motivation for marriage than having found the right life partner. Have you seen movies from the '50s? Often the plot is boy meets girl and after a whirlwind courtship of two weeks or so, they get married. Today it's boy meets girl and after a whirlwind courtship of two hours or so, they are in bed having sex while we watch. *Getting married* was the code image of the 1950s for having sex. The same ending, but in a dramatically different form. When I watch those '50s movies now, it often seems to me that those movie marriages, based on so little, are destined not to last.

Bridging Two Eras

In **Teresa's (1946)** interview we encounter two themes that did not appear in interviews with any of the women born before 1946: oral stimulation of her genitals before she first had intercourse (rare for women born before 1950), and access to birth control pills. She told me: "When I was a senior in high school I started going out with the guy I would marry three years later, when I was twenty. I think I felt obliged to marry him because I had gone so far with him. I didn't feel that I had a choice. I didn't have intercourse with him until after marriage but we did a lot of sexual experimentation and I became orgasmic with him doing oral sex to me. By the time we got married, we'd done just about everything except intercourse. The first intercourse was painful because he was very well-endowed, but he was very, very patient . . . very considerate, and very gentle, a real wedding night thing. It's still a nice memory. The night itself, the feeling of intimacy, was like a dream come true. The first year was fun because now I felt I could enjoy sex, and I did."

Beginning with Teresa's narrative (chronologically the first to mention availability of woman-controlled contraceptives), fear of pregnancy—mentioned as a theme by virtually every woman older than Teresa—recedes into the background dramatically. She continued, "Being Catholic we weren't supposed to use birth control. The priest we went to found ways around it. He said that if I was irregular I could take birth control pills for about six months to regulate myself so that I could bear God's children. So I went on the pill and went off after six months and got pregnant. Marriage was still fun. I was living it like one of the movies I watched; it was part of the 'happily ever after.' Now, looking back, I was as ready to have a child as a two-year-old is. But, at the time, I thought it was the second half of the movie. We were married about twelve years."

For Women Born at Mid-Century: A New Trend

Our data suggest that a new trend started with women born in 1949 and 1950. A woman in our Survey who was born *before 1950* would more likely than not have her first intercourse with a man she planned to marry or on her *wedding night*. A woman born *after 1950* would not be in the majority of women her age if her first intercourse was with someone she was planning to marry or had already married. **Sara**, born in **1949**, had a conversation with her mother that illustrates the beginning of this generational shift in values: "I lost my virginity to a boy's bicycle when I was about twelve. It slid in gravel and I just slammed on the bar. Ouch! I remember my mother telling me it wouldn't hurt *when I got married*. It took me a couple of days to figure out that she meant *when I lost my virginity*. It was like, to me they didn't go together, but for my mother they clearly did."

Coming of Age During the Sexual Revolution

Women who were born in the 1950s reached sexual maturity in the late 1960s and the 1970s, during the "sexual revolution." As these women entered sexual adulthood, they met with a number of significant social changes. The media told them that it was not only permissible, but also a good idea, to masturbate and learn about orgasms for themselves. Men were allowed in women's college dorms and some dorms became co-ed. Close-to-100 percent effective birth control pills became relatively easy to get; and, in the 70s, sexually transmitted diseases (STDs), then still often called venereal diseases or VD, weren't viewed as particularly serious. Most people believed that brief treatment with penicillin or other antibiotics could cure anything. In earlier years, before antibiotics became available, venereal diseases, particularly syphilis, which could cause insanity and be fatal, had been of great concern.

It's What You Do in College

For many women who were seeking higher education, intercourse became part of the curriculum, "what you do in college." When **Cindi (1952)**, casually mentioned her decision to "do it," she alluded neither to marriage nor to love. She was seventeen, in her first year of college: "We were both living in dorms with a roommate. He was a sophomore, a kind of odd-looking creature, very nice, very gentle, tall, thin. I was on birth control pills several months before we actually did it . . . in my dorm room, on my little single bed (not particularly comfortable) with the Indian bedspread. It was slightly painful, not very erotic. We both viewed it as a hurdle to get past, to get to the point where it would be enjoyable. We were then boyfriend and girlfriend, sexually active. I don't think I had an orgasm the very first time, but very shortly after I did, because I knew how to do that from masturbating. *My values?* It just seemed like a very natural and normal progression, what one did when one was in college; there was a kind of peer aspect to it. I left a community where my parents were well known, well regarded, and I was known because of who my parents were. I felt very on my own: independent, carefree, and able to wear what I pleased. This was 1970, just past the cusp of the free love movement, and hippies were much in evidence. There was the cultural wave that carried me and also this sense of individuation, getting away from the parents, becoming independent, becoming who I was going to be."

The 1960s and '70s were filled with dramatic challenges to cultural norms. Anna, who is Jewish, had her first intercourse with someone *very* experienced—and black—at a time when interracial dating was a provocative challenge to social mores. It was passion and the forbidden rather than the security of an ongoing relationship that left **Anna (1949)** feeling good about herself and the experience. In fact, her previous more long-term partners had *not* been sexually affirming: "The first high school boyfriend who fingered me always got up and washed his hands afterwards . . . not very positive feedback about my vagina. (I never considered having intercourse while in high school.) In college, I dated a very nice guy who was romantic but guilty about sex. We dated a month before he kissed me goodnight; then we slept together but didn't do anything. I remember crying because I thought something was wrong with me."

When Anna was twenty-one, a black classmate "seduced" her. "He invited me over to his room," she told me. "I went there thinking I was setting myself up but I didn't care. I had this lusty, passionate, glow-light dark experience with somebody who really turned me on. He informed me as we had intercourse, my first, that I was number ninety-three. This, for me, after being in a relationship with somebody who didn't even want to talk about it . . . was total lust; we weren't going to have a relationship, and I had to be totally secret about it because you shouldn't be seen with black men. I thought, *After all this talk about it, that's all intercourse was!* and *Where are my legs supposed to go and how am I supposed to move?* It was a real letdown. Looking back, someone experienced teaching you was sort of nice, although I'd give the foreplay much higher marks than the intercourse. Shortly after that I got involved with another guy and it turned out I was his first; we were together a long time."

Being in Love Replaces Marriage

Although not Anna's experience, for many women of her generation being in love replaced being married or planning to get married as the necessary prerequisite for sexual intercourse. As **Barb (1955)** said, "I lost my virginity at seventeen, in my first year of college, 1972. My values then were that you had to be in love with someone to have sex with him. After dating my first college boyfriend for a year, I felt that I was with the love of my life and so sex became justifiable. We talked about it. The first time was wonderful because I loved him, but I didn't really know what was happening. The first few times we made love, we used withdrawal. I knew I didn't want to get pregnant, so I saw a gynecologist and got myself a diaphragm."

Age of First Intercourse

Over the years, the average age of first intercourse has become younger and younger. If we consider all 2,405 women who gave that age in the Survey, the average age of first intercourse was 17.8. However, for the women born between 1905 and 1944 the average age was 19.4 and for the women born after 1964, the average age was 16.6.

It's What You Do in High School

In the second half of the twentieth century, sex gradually became not what you did when you got married or when you got to college, but what you did *in high school*. In earlier generations, peer pressure kept high school girls from even admitting to sexual behavior. These are some of the marginal notes written by women born from 1937 to 1949 in response to a Survey question asking them if, compared to their classmates, they were *about as*, *more*, or *less* sexually active during their adolescent years:

♀ We *never* talked about it in 1953-55 but later I discovered quite a few of us were sexual; ♀ This was *never* discussed even with the closest of friends; ♀ In the '50s everyone pretended they didn't do "it" and no one admitted to masturbating; ♀ We did not discuss each other's sexual experiences.

By the late 1960s, peer pressure in some high schools had begun to support and encourage early sexual experimentation, including intercourse; girls were talking and even bragging about their experiences. **Ronni (1955)** started to experiment sexually, petting, when she was around thirteen, in the late '60s. She said: "I felt very pressured to have sex early—socially, not from my family. I remember saying to a friend, *Boy, we're thirteen and still virgins!* I had sex for the first time just before my sixteenth birthday."

A daughter's perspective on her mother's reaction. Ronnie continued: "I brought it up with my mother because I was having trouble with my diaphragm; I'd gone to Planned Parenthood by myself. Then my messages from my mother switched. On the one hand, she was very open about things. But faced with an almost sixteen-year-old daughter who was having sex, she was clearly unhappy about it. (See Ronni's narrative in chapter 3.) But at a certain point, she said, *If you're going to have sex, I want you to be safe and comfortable.* So there was an awkward period for a while and then she accepted my high school boyfriend and even allowed him to sleep over during my senior year, which was unusual, to say the least. The only thing going for that first experience was the romance of it. It was not enjoyable; the physical sex was not very interesting at all and mildly painful. If I could live my life over again, I'd never have sex as early as I did."

We know there have been dramatic changes when we compare Ronni's experiences in 1970—going to Planned Parenthood at age fifteen for a diaphragm—with those of Carole who said of her experiences in 1950: "In those days you didn't go to a doctor to get a diaphragm unless you were married, and as far as I knew there was nothing else available."

In the 1960s and '70s girls still were worrying about maintaining their virginity, and boys and girls were still locked in the age-old giving-getting struggle in which boys push girls for as much as they can get while girls hold out for as little as they can give. But by the 1970s, girls were dancing this dance at fifteen instead of at twenty. This was not just a simple five-year difference. A twenty year old is a young adult; a fifteen year old is only beginning to leave her childhood behind (Rubin 1990).

Cynthia's (1954) first intercourse, like Ronni's, occurred at age fifteen; her partner was her first boyfriend: "It was awful. I cried, I felt bad that I had given in. I didn't have any physical arousal, it was very painful. He was just banging on me and I wanted to get it over with as fast I could. That's all it ever was with him. That was the late '60s and early '70s, the era of hippies and free love and 'Make Love, Not War.' I was getting a lot of stuff from the media but not really understanding what it was about. I was having sex with my boyfriend, not because I enjoyed it, but in order to keep him. He wasn't very good to me, but he was the most popular guy at school. I broke up with him in my junior year in high school and then I had sex with almost every boy who wanted to."

I was having sex with my boyfriend, not because I enjoyed it, but in order to keep him. Girls having sex, not because it gives them much physical pleasure, but for other kinds of benefits, such as the status of having a boyfriend, is a recurrent theme.

A mother's perspective on her daughter's experience. In the previous narrative, Ronnie reported to us *what her mother felt* when at

fifteen Ronni began having sex. Cynthia, who is of Ronni's generation, went on to tell us what she, *as a mother*, felt when *her daughter*
gave up her virginity, also at fifteen: "She gave up her virginity last
summer. I was so disappointed and really had to fight with myself
not to project that to her; I didn't want to make her feel bad. She had
sex for all the wrong reasons . . . mainly pressure and some curiosity.
All of her girlfriends were having sex and were pressuring her to do
it. I also try to respect her privacy. She's been real clear about where
the lines are. When she was thirteen and started menstruating, and
again when she was fourteen, I talked to her about sex and contraception. I tried to give her the information and support I never got. It
didn't turn out the way I wanted it to. For a year I'd stressed going to
Planned Parenthood, even gave her the phone number and the names
of some people there she could talk to, but she had her first sexual
experience without going there. But it turned out they used a condom, and it was just a one-time thing. I don't think she's sexually
active now."

This account is another example of the intergenerational barrier
that exists between parents and their children when it comes to talking about the specifics of sex. It may be that first intercourse—an act
that separates us from our childhood—is by psychological necessity a
sexual event that most sexually mature children do not immediately
reveal to or discuss with their parents. This privacy barrier may
reflect an inherent taboo, an aspect of that psychological limitation of
imagination: *Everybody has sex but our own parents and our own children.*

A daughter's perspective. Deanna (1971), who is about the age
of Cynthia's daughter, reflected, "My mom always stressed, *Make sure
you know the person.* I don't think I even told her the first time I had
sex. She probably wouldn't want to know. She was very concerned
that I used protection, and that the person I was with was okay. And
probably, that I was in love with him was what she preferred. I don't
think my friends were as concerned as my mom about being cautious
but just thought that it was a good thing for developing a relationship."

Women Attracted to Women

Not all women, of course, had their "first times" with men. **Beth
(1961)** had many opportunities to be sexually active with guys she
dated in high school and early college. She explained: "I was never
interested. Part of it was my Catholic upbringing; sex was saved for
marriage. I also didn't have a connection with these guys on a feeling
level. I knew sex was something I wanted to share with someone

special and they just weren't it. I did some necking, kissing, and light petting from the waist up, usually when I had been drinking. It was an altered state. It wasn't just me as I am. It was more like *Let's have a couple drinks* and *Oh, you took me out to a movie and to dinner—so I'm obligated.* It wasn't really enjoyable. I never had intercourse with men."

Beth continued: "In college I started having feelings for a close girlfriend. We never really talked about our relationship. We were just best friends, although, looking back, I know I was in love with her. We would touch in safe ways ... little things like rub each other's back, touch each other in places that didn't seem like they were sexual, not our breasts or vulvas. I was having feelings I'd never felt before. It was like *Wow, this is really great!* I continued to find myself really attracted to and falling in love with different girlfriends in college and grad school. Then, in my last year of grad school, five years ago, I met a woman who liked me back. That really surprised me and it was kind of scary. The first month we dated, we became progressively more and more sexual and eventually we made love. The *first time* was wonderful from what I knew, but later, having sex with her more, it just got better. It was amazing. We were together three years."

Unlike Beth, most of the lesbian women who took part in our research had at some time had intercourse with men. **Bonnie (1966)**, on the other hand, who described her orientation as heterosexual, had her first sexual relationship with a woman. She said, "I think that was an accident more than anything else. I was in an all-girls Catholic school and at seventeen had raging hormones with nowhere else to channel them. We were very close friends, would go to school together every morning, and it just happened. We both had feelings and we expressed our feelings and then we did something about them. When we were getting along, sex was great. I was always orgasmic, usually with oral sex. Then, after two years, we weren't getting along and broke up."

Finding Our Way—We Learned How—and It Got Good

Learning to enjoy sexual expression is an ongoing process. When we become intercourse-active, we are inexperienced and just beginning to find our way, doing the best we can with what we know and the skills we have. For most of us, like **Josephine (1913)**, sex gets better as we acquire more experience. A step at a time we learn about mutual erotic pleasure and how to create satisfaction with a partner: "My first intercourse was when I was twenty, with the man I later married. I'd waited for someone I could trust. . . . Our sex wasn't too satisfying in the beginning, but we learned and it got good. After about a year, I became orgasmic with him. I needed to learn about my body and teach my husband what felt good to me and what didn't. Then it got very good."

Lori (1969) had a relatively positive first intercourse experience with her best friend. Like Josephine, she mentions trust as important in her decision making. But unlike many of the women who came of age before the sexual revolution of the 1960s, Lori, in the late 1980s, was able to engage in sex with more than one partner before choosing the man she would marry: "I was nineteen, in college; he was my best friend, and this was a kind of progression of our relationship. We'd slept together a couple of times, but hadn't had sex. I'd been thinking about it . . . wondering, *When I do, who will it be?* I trusted him implicitly and was comfortable with him . . . it kind of progressed naturally . . . like this time I said, *Well, okay.* Emotionally, it was kind of a neat thing to do. I probably didn't enjoy it as much as I could have because I was thinking about what I was supposed to do, instead of what I really felt like doing. Sex was still such a mystery to me. But it was fun. I didn't have regrets."

Lori went on to say that for nearly a year she didn't know what she thought she needed to know. Then she met her current partner: "He was so open about it, and we just talked and talked and talked. In the four years we've been together, I've gradually become more comfortable with it, and with myself, sometimes more aggressive about sex, saying, *I want it,* and not having to wait for somebody else to say that. It's still an evolving process. Sex in general seems to be more and more fun and adventurous all the time. We're engaged and I'm looking forward to getting married. That'll be fun and add a whole new twist to things."

Which Comes First, a Relationship or Sex?

In addition to demonstrating how sex can get better over time, **Leslie's (1971)** narrative illustrates a frequent discrepancy in the expectations women and men have about sex. Her first intercourse was at eighteen, as a college freshman; her boyfriend was twenty, a junior. She said: "I'd been seeing him for three months, and he'd been adamant about wanting to have sex from day one. I had this very idealistic view that I wanted to wait, and he did understand, because I was a virgin. I assume he had feelings for me, but there was also this pressure on me to have sex. I wanted to make sure that I was in a relationship, that this wasn't fleeting. I remember I was a little drunk, and I was kind of restless, and kind of excited, and all of a sudden I just really wanted to have sex. I was over at his dorm, and I told him to meet me back at my dorm and to bring a condom. He came sprinting over and we had sex in my room. I remember being completely terrified when he was naked and he had an erection, thinking that this huge penis was going to be going inside of me. Afterward, I think I cried a little bit. I don't know why, but I did. And then, we had sex probably every day for the next week. And I couldn't really walk too much. And then it got better. And then I learned to enjoy it."

Leslie wanted the relationship to mature before engaging in sex; her boyfriend wanted sex even before the relationship had been established. Although Leslie doesn't know why she cried, she may be reassured to know that tears that don't seem to be about anything in particular are not unusual after the release of sex.

Rite of Passage

Although self-realization is a lifelong project, the process of acquiring a clearer sense of self—and of a sexual self—is particularly significant in our adolescent and young adulthood years. A young woman in her teens may not yet know what she wants sexually, but she may be quite actively trying to figure out her answers to the question, *How does your sexuality fit into who you are?* As we saw in the first part of this chapter, unless she finds herself more attracted to girls than to boys, a girl in her early teens is likely to find her attention frequently occupied by thoughts and curiosity about giving up her virginity. Like **Joan (1944)**, she may consider actually "doing it" a significant rite of passage. "My first sexual intercourse was exciting. It was the first time and we were doing something naughty, which always makes it more fun, and I was fulfilling some kind of fantasy about my own growing up, a rite of passage. One of my girlfriends beat me to it; she said she'd gone all the way with someone, so that was one of the reasons I decided to try it, so I could keep up with her. I was sixteen."

From earliest childhood most people feel freest to explore when they are in situations in which they feel confident and secure. A woman's desire for excitement, a new experience, taking a risk, and initiation into one of life's mysteries is one side of the coin. On the other side we find her desire for safety, the familiar, security, and continuity with a partner she can trust.

All societies have rituals to denote significant rites of passage. Before women themselves could reliably prevent pregnancy, the ritual of marriage was the rite of passage that sanctioned a woman's first intercourse. Marriage created the structure of a continuing relationship in which intercourse—and pregnancy—could safely take place. Once women gained relatively easy access to reliable ways of preventing pregnancy, that age-old custom changed.

Young Women in the 1990s

Unfortunately, without ritual, and without clear societal expectations, many young women who came of age in the 1990s seemed to be floundering. Many did not even consider reserving intercourse for marriage, engagement, or a strong relationship. They had to find their way without clear guidelines. Too often their rite of passage became the sex act itself instead of—as it always had been historically—the creation of a context of safety. **Olga (1971)** was sixteen. "I'd been going out with this guy for about a month and I don't think I was pressured into it in any way. For me, it was kind of like *Well I'll do it and just see what it's like.* In that sense, I feel almost as if I used him, because I knew that he would sleep with me if I wanted him to. We only had sex once and then we went out for another month and the relationship ended. But, for me, it was like no big deal. You know it's like trying drugs once—no big deal. And I didn't have sex again until about a year and a half later when I got into college. The funny thing is I can't even remember a lot about that night. Not that I was drunk—it was just so meaningless to me. I knew he cared, but there really wasn't a whole lot of like foreplay or passion to it. It was just like kind of *Do it, get it done* . . . nice in the sense that I didn't feel dirty about it. I didn't really regret it or anything . . . but in terms of being turned on or sexually excited, I didn't feel very much. . . . I don't remember very much."

We see that for some women of Olga's generation, clearly virginity and a woman's first intercourse were no longer highly valued and to be saved for the one she loved.

Getting It Over With: Alcohol, and Doing It for Him

Many of the young women born in the late 1960s and early 1970s seem to have been motivated more by eagerness to "get it over with," to be rid of their virginity, even in far from ideal circumstances, than was the case for the majority of women in previous generations. Alcohol as a significant factor was mentioned in the interviews of a number of women in this age group, whereas it was mentioned rarely in conjunction with the first times of older women. Also, these younger women frequently express regret in retrospect for having engaged in intercourse so early.

With the exception of Madeline's narrative, the excerpts that follow are from a series of twenty interviews of college women born between 1969 and 1972; the interviewer was Michaelle Davis. For **Michele (1972)**, doing it the first time just to get it over with—the rite of passage—took precedence over being in a relationship or being in love. Alcohol also played a significant role in an experience that involved ambivalent consent and virtually no satisfaction. "I was sixteen, and he was fifteen, from another state, visiting his mom. We were camping, and my relatives were around, and we got really, really drunk. And I don't know what happened. We ended up in a tent buck naked and 'doing it.' I was attracted to him. We'd fooled around, kissed, before. Kissing him while I was drunk was okay. But when we did that, it was just, *Oh my gosh, what are we doing?* And then I felt like I kind of had to because I had taken it so far. We took off all our clothes and I was like, *Do I really want to do this?* And I was like, *I may as well.* I felt like I kind of had to or else I'd let him down. And it was also, *If I do it now, then I can just tell my friends I did it.* It was just stupid! And I didn't like it. I thought I was supposed to like it. It didn't hurt as much as everyone told me, and I didn't bleed or anything, but I really didn't see the big deal everyone was talking about until later, when I was eighteen. It was totally unplanned, we didn't use anything. It was just stupid. I cried until I got my period the next month, because I was so worried. Satisfaction, zero!"

I felt like I kind of had to or else I'd let him down. Michele shares this recurring theme with women of all ages. In Michele we see a young woman having intercourse, not because it is right for her or what she really wants to do, but because that is what she perceives her partner wants or expects. This theme also appeared in **Madeline's (1915)** narrative and in some of the narratives that follow. Madeline was born nearly sixty years before Michele and her contemporaries. She said, "In 1936, when I was a junior in college, I met the man I later married. I don't remember any great urgency on my part to have intercourse, but he wanted to do it, we were in love and engaged, all that. Love was required; you had to be in love. So we began to have intercourse. I was not particularly happy about the whole thing. In fact, I was scared and I was unsure and felt totally out of my depths. I didn't really enjoy it that much. It was very much a business of making him happy, doing what he wanted to do. It had not very much to do with me. I do remember that I missed a period after and I feared I was pregnant. I resented the fact that I had to worry about this. As a matter of fact, I probably wasn't, but I did miss a couple of periods."

As young women not only do many of us think we have to sacrifice our own needs and wants for the men we are with, we also often think that we are at fault if sex doesn't work out, even if the man—like **Chris' (1970)** boyfriend when she was almost eighteen—doesn't know any more about sex than we do. "He was my third boyfriend; I'd finally decided that I was ready and I wanted to. It was very planned, a day his parents weren't going to be home, going over to the house knowing what was going to happen . . . not at all romantic. Now, I realize how much it wasn't really a good experience. I had all these romantic ideas about how it would be so wonderful, but it was really painful and there was a lot of shame around it. I don't feel like I was really pressured into it, but in some ways I was, because I knew that he really wanted to, and he had before and I hadn't. I wanted to, but I was also a little nervous. I don't think either of us was really skilled enough at foreplay, so I just wasn't ready; we didn't even go all the way. He didn't ejaculate; I didn't reach orgasm. He stopped because I was in pain. I felt really awful about it . . . like I'd disappointed him, let him down. I sort of know intellectually it could be a lot better now. We had oral sex, but not intercourse again. That was the only time I ever had intercourse, because I haven't had a boyfriend since then."

Chris and her boyfriend wisely stopped when their attempt became too painful for her. She mentions their mutual inexperience, and from my perspective—and probably hers now, too—she didn't "let him down" at all. She did the best she could given the circumstances and what she knew—and what he knew—because it takes two to create satisfying sex; her boyfriend wasn't a skilled lover yet, either.

The TV Generation

As we saw in chapter 3, the media—television, movies, magazines, and the like—were the number one source of misleading or harmful sex information. **Lisa (1970)**, a member of the TV Generation—those born in the 1960s and later—demonstrates some of the distorted images of sex and sexual values the media can create.

By the time she was fifteen, Lisa believed that getting her first sexual intercourse over with was one of the *"stupid shitty prelim-*

inaries" to having a boyfriend. This image is unlike any that we heard from women born before 1970, who more typically thought that they would have a boyfriend and then, after a time of mutual sexual exploration and experimentation, sexual intercourse would occur within a context of commitment.

Lisa's attitude reflects a significant cultural change. She herself mentions the influence of television. What Lisa—an only child—remembers as starting her thinking about sex or sexuality in the first place were the hours she spent at ages seven and eight in her room alone "... watching my little black and white TV and having crushes on young guys who were on these shows, and creating these little fantasies of being kissed for the first time, or someone saving me, or some hero situation." Some of her actual life experiences—rites of passage—had the quality of TV images—brief moments of intense contact without ongoing physical or emotional connection. For example, at a mall when she was about fourteen: "... someone dared this guy who was sixteen and kind of flirting with me to kiss me; and I acted like I was all experienced and I kissed him. I was very innocent. I'd never kissed anyone or done anything except thought a lot about things. I didn't know what I was doing. I had the feeling like, *Well, I know that I had to do this sometime, so I'm just going to get over it with this idiot.* And I was so excited, and I wanted to tell everyone: *I French kissed!* I felt so old already. I'd just started being flirted with, so it was new, and I liked that a lot. And I was very excited when people started giving me attention that way."

Lisa related to the experience, not the person (*this idiot*). Her first intercourse at the age of fifteen was similar: "I liked this seventeen-year-old guy, sort of. I wasn't even dating him seriously. It was another one of those *I just want to get it over with* experiences." Since Lisa has been in college, having sex and having a relationship have come together for her. She has been with her current boyfriend for over a year and describes theirs as "a *very* close relationship—it's like I'm married."

First-Time Experiences Without Consent

Even though most of the Survey respondents consented to their first intercourse, at least 12 percent—more than one in ten—who had engaged in sexual intercourse indicated that their first time was without their consent. Actually, there are more women whose first intercourse was without their consent than the numerical statistics show.

As we saw in chapter 4 and with Pam earlier in this chapter, women may not consider experiences that they don't choose and consent to as "sexual" ones. Some women who were physically misused entered their first *consensual* intercourse to be statistically counted; they strongly asserted that for them an experience wasn't a sexual one *without their consensual participation*. For example, one Survey respondent wrote: "My very first intercourse was committed *on* me at age fifteen, when I was drunk, by an ex-boyfriend, age twenty, with some serious problems. I consider this rape, not sex. My *sex* life started at age seventeen. I'm answering this question about my first intercourse as of that consensual experience." Because we honored the answers women gave us, this woman was counted in the statistics as someone whose first intercourse was consensual with a peer at age seventeen.

Another Look at a Danger Zone: High School Girls and Older Boys

As we noted earlier in this chapter, when high school girl-women date older boy-men, they enter a *danger zone*. **Mary Jo (1947)** whose teenage experiences with "the guys" were described at length in the section above entitled "Coming of Age," related the circumstances of her first intercourse: "I was always raised that you didn't have sex before marriage, but it was sort of everything else went. Apart from being raped one time, I didn't have sex (i.e., intercourse) before marriage. When I was seventeen, I met this guy at the beach who was twenty-seven . . . a teacher. I'd given him my phone number in the waves and he'd remembered it; I thought this was exciting and romantic. He took me to a drive-in movie and gave me alcohol . . . I was very impressed. I never drank before, so I got loaded; he thought I was faking until I threw up. But, you know, I was used to guys who when you told them to stop, at a certain point they would stop. But he wouldn't. He knew I was a virgin. It was not a good way to experience your first sexual encounter. I didn't tell anybody. When I look back on it, I realize I just got really depressed. But I didn't know that then. Nobody knew about the rape until I told my mother fifteen years later. I got married when I was eighteen, shortly after it happened, to a guy I met when I went to college. He's the father of my children and, although we're now divorced, he is still a good friend."

Mary Jo tells us: "*I was used to guys who when you told them to stop, at a certain point they would stop.*" Pam, more than twenty years younger, who told us about being raped by a college friend of her sister's, in the section above entitled, "Danger Zone: High School Girl-

Women and Older Boy-Men," described her experiences with her high school friends: *"I would only go so far . . . and would never do intercourse with any of these guys. I definitely lived the notion that there's a lot you could do without having intercourse."* Older boys and men play by different rules than a girl's high school peers. Those of us who are older and more experienced must find ways to convey that to teenagers when we have opportunities to talk with them about sexuality.

Mary Jo also tells us: *"I didn't tell anybody. When I look back on it, I realize I just got really depressed."* You may recall from chapter 4 that a girl or woman can begin to heal and neutralize a traumatic experience almost at once if she is immediately able to tell someone about what happened, she is believed, and the person she tells is able to help her understand that the person who violated her is the one who was responsible and wrong. Unfortunately, this didn't happen for Mary Jo until fifteen years later. It is only in retrospect that we can consider what we might have done differently or would do exactly the same if we could live through an experience again.

Healing First Times for Women Who Were Sexually Abused

Sara (1949), who, you may remember from chapter 4, was abused by her father before she was four, hitchhiked with a girlfriend when she was seventeen in the mid-sixties from New England to New York City. There she met Dan, an artist; he was twenty-eight.

> The man who took my virginity was very decent. Thank you, Dan. We went to his house, smoked some weed, and he started to make a pass at me, which freaked me out. I hadn't had any kind of erotic encounter since my father had returned when I was twelve, so I immediately flashed back to my father. Dan could tell that I was very upset, and asked me what was going on, so I told him . . . about my father, that I'd never dated, never kissed anybody. (I didn't remember then what my father did to me when I was four.) And he said, *Well, I'm not going to tell you to do anything with me. But . . . I think you have no experience except with your father, and you're scared to death of something you've never really experienced.* That seemed true. All I knew was what happened with my father when I was twelve. I thought *That was then; this is now. Well, let's find out.*
>
> So we got up on his huge king-size bed with orange sheets and he started giving me a massage. And I started to

get turned on. He kissed me, and I liked it. And then I thought about the books I'd read [her neighbor's porn collection she found in the trash when she was around twelve], and I thought, *Thousands of people are doing this all over the world, all the time. Why not me?* Next, he went down on me. I liked that a lot. I don't know if I had an orgasm, but I was really turned on. He entered me and it felt good. The funny thing is, I thought that you were supposed to, like, keep pace with him. I didn't understand about friction. So when he would pull back, I would raise my hips up with him. And he'd push forward, I'd back up. Finally he grabbed my hips and said, *Hold still.* And he fucked me. And I was like *Oh-h-h-h-h! I get it now.* Then we were in sync and everything worked really well. And then I wanted to do it again. So we did it again. And then I wanted to do it again, and we did it again. So I had a very good introduction to sex. And I had a little crush on him, of course, but I never saw him again after I returned home. That was without birth control. I was lucky.

Pam (1968), who was raped by a friend of her sister's when she went East to check out colleges while in high school, continued her narrative with these comments:

After the rape surfaced, I had this need to be with men . . . trying to heal some of that stuff by having these two- and three-week relationships with men and yet still feeling uncertain and scared. By the time I was a senior in high school I'd had many of those kinds of experiences and then finally I fell in love with my best male friend. My first intercourse was with him, just after I turned seventeen. It was a very loving, gentle, and nurturing kind of sexual experience. [Notice how Pam acknowledges ownership of her first *consensual* intercourse; she does not count the rape.] I wanted this to be with someone I love, and that's what it was. I don't think it was very good sex now that I know what sex is, but at the time it was exactly what I needed. It was very calculated. We went out for months and did lots of touchy-feely things, kissing, and petting. It was very romantic. His parents were gone the night of our senior prom, so we were all prepared, we bought all of the things, came home and had this very romantic, wonderful evening. It was awkward. I think first sex is always awkward; I'd never dealt with an erect penis before and putting on a condom. With him it was a very conscious thing for me, wanting to be present, wanting to really enjoy this. And we did, we laughed about it. We're still good friends, and we still talk about it.

Guidelines for the 21st Century: Optimizing Pleasure, Confidence, and Self-Esteem

Kirsten and Jessica, the two women discussed in this section, each had a first experience that was satisfying and enhanced her self-esteem. Both were born in **1970**. Kirsten was twenty when she first had intercourse, Jessica was seventeen. The experiences they describe—and those of the other women in this chapter—provide us with clues to the conditions that make sexual satisfaction and enhanced self-esteem most likely to result from first intercourse.

Two Women Born in 1970

Kirsten was the older of the two when she had her first sexual intercourse. The values she'd learned from her parents helped her to defer her first time until she found someone she really wanted to be with: "Until then I had always held back, basically because I'd held my mom's view of 'no sex before marriage' . . . not really my own view, but I hadn't found somebody who I really wanted to be with." Then, when she was twenty, she ". . . fell in love . . . I felt I was going to marry him someday. We'd been going out about two months . . . had slept in the same bed . . . been pretty much naked with each other, until I just eventually came to the point where I wanted to share this experience with him. Never once did he pressure me. We'd been at a party in one of the dorms, done some dirty dancing, which had turned us both on. We went back to my room (a usual thing; either he spent the night at my dorm, or I spent the night at his). We got ready for bed, started kissing, doing what we usually did. He kind of got on top of me, and then we were just kissing and hugging and touching each other. And then I started kind of grabbing onto him. And when I realized he was aroused, I just kind of encouraged him a little bit. And then he got to the point where he was getting closer and closer to actually having sex with me. So at that point, he's all, *Do you want me to stop? Do you want me to stop?* And I said, *No.* It was a great night. I don't think that I'll ever forget it. It hurt a little bit at first, but the feeling I had for this person, it was a great, great experience. We're still together."

Jessica was seventeen; she and her boyfriend had planned ahead. "He was my first boyfriend and we'd been going out, kissing, for two months ... discussing it, 'cause he was a virgin, too. His parents weren't home, we were watching movies on his bed, had been kissing for half an hour. And we were both like, *Are you ready?* I reached for a condom and put it on him, and we just had sex. It was more or less planned. Maybe not for that day necessarily, but we'd bought the condoms because we thought we might soon. The first time it was good because he was responsive and nice about it, but I thought kind of, *This is it? I hope there's more to it.* But it got better. *The decision to do it?* I never received any pressure. He and I had a mutual respect. And we knew each other and had all these feelings for each other."

What These Experiences Had in Common

The first time experiences that were sexually satisfying and enhanced the self-esteem of these two women and their partners had the following qualities in common. Furthermore, these qualities clearly create conditions that make such good outcomes likely:

- Neither of these women felt pressured by her partner.

- Sexual intercourse was discussed ahead of time.

- Each experience involved mutual consent and felt shared.

- "Doing it" was preceded by several months of physical exploration and sex play.

- Sexual intercourse took place in a safe, comfortable setting.

- Sexual intercourse occurred in a relationship that continued.

Another important condition is protection against pregnancy and, if with a man who has had a previous partner, against sexually transmitted diseases. Jessica used condoms her first time; Kirsten didn't, although subsequently she did use them. Later, both Kirsten and Jessica switched to birth control pills.

Still Waiting

When **Andrea (1972)** was interviewed at age twenty, she had recently engaged in some clothed sexual exploration with a male friend but nothing more; she was still waiting, and she had thought a lot about what she wanted: "My friends are a lot more sexually active than I am, so it gives me a chance to hear from them what their experiences are to see if that's kind of the path I want to go or not. And it's not particularly. Hearing about their sexual experiences has really shown me what I don't want to do."

I end this chapter with the advice that three of Andrea's sexually active peers, college women who came into adulthood in the 1990s, would give their daughters about conditions for *"having sex."*

Lori (1969): "If you think that you're going to have sex with someone, it's something you should definitely discuss rationally outside of a sexual setting. You should talk about it over coffee, instead of talking about it during foreplay."

Katy (1970): "It's not something that you have to do or should do. It's something that should be shared with someone who you care about very deeply."

Angela (1971): "Even though the world on the outside puts a lot of emphasis on sex, and on defining yourself as being sexual, you don't have to feel pressured to conform right away. It's okay if you're putting your energy toward reading books or doing things that you like; you don't have to grow up so quickly concerning that."

What Does This Mean to You?

Now, if you wish, pick up your notebook and express the thoughts and feelings you're having about your *first time.* Here are some questions you might want to consider after you've done that.

- If you are not committed to celibacy, how did you (or will you) decide when, where, and with whom to have intercourse or woman-woman genital sex for the first time?

- If you've had intercourse or woman-woman genital sex:

  - What guidelines and sources of information and advice were helpful to you?

  - What were harmful or misleading?

  - Is there anything you wish someone had told you?

- What decision-making guidelines would you offer to women who have not yet had their *first time*?

- Would you suggest the same guidelines to a sexually experienced woman thinking about whether to have intercourse or woman-woman genital sex for the first time with a new partner?

- If you are recalling experiences that you now regret, consider the circumstances, the roles of others, and how you saw your options at the time. Then, sit quietly with your eyes closed and imagine what you could now gently and lovingly tell your younger self that would be healing and would lead to greater self-acceptance.

Part 3

Sexual Partners: Licit and Illicit

6

Partners and Contexts

The variety of contexts in which women experience and express their sexuality is fascinating to me. Of those women who provided information, about 40 percent had at some time lived with a sex partner she did not later marry, about 6 percent of those who provided information had lived with more than two partners; 66 percent had been married, 15 percent twice, 3 percent more than twice; 35 percent had divorced, 7 percent twice, about 1 percent more than twice; 4 percent had been widowed, four women twice, one six times.

Living Arrangements

The Survey asked about a woman's current relationship and living situation. A respondent could check: 1) No sex partner now; 2) Seeing but not living with my sex partner(s); 3) Living with a sex partner, without marriage or life commitment; 4) Living with a sex partner, with marriage or life commitment; or 5) Other (Please Specify).

Living with a Sex Partner, with Marriage or Life Commitment

The circumstances of the 1,205 women in this category covered a variety of circumstances that ranged from being married a long time to being engaged or semi-engaged. Respondents ranging in age from late teens to nearly eighty wrote of planning to marry. One lesbian noted she was "working toward marriage," and one heterosexual described how she was committed to life partnership—but done with marriage and wifeliness: "We're not married, but we own a home together and are committed—possibly even probably for life; one marriage and one divorce—too many!" A young woman noted: "For us, life commitment is a description rather than a prescription, an intent and desire rather than a decisive promise."

Living with a Sex Partner, Without Marriage or Life Commitment

The 150 women *living with a sex partner, without marriage or life commitment* also represented a variety of situations. A few wrote of *almost* living with their partners: ♀ I live next door with/to a sex partner *without* marriage; ♀ I practically live with him—see him almost every day and we stay at one of our places; ♀ My body lives at my partner's home but I keep up a separate residence with friends; ♀ I live with my partner part-time; during school I live with my mother. Some in this category were ambivalent about marriage or thought they might be getting married—someday: ♀ It *could* be for life; ♀ He wants marriage—I'm scared, but see myself with him.

Seeing but Not Living with My Sex Partner(s)

Among the variety of arrangements for meeting sexual needs of the 605 who were *seeing but not living with their sex partner(s)* were: occasional sex; sex with a friend who was not a partner; intermittent sex as part of dating; twice-a-month sex with an old friend; and a "casual" sexual partner. One woman was sexually active without one specific partner; another rarely saw her sex partner.

Some respondents emphasized that although they weren't living with their sex partners, there was indeed commitment. One said she was seeing but not living with her partner "*with* marriage commitment"; they had a one-year-old son (1974). A lesbian noted that she had a sex partner she didn't live with and added, "plus I'm living with a gay man."

Some women lived at a distance from their partners. Among their situations were a partner out of the area, so sex was occasional (1929); a husband who was working overseas ("but we'll be reunited soon"); female partners living in other states; a male partner in California when the respondent was in Florida; and a partner who lived in England.

No Sex Partner Now

The 599 women with *no sex partner now* included a retired teacher with a graduate degree, born in 1910, who strongly agreed with the statement: *On the whole, I have been satisfied with my sexual life* and said she had had "no sex partner ever." Another woman who had never had sexual intercourse said: "I'm seeing someone but he is not my sex partner" (1958).

About 1 percent of the respondents, most but not all over forty, indicated that they were *married and living with their husbands but not having sex:* ♀ Our last sex was ten years ago (1912); ♀ No sex for eight years (1927); ♀ My husband had prostate surgery two years ago, says he can't achieve erection (1936); ♀ I have a husband, no sex; we've been together thirty-five years, last had sex eight years ago (1939); ♀ I'm living with my husband in the same house but we've been separated since April '93. He retired three years ago; he sits and reads and watches TV a lot (1939); ♀ I have a dysfunctional/disengaged sex life; I've had sex two times in fifteen months, maybe ten times in three years (1950). Two women in this category who were younger than forty said: ♀ I'm married/living with my husband, not sexually active; ♀ I'm living with the father of my children—no sex.

Separated from husband or boyfriend. Some women who had no current sex partner were in various stages of separating from a partner or ending a relationship: ♀ Until three months ago, I was regularly seeing, and having sex once a month with two men, both married to someone else. These relationships ceased being convenient for me, otherwise they would still be going on. Both men knew of the other's existence; ♀ Just broke up!; ♀ Divorced after twenty-six years of marriage; ♀ Separated from my husband and living with my parents.

At least four respondents had partners who were incarcerated: ♀ My husband has been in prison for five years—no sex partner; ♀ My boyfriend is in jail.

Others noted: ♀ I'm committed to writing letters for the moment; ♀ I'm dating various people; ♀ No partners, I live with my parents. One Survey respondent provided a glimpse of a relationship taking off. On page two of her questionnaire she wrote: "I am dating three men but not sexually involved with any of them (yet!)." She must have set the questionnaire aside for a while before finishing it, because by the time she got to page seven, her situation had changed: "I have a new lover as of two days ago!"

Widowed. Of the 2,632 respondents to the Survey, eighty-nine indicated they had at some time been widowed, five of these more than once. A few described their current status as *Widow* rather than *No sex partner now.* One woman, born in 1920, gave her occupation as *Widow*; perhaps while her husband was alive she thought of her primary life work as being *wife* and *homemaker.*

Multiple partners. Only a few women indicated that they had multiple partners, but they covered a wide age range and the spectrum of possibilities: two male partners, two female partners, one of each, and more than two partners. One respondent, who described herself as *bisexual,* noted that she was living with her husband and "looking for a girlfriend." The topic of nonmonogamy is addressed in the next chapter.

Among those in the miscellaneous category were a sexual surrogate who works with men in the process of sex therapy and also has a private life sex partner with whom she doesn't live; a nurse who is remaining celibate until marriage; and a student who said: "I have a boyfriend but I'm not sexually active."

Sex Outside the Safety and Structure of Commitment

Since the sexual revolution of the 1960s, young women may become sexually active many years before they marry, if they marry at all. Many of the women born in the 1950s or later had sexual relationships they didn't expect to last or episodes of casual sexual dating before ever having a committed long-term relationship. Women of all ages had such experiences between or in lieu of long-term relationships. For some, such as this Survey respondent, there was a period of time when their liaisons were based more on sex than on appropriateness for life partnership: "I've had over thirty sexual partners, more than ten casual. I was very sexually active in college, but began to understand the risks, physically and emotionally, at age twenty-one. I've had only monogamy after age twenty-two." **Mindy (1965)** lived and worked at a ski resort for a winter between high school and college. She said: "I began hanging out socially with a guy I'd actually known for a long time; he'd given me ski lessons when I was younger. We became involved in a very lustful relationship. One of the biggest things we had in common was sleeping together. I was just eighteen, free and on my own for the first time, doing what I wanted to do. Sex with him was a big part of it. At the time, it was great. I recall it being really nice. I still keep in contact with him and sometimes fantasize about him."

Casual Sex: Commitment Only to the Here and Now

In the three months before they filled out their questionnaires, 149 Survey respondents engaged in sexual activity with someone they had known at the time for less than seven days. Forty-eight of these 149 women had known their partner for less than twenty-four hours.

When **Deanna (1971)** told of an experience of casual sex, a one-night stand she had, she said, "I've had casual sex once. I felt fairly comfortable because I knew I probably wouldn't see him again. I had nothing to lose." **Michele (1972)** reacted quite differently to her experience. She described what happened as "a very traumatic one-night stand" and went on to say, "You sleep with somebody you don't even know. And it's like I really wanted to, and I did. And then the next day, I felt like a *slut*. I went up to my room, and I took a hot, hot shower. I just felt awful. I said to myself, *Why did you do that?* "Cause I wanted to. It felt really good.' *But that's wrong. You're never going to see that person again* . . . a constant inner battle. I really wanted to do it in the spur of the moment . . . but I knew it was morally wrong and I'm not going to see that person again. And it was just bad, really traumatic, this one-night stand. But it ended up that we became really good friends. He called me the next day, and I said, *Can you come up?* And we talked about it. I felt guilty because I enjoyed it. If I hadn't enjoyed it, maybe I would have felt better."

Self-Acceptance

With respect to values about what was appropriate for her in sexual relating, Michele was still "finding her way." The tension between her urge to do and explore and her long-standing values is obvious. Throughout our lives, we continue at times to wonder *Should I be doing this?* Not everyone agrees on the acceptability and value of casual sex. As with other issues, we have to consider conflicting views when trying to determine our own values. Unless yours are well established in your teens and early twenties—and usually they're not in those years—you're likely to experiment with what your peers are doing, with what's available to you. I hope Michele can now say, "From this experience I learned a lot about what I wouldn't do again, but I also enjoyed it; that's how it was." That would be a statement of self-acceptance.

Finding Our Way

In her late teens **Ronni (1955)** went through what she described as "a very promiscuous phase" while she was in college in the early 1970s. She said, "At the time I was very guilt-ridden about that. When I look back on it, I'm glad that I did it. However, I've had more sexual experiences with more strangers than I would have liked, and I think emotionally it didn't add to my self-esteem. I believe I would have grown more quickly emotionally or come to a better sense of self if I had sat with my loneliness instead of taking the easy way out and going out and picking somebody up. I do regret that."

In looking back over their entire sex lives, close to half of the Survey respondents said that they regretted that *I had sex with partners I should have turned down.* Nearly one in four regretted that *I got into sex when I was too young.*

Are there conditions under which sex without commitment, what I'm calling "casual sex," can be a validating and healthy expression of one's sexuality? One measure I apply in evaluating interactions such as these is that afterwards each person involved feels good about herself or himself and the other or others. One key to success in casual sexual encounters is that there is a mutual understanding, an implicit or explicit "contract," about what having sex means—that each person thinks it means more or less the same thing. And, of course, it is crucial for mutual well-being that there is protection against such unwanted consequences as pregnancy, disease, and irate other partners. **Amanda (1970)** put it this way: "I feel okay about casual sex if it's been discussed, if you know that that's what it's going to be, that you're just gonna have sex."

Once-Again-Single

A time in their lives when women may engage in sex without a long-term commitment is after a relationship ends. **Donna (1949)** described what happened when she became once-again-single: "I was selective sexually, but early on after my marriage I did experiment. Part of me would say, *Well by some standards as long as a person is a good person there's nothing wrong with going to bed on the first date.* Yet there were times I would think about being more traditional and say, *That's not good.* I tried it both ways and on the whole it went well. I am friends with every person I've been to bed with except for one. I went out with him, we went to bed, and two days later I got this angry call at work from a woman who claimed to be his fiancée."

Unfulfilling One-Night Stands

Motivations for casual encounters may include feelings that are experienced as the need for closeness, affection, and for affirmation that one is attractive and sexually desirable. **Judith (1940)**, who was currently happily married, talked about a four-year period in her late twenties, after she had divorced the man she married at eighteen. In looking back, she realized that her one-night stands devalued her because she and her partners did not see sex in the same way. They had no mutual agreements about what having sex would mean:

> There was a lot of experimenting, a seedy side, one-night stands. It could be someone I knew and liked ... in the same social circle ... and you'd end up going to bed with them. My sexuality was out of control. I realize now that I didn't need sex but that's how I got closeness. I wasn't aware of what I was doing. I deceived myself into thinking these guys liked me and what they really wanted was sex. In hindsight I see that they got what they wanted and left. I would merge and they wouldn't, and then I would feel devastated because afterwards it felt like abandonment. I would wake up the next morning filled with guilt and shame, thinking: *Holy shit, what have I done?* I would see these guys again socially and they would act as if nothing happened. That feels terrible. It was when I invited a man I knew socially but not sexually to a Christmas party and that night we had sex and then I didn't hear from him that I finally became conscious and able to say, *It's as if I don't matter. If it didn't mean anything, then why did we do it?*

Over time Judith became able to consider *What am I doing?* As she became more and more conscious of her own Observing Inner Self, protective and watching out for her well-being, she became aware of what made sex satisfying and successful for her. Gradually, she found her way to the realization that it wasn't really sex she needed; she was looking for closeness through sex. Even though it was difficult to change her long-standing ways of doing things, over time, she became able to stop having sex with men who were looking only for sex.

Leslie (1971), a much younger woman, talked about "finding her way" to understanding that one-night stands didn't give her what she wanted. She'd had seven intercourse partners, including three one-night stands that "involved large amounts of alcohol"; she had had no ongoing relationship for two years. She said: "I've had three one-night stands with complete strangers I never saw again. I met them on vacation, in bars, at parties. Each time I was definitely drunk. They'd go through all their motions of mating, as far as flirting. Once we decided to go home together, I always in my mind presumed that I should sleep with them, that if I didn't sleep with them, they would think that I was kind of a tease. So most of the reason that I would sleep with them is that once you do go home with someone, it's presumed that you will. They would initiate having sex."

Leslie provides us with examples of some beliefs that many women have about appropriate dating behavior. These are not beliefs we create by ourselves. We are socialized into believing them through the messages the culture we live in sends to us. How are we, as women, misled into the belief that we should put the feelings and needs of a man we don't even know over and above our own feelings, needs, and well-being?

Perhaps part of the answer lies in the fact that many of us learn as we're growing up that we should take care of a man's needs before our own, whether it is our father, brother, date, or husband. We learn, *When I please a man, I'm successful as a woman.* That can lead to the sexual script that Leslie was following. And she is not alone; many other women follow it, too. It goes something like this: *Once you go home with a man you should take care of his needs. You should sleep with him so he won't think you're a tease or, worse, a prick tease. You can't leave him sexually unsatisfied. You should put his feelings and needs before your own.*

But it's okay to put your own safety and your own needs—pleasing and taking care of yourself—first. If this were a mature ongoing relationship, you would watch out for your needs and he would watch out for his—while at the same time you would consider and care for each other. If Leslie had understood that her well-being is more important than appearances, she might have considered *Will this experience enhance me? Will I feel good about myself afterwards? About him? Do I want to say "No" or go ahead?*

It is perfectly okay to say something like, *I think I'd like to go to sleep now and see what we want to do in the morning* or *I'd like to stop (or leave) now.* It is okay to sober up a bit and change your mind. In fact, there are some men who would be relieved if you did. I've talked to men who have gotten into similar situations and have gone ahead only because they thought the woman they were with expected them to.

One caution, though, about watching out for yourself. There are some men who react with violence when they are expecting sex and then the woman realizes she doesn't want to continue. This is one of the risks in going home with a man you don't know or with whom you don't have a clear understanding about sex and what having sex means. You may be forced by such circumstances to make a choice from options that all seem undesirable.

Through trial and error Leslie was "finding her way." Lamentably, what made her more aware of her choices was a sexually transmitted disease. The previous summer a man she "slept with" had given her venereal warts. She said: "I'm still dealing with getting rid of those, and the whole guilt factor that comes along with sleeping with strangers. The whole process of seeing doctors and getting treated has really made me feel guilty, ashamed, and dirty about my sexuality. I haven't been with anyone since getting warts. There was this one boy that I really liked, and we kissed one night, but I was terrified to do anything else. I didn't want to."

These difficulties helped Leslie become clearer about her values and what she wanted for herself: "Since I slept with the man who gave me warts, I'm much more reserved about my body. A positive effect has been reclaiming my body. But I have a relatively negative view of my sexuality at this point in my life. I just haven't had a very positive sexual experience so far. But I do know it'll get better." Leslie also talked about her hopes for the future: "I think a lot of developing my sexuality has to do with meeting someone who I feel comfortable around, who I know respects me . . . having a long-term relationship. But I just haven't met that person yet. I think I have to wait for some type of permanence." When asked about changes she might make in herself to make sex better, Leslie replied: "I probably wouldn't be drunk," and added that she hadn't regularly used alcohol during sex with the three boyfriends with whom she'd had ongoing relationships. I wish her well.

Further Thoughts on Love and Connection

Maria (1965) talked of some of her casual encounters and the conclusions she's reached about the importance for her of having an emotional connection or love before having sex. "Several of the men I picked weren't very affectionate or open and the only way I got any sense of affection or caring was through sex. So, with them, that seemed the way to do it; the sex was proof that they really liked me. Which I now know is backwards. You should first find somebody who likes you and then you have sex. In the past I used to think, *Well I'm an adult and I like this person so it's okay to have sex.* But now I think for it to be really good there has to be a bond, a connection, with the other person. If you love the person or really care for him, that's the emotional side; then there can be the opening and the sharing and touching and the spiritual side."

What Does This Mean to You?

Now, if you wish, pick up your notebook and express the thoughts and feelings you're having about partners and commitment or casual sex. Here are some questions you might want to consider after you've done that:

- What are your values about living with a sex partner without marriage or life commitment?

- What are your values about casual sex? How would you advise a younger woman who sought your advice about engaging in sex outside of a committed relationship?

- If you are recalling experiences that you now regret, consider the circumstances, the roles of others, and how you saw your options at that time. Then, sit quietly with your eyes closed and imagine what you could gently and lovingly tell your younger self that would be healing and would lead to greater self-acceptance.

7

Consensual Nonmonogamy and Affairs

Consensual Nonmonogamy

Can you be attracted to more than one person? Emotionally intimate with others than your primary partner? Can you love more than one person? Have sex with someone else and not threaten the commitment of your primary relationship? Some people—although they are in the minority—consider these questions and conclude *Yes, I can*, or at least, *I'll see if I can.* They renegotiate their initial relationship contract of monogamy, or they may never agree to have an exclusive relationship in the first place. They make partnership agreements that specifically permit sex with certain others.

If you never have had a nonmonogamous arrangement, could you accept a relationship agreement like one of these? ♀ For us outside sex is okay; ♀ My primary partner is a woman. Both of us have had sex with men during this time together; we don't see this as having an "affair"; ♀ I have been in an *open* marriage. Of my thirty-one years of marriage, all but the first seven were open; ♀ We have a "nonmonogamous, poly-intimate agreement" = safe sex with any others; ♀ The relationship is "OPEN." I have sex with others often, but it is not considered an "affair."

About 1 percent of the Survey respondents had mutual agreements of consensual nonmonogamy—having more than one partner—also called, in some variations, *swinging, open marriage* or *open relationship,* and *in the couples' lifestyle.* In their relationships, sex with others was okay under certain conditions. Some of these women requested a questionnaire after our survey was mentioned in a newsletter for people interested in practicing consensual nonmonogamy. Although about 1 percent of this Survey's respondents were currently involved in consensual nonmonogamy, this describes only the group of women we surveyed and does not imply that this is the percentage for all American women. One Survey respondent noted that the Survey left out "a whole category of sexual experience: group experiences. . . . While I have never had 'affairs' or 'one-night-stands,' I have had groups of friends where sexual rules were 'relaxed,' i.e., hot tub parties that resulted in heavy petting or intercourse, date swapping, etc."

Some of the women I interviewed who were not currently in open relationships had been in the past, usually in the 1960s and '70s when such arrangements were talked about more and were more customary than they are now. When I asked **Pat (1945)** if she had ever had an affair, what she described was *not* a liaison that was secret or in violation of her relationship's rules. She and her husband had agreed to a partner exchange with another couple who were very much into open relationships. This was after ten years of marriage at a time when, Pat said, she was *feeling dead inside* and her self-esteem was low. It was the mid-1970s. "Not so much happened between my husband and his wife, but I really fell in love with the other guy. The couple didn't intend to separate our marriage, but they felt that people could love more than one person. They really validated who I was. It was very painful for my husband because the man and I had intercourse. My relationship with this man was very spiritual . . . soul oriented, nurturing. The arousal with him was better, maybe because we spent more time getting aroused, but he had a little more difficulty coming to orgasm, so I actually found sex better with my husband. Sex for my husband and me became very good at that point; I could orgasm with him in the morning and again in the afternoon."

Jealousy in Open Relationships

In the late 1960s and the 1970s, people were imagining, writing, and talking about "open marriage" as a lifestyle and experimenting with communal living much more openly than they are today. *Open Marriage* by Nena and George O'Neill (1972) hit the best-seller list and people were reading novels by Robert Rimmer that addressed various permutations of nonmonogamy. Although I was a fan of Rimmer's and admired his consideration of nontraditional relationships, I did think that real-life experiences were probably not always as idyllic as his fictional ones, because he almost totally ignored the emotion of jealousy. An author of that era who did thoughtfully consider jealously was Ronald Mazur in his *The New Intimacy: Open-ended Marriage and Alternative Lifestyles* (1973).

One of the biggest challenges of consensual nonmonogamy is how to deal with feelings of jealousy, the emotion that alerts us to: *Wake up! The bond of an emotional attachment important to you is in danger.* In multiple-partner situations, jealously is almost always experienced at some time by some or all of the parties involved. Pat's husband was jealous when she had intercourse and fell in love with another man. When he met another woman, their positions reversed: "During the time we had an open relationship, my husband met another woman. I knew who she was, and he did have sex with her. As far as I know, that's the only other relationship he's had. There was a lot of jealousy on my part."

Looking back, Pat evaluated her own affair as essentially positive. "I grew a lot because of the affair. I came to see myself as a valuable person. I started standing up for myself, became more of an individual and respected myself more. George and I have now been married for twenty-three years."

One or both partners experiencing jealousy is not necessarily a reason to avoid an open relationship, but the emotion must be addressed if the feelings and sensitivities of everyone involved are to be considered and honored. Having multiple partners—even with mutual consent—can take a relationship to the "edge" we have seen in other contexts, that limit where curiosity, danger, excitement, and the forbidden meet. There is always some danger that switching partners will end a marriage or relationship. For example, a Survey respondent wrote, "While I was married my husband agreed to a 'partner switch.' He then backed out but I didn't. We divorced and I married that other partner."

Even if the marriage doesn't end, swinging relationships aren't always enjoyable. Each person involved has her or his own experience, and not all necessarily end up feeling good about themselves and the others. **Roberta (1943)** described what happened when she and her husband got involved in "a swinging kind of thing" in the early and mid-1970s: "That was 'open marriage' time and all that stuff was going on. To me, it had a negative impact on the relationship. My husband always wanted other women; he talked a lot about open marriage. The only time that was positive for me was a time where we swapped with another couple, and that was because there wasn't jealousy. But when we got into the swinging part with other couples, I didn't like that at all. I did it for him; I would rather have been making love with him. To me, it was mixed up in my mind and to me it's a sex act versus the total person. *Diseases?* At that time, we weren't concerned about condoms and everything else and we didn't get any diseases either. It wasn't like it was wholesale; in the swinging scene we had a very closed group."

Women and men tend to approach nonmonogamy differently. "To me it's a sex act versus the total person," said Roberta, and when Pat and her husband exchanged partners, Pat *"really fell in love with the other guy."* More women than men want the sex within the context of relationship; more men than women are looking to just have sex. For **Mary Jo (1947)**, *nonmonogamy* meant having more than one relationship: *"Jealousy?* Oh, yes. I've experimented with lots of different lifestyles but I wouldn't say that I've ever had casual sex. In my experience with open relationships, the men's idea of *nonmonogamy* means—at least the ones that I was with—that they have a relationship where they get to have *occasional flings* on the side, maybe with overnights or one-night stands. My idea of nonmonogamy, as it worked out, is I had a *relationship* with a man with whom I was living and a *relationship* with another man. Now the men I lived with didn't think that was very cool. They wanted me to do it their way. But I couldn't see the point."

Most couples do not so easily embrace nonmonogamy, however. Alice, close in age to Mary Jo, represents a set of values at the other end of the monogamy/consensual nonmonogamy spectrum. Alice and Ron were so committed to their value that marriage is a sacred contract that, for them, just the fact of Alice having a strong attraction to another man was enough to create emotional and marital turmoil. **Alice (1938)** married Ron when she was twenty and he is still the only sex partner she has ever had, but eight years into their marriage she attended a week-long seminar sponsored by her Protestant church:

> I was drawn to one of the men in the group and had to deal with having really strong feelings—sexual feelings—for a man other than my husband. I was into fidelity but that didn't take away the feelings. I knew I had to go home and tell Ron about them. It was really difficult. I didn't know how it would affect him but I couldn't not tell him because

it really had affected me. It really threw him into a tailspin. We had very long conversations about what the words "love" and "marriage" meant and what it meant to have the same feelings for two people. Your values come into play. What do your marriage vows mean? Does it mean you don't look at another person, that you're not friends with other people? I'd always had men friends but I'd never had to deal with being drawn to someone at that level. Looking back almost thirty years later, we regard this whole crisis as having strengthened us and our marriage, but at the time it was very traumatic.

Your values come into play. What do your marriage vows mean? What does it mean when you pledge to *forsake all others 'til death*? Today, when so many people write their own wedding vows or live together with a less formal commitment, not all ceremonies contain these words, but for centuries most couples who married agreed to some version of this promise. Alice and her husband Ron had made this vow and took it literally and very seriously.

Thinking about it now, *where do your values fall on the continuum between monogamy and consensual nonmonogamy?*

Affairs

Nonmonogamy that is not mutually consensual has a very different quality than that involving consent. An affair, sex outside of the primary relationship without prior agreement, involves a violation of mutual trust. In the Survey, we defined "affair" for the purposes of the questions we asked as "you having sex outside of your relationship in a way that violates rules of the relationship against it. If you and your partner have agreed that outside sex is OK, then it's not an affair. If you are single and having sex with someone who is married, that is *not* an affair for you."

Of those women responding to the Survey questions on affairs, 43 percent said they had at some time had at least one affair. This means, though, that more than half, 57 percent, had no affairs. Of the women who had had an affair, nearly half had had only one; about half that many had had two affairs and half as many again had had three; 13 percent of those who reported outside-of-relationship sex had had five or more partners.

Two factors contributing to the quite large percentage of women who said they had had an affair were (1) that the relationship context wasn't necessarily a marriage or a serious commitment and (2) that "having *sex*" did not necessarily mean having *sexual intercourse*: ♀ I went to bed with someone, but there was no penetration because of impotence; ♀ I've had five affairs, but these were not necessarily major sexual activity; ♀ In the second of my two affairs, no sex—no intercourse—happened.

Three Affairs

Here are three women who have had affairs. Each entered into her affair for different reasons. Emily, Second Chance, and Mindy provide us with further examples of the great variability in women's sexualities.

Emily

Emily (1919), whom we have met in other chapters, was married in 1940, when she was twenty-one. Her husband was her first intercourse partner, and sex was satisfying at first. "When it was good it was very good, because he had such a sensitive touch," she said. But over the years, problems developed:

> Over time he became a heavy drinker of alcohol and a heavy smoker. Sex became less frequent. In our first year we had sex about three times a week, after that never as often again. When I was thirty-five, we once went six months without sex and I got very angry. I would work very hard and go to bed exhausted so I wouldn't think about sex, so I wouldn't feel rejected. I felt unattractive and I was repressing my sexual urges. His sex drive wasn't enough for me. Also, he had a problem controlling his anger when he had been drinking and that was very hard for me.
>
> Toward the end of that six-month period without sex, when I was feeling like *a keeper of children, including my husband*, I met a man who found me very attractive. When he kissed me, I felt like all my controls were gone. I felt I was totally available and it scared the hell out of me and I ran away from him. I realized I was sexually attracted to him, but I couldn't agree to have sex with him. I wasn't brought up that way. Men are allowed to sow their wild oats but a good woman can't do that. The idea of having sex extramaritally brought up tremendous waves of guilt, yet the charge remained strong between us. This struggle went on for a good while. I even saw a therapist. I realized I was

following my father's rules. He had laid the law down about being a virgin until marriage and staying faithful.

Finally, one very hot summer day, I was home alone ... so tired of thinking about it ... of the waves of guilt every time I thought about it. I put down what I was doing in the kitchen, ran into the bedroom and laid across the bed and did a relaxing exercise I'd read about, imagining falling through black space. And in the midst of that blackness suddenly my father's face appeared, like a portrait. I knew nothing about psychology then, but I talked to my father's image. I said, *Daddy, I'm not your little girl anymore.*

Emily went on to have a dialogue with the image of her father in which his face appeared and disappeared several times. She also had a fantasy of having sex with the man she found so attractive. Finally, her father's face broke up and disappeared:

I couldn't bring it up again, and I got this tremendous sense of relief—lightning hadn't struck me dead. At that moment I began to feel energy moving up through my body. It felt like it shot out of the top of my head and then settled down again. It was so strong that I jumped up and I ran out into the front yard under a big tree with many branches; it was a very hot day, and I just rolled around in the cool grass. And I felt great! *Oh, I love life! Oh, it's wonderful!* I was in this ecstasy of relief.

I arranged a rendezvous in a hotel with this man, exactly as it had been in my fantasy, and everything went just the way I wanted it to. Two days later, my husband approached me and we had sex. When I went into orgasm, I cried and cried and cried ... in sadness for what we had had and because I knew I would never be monogamous with him again. From then on I always had lovers. I did try once to give up on all this because I really wanted to have it all with my husband, but it wasn't possible because he had so many psychological problems. By the summer of 1966 I knew I had to end the marriage; we'd been married twenty-six years.

That decision sent Emily into panic, because she had no preparation for entering the marketplace to find work, and she had no idea of how she would support herself. A therapist who told her, *"One step at a time"* helped her to become focused, and Emily started a very successful career. She had a number of long relationships and engaged in a good deal of sexual and relationship experimentation in the years that followed. Many years later, when she was sixty-nine, she married again. In that marriage, she returned to monogamy: "That was something we both agreed we wanted. With the circumstances as they are these days, I'm not willing to take those kinds of risks anymore."

Second Chance

A one-night affair that helped one woman reclaim her sense of self and strengthened her marriage, at least temporarily, was described in this note attached to a Survey questionnaire. Did the marriage survive? I don't know. But the affair gave it another chance. To protect the woman's identity I have omitted identifying details. I will call her "Second Chance."

> After a year of couples' therapy and medication for my husband, we were on the road to a better understanding of each other. Our sex life had improved even though he was not always able to have an erection; we were growing closer again. Previously we had not made love more than four or five times in four years. So we stopped therapy and I lost thirty-five pounds and I was feeling good. Within a month, my husband stopped paying any attention to what we had learned and discovered we needed. We were sliding backwards. I became angry and hopeless, and he did not want to go back to therapy. In mid-summer I told a male family friend of fifteen years about my problems. We ended up on a beach kissing and having oral sex. We didn't have intercourse. This one-night affair has turned my life upside down.
>
> I'm back in therapy by myself, trying to understand who I am, what I want and need. Therapy has helped me make it clear to my husband that he has to make an effort to work on our marriage and sex life or I will leave the marriage. He has been making an effort, our sex life is better, and I feel closer to him. He doesn't know what happened with our friend and I plan to keep it that way. My friend and I are trying to put behind us what happened between us and remain friends.

Mindy

Mindy (1965) had been living a completely heterosexual life until she fell in love with Jody, the woman with whom she was living when I interviewed her. During her three years with Jody she'd had two short affairs with men.

> They really satisfied a need in me that had nothing to do with Jody. There was no way she could have satisfied that. There's something really different about it. I really like the feeling of a man being inside of me. It's hard to describe. There's sort of a depth at which that feels greater to me than Jody's finger inside of me. I also like the feel of men's bodies. The sex was great and I really enjoyed it. The biggest discomfort that I had to work through was that Jody would probably interpret this as cheating on her. She knows I've been attracted to men and enjoy being with them, but she can't imagine it herself, can't understand it, and finds it real threatening. She knew about the first affair and it really bothered her, so I haven't told her about the second one. I wish she could understand that it really isn't a threat, that it really has nothing to do with her or with our relationship. It's just something different I want or need occasionally.

Why Do Women Have Affairs?

Three women, three affairs—different reasons, different outcomes. Women do not generally enter into affairs lightly or for just one reason. Let us consider Emily, Second Chance, and Mindy in more detail.

The stage is set for an "affair" when an outward attraction meets strong dissatisfaction within a relationship. Within her primary relationship, Emily's husband had become an angry user of alcohol, and they stopped having sex. Emily was repressing her sexual urges and feeling rejected, unattractive, and like *a keeper of children.* When a man from outside her marriage who found her very attractive appeared on the scene, Emily went through a time of ambivalence, clarification of her values, and decision making; she struggled with a huge amount of guilt.

Throughout our lives we confront and resolve over and over again the tensions between a *wish to do* on one hand and *prohibitions against doing* or *reasons not to do* on the other. We move toward exploration and self-development, and at the same time we are influenced by the external values and limits imposed by the important people in our lives and the society in which we live. As adults, when we experience shame or guilt, we can understand that these emotions mean that we are breaking some internalized rule. As adults we are able to consider, as Emily did: *Whose rule is it? Where did I get it? Does it make sense for me to follow it?* Emily did decide to have the affair. For her, this became a way to reindividuate, to reclaim her separate sense of self. Eventually, she and her husband divorced.

Second Chance found that inside her relationship, the more successfully she reclaimed her individuality, the more her husband seemed to slide backwards, trying to get her to "change back" (Lerner 1985); she then responded with feelings of anger and hopelessness. The brief affirmation of her sexual attractiveness from another man—from the outside—led her to value her own potential for relationship satisfaction enough to inform her husband that she would not continue in the marriage unless he made efforts to improve it and their sex life.

Mindy's situation is somewhat different; Mindy is not so much dissatisfied inside of her relationship with Jody as wanting to have sex with a man sometimes. Mindy chose to take the path of an affair rather than directly addressing what might distress Jody and prove to be an irreconcilable difference between them.

Of the 2,632 Survey respondents, 1,087 gave *most important reasons* for their *first* affairs. Their responses demonstrated how immeasurably complex such experiences can be. Most women gave more than one reason, and even though we asked for only *up to three reasons*, 20 percent gave four or more reasons. Conceding to this complexity, we counted up to five reasons from each questionnaire; even then, thirty-five women provided more than five reasons and these responses are not included in the table below.

N of ♀♀ = 1,087 **The most important reason(s) for my first affair were:**	**N of ♀♀ marking this reason**
Strong attraction to the other person	776
Not enough closeness in my primary relationship	599
Desire for something different	352
Curiosity	303
The affair provided a way out of an unsatisfactory relationship	270
Not enough sex in my primary relationship	213

To get back at my partner for something done to me	125
To make my partner jealous	36
My partner is/was unable to engage in sex (e.g., due to a medical problem)	21
Trying to get pregnant (I couldn't get pregnant with my partner)	2

These are the numbers. Interviews and marginal comments added more about how women experience the tensions that lead them to affairs. It may be that for some of the women who have had more than one affair, their reasons for affairs after their first one changed and were different than the reasons that led to the first affair.

Attraction Outward Meets Dissatisfaction Within

Of the choices we provided, *strong attraction to the other person* was the most frequently selected characteristic of first affairs. The initial attraction to another may be specifically sexual, but not always. For example, one Survey respondent said she "formed a strong spiritual bond with the other person."

Strong attraction to another is usually not the only factor that leads a woman to have an affair; typically there are a number of inter-acting reasons in which attraction outward meets dissatisfaction within the relationship. The second most-checked reason was *not enough closeness in my primary relationship*. Most women who act on a strong attraction outward do so at a time when they are feeling unfulfilled and not valued within their primary relationship: ♀ Not enough good sex with my spouse; he was unwilling to try to please me; ♀ My partner was an alcoholic; I didn't respect him enough to want to sleep with him; ♀ My partner at the time was not a "nice guy"; the man I cheated with was very nice and attentive.

An affair can be an attempt to meet needs not met by what is otherwise a very satisfying relationship. A woman born in the 1940s, who appended a note to her Survey, had no desire to destroy her marriage. For her, affairs of which her husband is unaware both provided a solution to the absence of sex in her primary relationship and enhanced her regard for her husband and her marriage. She wrote:

"I've been married for over twenty years, the last four of which have been celibate within the marriage. Four months ago I took a lover (a friend for several years) and twice have made love to another long-time male friend. I have no desire to terminate my marriage and in a strange way having my sexual needs met has even made me more certain about not divorcing. I've examined my values and know that my husband gives me other things I desire—financial security, prestige, travel, and belief in my abilities. We respect each other tremendously and are affectionate. Our children are all grown. We have much history and ease with each other and do share the same bed. He travels often in his job and sometimes I go with him."

Feeling Like a Mommy Person

Clearly, if a mutual attraction develops when a woman feels badly treated or neglected by her primary partner, she can feel strongly tempted to have an affair. Having young children can be a compounding factor. **Emily (1919)**, who described her affair earlier, told me that at the time she met the man with whom she had her affair, she was feeling both neglected by her husband and like "*a keeper of children, including my husband.*" **Deborah (1949)**, thirty years younger than Emily, was feeling like a *mommy person* when she met someone new and exciting:

My ex-husband and I had an active and satisfying sex life when we were dating, but after we got married and he went back to school, it dwindled to almost nothing. I would want to make love and he said he had to study. My sexual needs were not being met. I knew he was masturbating regularly in the shower and that didn't help. Over the years I begged him to spend more time with me, to take some trips without the kids. Later, as I grew more desperate, I asked him to go to counseling. I told him repeatedly, *We have to nurture this relationship or we're not going to have one.* It didn't help. I felt totally like a *mommy person*, not a sexual woman. I thought that I wasn't okay. Then I met Yalom; and I was primed. He was exciting, open, and had a beautiful body. I didn't hesitate for a moment. We made love more in one weekend than I had with my husband in the last five years. Sex was terrific . . . expressive, free, comfortable. Meeting him complicated my life and it was very painful when he moved away, but I will always thank him for bringing me back to life sexually and making me realize I could be both a sexual woman and a mother. The affair showed me that I was okay.

A Desire for Something Different

The desire for something different, which seems fueled by her dissatisfaction with the sex in her marriage, is what leads **Anna (1949)** to sometimes wonder about having an affair. She married late in life after many years of dating and passionate sex. The man she married is "a wonderful husband and father." In fact, marrying him allowed her to have, in her late thirties and early forties, the children she wanted. But the lovemaking in her marriage is not like that she remembers from her single life: "I find myself wondering if I could have an affair and handle what I know would be tremendous guilt. I have a lot of years left in my life. Sometimes I miss the sort of spontaneous lusting and fucking that you did at times. That doesn't seem to be something I'm doing in my marriage. It's just much more of a tender, caring, affectionate, and a mothering wifely kind of thing. And I think: *Is that what marriage is? Is that what people evolve to? Or is that a rut we're in?*"

Anna experiences the interplay between her opposing needs and desires: marriage, children, and security in contrast to the exciting spontaneity she remembers from before. We also find the allure of something new or different in the reasons the following women gave for their first affairs: ♀ For fun, escape; ♀ Desire for someone different; ♀ For excitement, danger; ♀ I'm slightly addicted to the illicit and forbidden; ♀ To explore my sexuality.

Trying to Get Pregnant

The urge to conceive can be powerful. In a primary relationship a partner's infertility can be experienced as a very specific deficit. Although *trying to get pregnant (I couldn't get pregnant with my partner)* was a rare reason for a first affair among the women we surveyed— only two women marked it—it can be a powerful motivator for a woman who sees her partner as responsible for her inability to conceive.

In an interview, in which long-standing infertility was a very significant theme, a woman born in the 1950s told me that she had engaged in her first affair just a few months previously. I'm omitting her name to protect her anonymity. Like so many other women, she struggled with strong ambivalence before making the decision to go ahead. In fact, when I interviewed her, she was still experiencing tension between the excitement of being with someone new and the risk of wrecking the familiar life she had. Specific to her situation was the added complication of the possibility of conceiving a much-desired child in circumstances that would have very complex consequences.

At the time of her affair she and her husband had been dealing medically with a diagnosis of "unexplained infertility" for more than six years. She had had repeated injections to produce multiple eggs and had undergone numerous other painful procedures. She said, "Meanwhile, I have a sister who is having one baby after another, and he has a sister who is infertile. So I'm thinking: *It's his fault. I'm ovulating, I'm having eggs. It's got to be him.* So I went through a whole phase where I just wanted sperm. That changed how I perceived my husband; he's very against using someone's sperm other than his. I was trying to figure out how to get someone else's sperm and get pregnant and have him not know that this was how I conceived."

About that time, this woman and a long-time male friend of hers began to experience a strong mutual sexual attraction and she realized that there were other issues to consider besides her desire for another man's sperm: "We did nothing about it for the longest time, because we're both married. But a few months ago we were away at the same conference and, after being in love for over a year, we made love. Several months previously we'd had another opportunity to be together and chose not to have intercourse but did very heavy petting and necking. I was amazed that I could almost orgasm from that; I didn't know that was possible." She described her ambivalence:

"Once I'd been to that point I realized that this was out there and I could have it. Or not have it. I got to a point of *I don't want to be thirty-five-years old—or seventy-years old—and not have had what I know would be a great experience.* So I went for it, and it was incredibly great. We had unprotected sex over a four-day period, theoretically close to an appropriate time, but I didn't become pregnant. My body used to be completely like clockwork, but this whole infertility process with the real intensive medication changed my cycles. I haven't been able to read my body the way I used to. When he said he didn't want to use protection, I thought, *What do I have to lose? If this is the only way that I can have a child, then I'll deal with the consequences later.* It's like your life hangs in the balance. . . . It was probably one of the biggest risks I've ever taken in my life. We haven't had another encounter since then, because we can't work this in and we don't want to train-wreck our respective lives. I never understood before how people had affairs or why they did them. I always thought they were all stupid for doing it. Then I found myself in this situation."

Other Reasons

More than 200 women wrote in reasons for their first affairs that were different from the ones we listed. Some representative examples of these follow, categorized by various themes and arranged in order from the most frequently mentioned to the least. Each group of reasons begins with the oldest respondent and ends with the youngest.

1. **Being away from her primary partner** was the most frequent theme, with forty-one comments. Women of every generation have had to deal with a boyfriend or husband being away because of military service: ♀ My boyfriend was in the Navy during World War II (1921); ♀ My partner was in another country (1942); ♀ My husband was overseas in the military (1961); ♀ I was apart from my husband for seven months; he was at war for our country (1970).

   Work and being away at school are other reasons for separation: ♀ My husband had a traveling job; I was lonely and temptation was easy to give in to then; ♀ I rarely get to see my boyfriend from home, so I started dating someone at my school. I'm going to end my school relationship soon so I can be exclusive with my boyfriend from home again. I feel guilty about my other boyfriend.

2. **Wanting to feel desirable, to feel okay about herself, and/or to get emotional support** was the next most frequent theme. Often a shortcoming in the primary relationship is asserted or implied: ♀ My husband was unable to achieve an erection due to his own problems; he felt I was an incomplete woman (mutilated) because of the hysterectomy; ♀ My husband was abusive and the affair provided me with emotional support and validation; ♀ It helped me through an emotionally tough time; ♀ I was very lonely in my marriage due to an often absent and/or unavailable spouse. He abused alcohol and drugs, and hunted in any spare time; ♀ My partner and I were fighting all the time. My affair was with a close friend who comforted me; I was very sad at the time.

3. **The ending of the primary relationship** was the occasion for some affairs: ♀ The marriage was going bad; ♀ My partner was ready to leave; ♀ I'd been thinking about ending the relationship but wanted to find someone else first; ♀ I hated my husband, but was afraid of divorce; ♀ The primary relationship was clearly ending—the affair was with my current husband; ♀ I was in love with someone else.

4. **Sex with a friend or an old flame** was a theme addressed in other comments; a pre-existing bond was revisited: ♀ I gave up this man to marry, but I always felt I should have had a relationship with him before choosing; ♀ I sought out an earlier serious boyfriend during a period of extreme unhappiness in my marriage. We had spoken of marriage when young; ♀ I really think I was bored. We had just moved to a new city and he had friends at work and I knew no one, so I called an old "flame"; ♀ My ex-boyfriend came to visit; ♀ I loved the other guy—he had been a former lover—we needed each other—no one ever found out.

5. **Drugs and/or alcohol** were mentioned by a few women: ♀ It had to do with alcohol and being depressed and unhappy in my marriage. At the end of my first marriage when I was drinking heavily, I had two isolated incidents of sexual contact with two separate men. One was oral sex, one was failed intercourse. Both times I was very drunk.

6. **A partner having an affair or paying a lot of attention to other women** also was occasionally mentioned: ♀ I had low self-esteem because my husband had been engaging in an affair; ♀ I was married to a man who spent his time gambling and socializing without me so I got love from others; ♀ My husband was in jail; he committed bigamy. I was angry and used sex as a weapon to hurt him. I was seventeen; ♀ I felt hurt by his "open" attitude and actions toward other women; ♀ My partner was having an affair.

7. **Sex with a female partner** was mentioned by eight women, the youngest born in 1965: ♀ My affair partner was female. (This is not uncommon for married women, especially at mid-life); ♀ It was experimenting with another woman (just once); ♀ I did it to change my sexual identity; I'm a lesbian.

8. **Youth or immaturity** was mentioned by a few women: ♀ I was young and stupid; ♀ It was due to my immaturity, dissatisfaction, unwillingness to commit, my lack of clarity; ♀ I was too young (13-17) to be in a serious, monogamous relationship; ♀ I had no real concept of what an affair would do to my partner; I was young.

9. **Other reasons** mentioned included: ♀ My husband was dying and the emotional release was extremely welcome; ♀ To have an orgasm; ♀ I couldn't decide who I liked best.

Affair-Prone Women

Among our interview and Survey respondents is a small group of women who have had affairs in most or all of their relationships. They experience problems with trust and emotional intimacy as well as with sex. Usually these women grew up in an atmosphere where they were aware of someone—often a parent—engaging in affairs. Many also had personally suffered childhood sexual abuse.

As we saw in chapter 4, one aspect of developing one's sexual self is to explore, in early childhood, the belief that *I have the right to love and to be sexual*. When the adults around her overfocus on the sexual components of love, a girl may identify with her sexuality and adopt the belief that *Love is, in reality, sexual need; life is sexuality; sex makes the world go round* as part of her sexual self-image. A Survey respondent **(1940)** whose answer to *number of affairs* was "Many" added this: "My mother was promiscuous, and married multiple times, and I grew up believing this was *normal*. So I imitated her behavior. The term 'affair' hardly has meaning in this context. I drank alcoholically until age forty, and don't even *remember* some of my one-nighters!" Of the reasons for her first affair she wrote: "I had a desperate need for feeling wanted. My sexual life was mostly looking for Mr. Goodbar. My problems are more with trust and emotional intimacy rather than pure sex."

Cecile (1952) was first aware that her father was having an affair when she was six years old. Once she and her sisters reached puberty, he violated their sexual boundaries both verbally and physically by, for example, occasionally touching their genitals through their clothing and "coming on" to their friends. Cecile, who is bisexual, has acted out her feelings sexually most of her life. Most of her partners now are male. She said, "I used to heavily criticize my father for his philandering and then I found my own self not being able to really be true to my partners. And I thought, well, you know, kind of *like father, like daughter*. When I would get emotionally frustrated, I would act out by flirting with someone or being sexual with someone and I would just say, *Well, I guess that's just how I was raised.* And as much as I hated and resisted it, it's what I was brought up with."

Maggie (1965) also was sexualized by others from early childhood and she began engaging in adult-like sexual behavior by age ten (see chapter 4). As is true for all of us, her pattern was shaped by her sexual history. She acknowledges: "I've never been completely faithful, which bothers me; I've always had some extracurricular activity here and there." When she was fourteen, her first intercourse partner informed her "that *the only way that guys would find me attractive was in* *bed.*" She went on: "I can't even begin to tell you how many partners, all male, I had my last year in high school. . . . often guys I brought home from bars. Some were my age, some were much older, in their forties. A lot of it was at my house. My parents were away weekends a lot."

When she was seventeen, Maggie had her first sexual experience with a female partner, a woman who was twenty-three. Since then, most of her partners have been women, including a five-year relationship. Age twenty-seven when I interviewed her, she said, "This past year was the first time since age ten I've been on my own. I'm with someone now, a long-distance relationship which is non-monogamous in theory and somewhat in practice, but I'm not really looking too much."

Maggie recognizes that one reason she has affairs is to feel good about herself: "When I'm in a relationship and feeling I want to sleep with other people, it's because of something in the relationship that's not working. My way of coping with feeling shitty about myself is to go out and have sex with somebody. Not that I always act on it, but that's my old way of feeling better about myself. When I'm feeling undesired or frustrated about life, I want to know that somebody wants me. It's much more that than the actual act."

The Survey respondent "looking for Mr. Goodbar," Cecile, and Maggie are more inclined than most to use sex with outside partners as a way of dealing with personal as well as relationship frustrations and problems. The inclination to seek sex outside of a primary relationship was modeled for them when they were growing up; as adults they carry the inclination within themselves.

Decision Making: Thinking About Having Affairs

Although some women act impulsively, others think long and hard before engaging in an affair. And some women have such strong values against affairs that they wouldn't even consider having one. Some noted on their questionnaires: ♀ An affair is against God's commands; ♀ God believes it is wrong, so I do also; ♀ I would never consider it. It is wrong! [a Catholic *housewife* pregnant with her fifth child]; ♀ I've never had a long-term relationship where this would be an issue. It would be against my morals; ♀ I am more mature and have regard for my values.

Others who have definitely decided not to have an affair wrote of their reasons: ♀ I could speak it now, instead of acting it out; ♀ There would be no long-term value; ♀ I value too highly the pleasure that comes from honesty in a relationship and peace/simplicity in my life; ♀ I didn't want that to be the way to deal with the problems in the relationship. I've thought about having an affair but decided against it.

We have seen that when partners are separated for an extended period of time, by war, work, or school, for example, some women do engage in affairs. Here is how another woman (1950) decided what to do about her sexual needs under similar circumstances. She attached the following note to her questionnaire:

> My husband and I were friends for about two years before becoming romantically involved, then courted four months and were married. I had had a few other intimate relationships, but I was rather inhibited in my sexual experiences. I can truly say my husband awakened my sexuality. . . . Sex just got better and better over the years. He is a gentle, encouraging, exciting lover. Now . . . the present. My husband has been in prison for the last five years. Our sexual relationship consists of brief embraces and kisses at visits and our fantasies and remembrances. Interestingly, we talked about sex a lot more our first year of separation than we do now. But—my favorite fantasy is about the day he gets out! For the past five years I've led a basically celibate life—but temptation and opportunity have been there. About a year ago I kissed a man in a sexual way. And in the past five years I've had half a dozen encounters with another man involving kissing and hand-holding and twice some groping and touching of sexual body parts (he touched mine).
>
> Basically, sex and this single girl was rather inhibited, sex as a married woman was wonderful—I was secure, uninhibited, and loved. Sex now, as long as I remain married, will just have to wait for my husband's return.

Those for whom an affair is a carefully considered choice may spend a period of time seriously questioning their values. This was true of Emily, who in an earlier narrative in this chapter, had to separate her own values from those of her father before she was able to act on her own desires.

Although one might hold a value about having affairs that would help to counterbalance a strong attraction to a potential outside partner, not all affairs are entered into as considered choices. Some women began affairs spontaneously or on impulse. **Cecile**

(1952), whose difficulties with monogamy were noted above, took a workshop after being married only a short time. She told me, "I heavily flirted with the instructor and allowed him to photograph me nude. We ended up being sexual. We didn't have intercourse but I gave him a blow job in the back of his van and I thought, *Oh, my God, what am I doing? I've only been married a year and a half.*"

Reasons for Not Having an Affair

Slightly over half of the women who filled out Survey questionnaires had never had affairs, and 70 percent had either never had an affair or not had one in their current relationship. Here are the reasons they gave (from a list we provided) for not doing so. These were the responses marked by 1,849 women. The question asked for "up to three reasons." So many women marked more than three that we counted up to four; the responses of sixty-two other women who designated more than four are not included.

N of ♀ = 1,849 The most important reason(s) I have *never* had an affair or *not* had an affair in my current relationship are . . .	N of ♀ marking this reason
I've had no desire to do so	1,263
Having an affair is against my values	1,197
An affair would destroy my relationship	915
I don't/didn't believe I could deal with the guilt	408
I am/was afraid of catching a disease	262
I've had no opportunity	137
I am/was afraid of getting caught by my partner	80

Women frequently added comments expanding upon their reasons for not having an affair. The reason checked most frequently for not having an affair was having no desire for one. Some added: ♀ I have affairs with my husband!; ♀ If your needs are being met, you don't need it; ♀ I'm very happy and satisfied. These women feel *fulfilled* in their partnerships.

We saw earlier some of the strong statements women made about sex outside of marriage or committed relationships being **against their values**. Nevertheless, some women gained greater clarity about their values as a result of having had affairs. One wrote: *"Having an affair is against my values* means not *morally,* but psychologically. Currently, I would want and need to talk with my partner about feelings of attraction to someone else before acting on those feelings. I don't necessarily believe affairs are *bad,* but they have been bad—stressful, etc.—*for me* in the past."

There is always the risk that an affair **will destroy the primary relationship**: ♀ He would never forgive or forget—the marriage would be over; ♀ I loved my partner and did not want to destroy the relationship.

Some women avoided affairs both because they feared **getting a sexually transmitted disease** and because they feared transmitting their disease to someone else: ♀ I would not want to expose my current partner unwittingly to an STD; ♀ With AIDS around it is crazy!

Among the reasons offered for avoiding affairs in addition to those the Survey listed were the honoring of **agreements, commitment, and trust**: ♀ We have agreed not to; ♀ We agreed we would be monogamous; ♀ It would break the trust between us and I would never do that.

Some would **end the primary relationship first, or talk over their attraction to another rather than engaging in an affair**: ♀ If I wanted someone other than my husband I would not stay with my husband; ♀ I'd end the relationship first—or declare my intentions; ♀ I would focus on my current relationship and try to understand the urge to go outside of it; ♀ I would break off the current relationship if I was that interested in another person or at least (if I wanted the relationship to continue) talk to my partner about my feelings.

The comments of others essentially reflected the Golden Rule: **"Do unto others as you would have them do unto you"**: ♀ It hurts too much. I wouldn't put the pain on someone else; ♀ I wouldn't want to find out he was having an affair—so I wouldn't want him to have to find out I was—I guess I figure *If I won't he won't;* ♀ I've been cheated on and it sucks; ♀ It's been done to my mother and to me. I can't give that much pain to anyone else.

Several women mentioned **not wanting to hurt their partners**: ♀ I love my husband too much to want to hurt him; ♀ I wouldn't want to hurt the person I'm with because I love him.

A discovered affair can cause tremendous pain and turmoil for both partners. Often, an affair is experienced as a violation of sacred promises, a breach of trust. The partner who did not have the affair can feel so personally violated that a reactive loss of desire for sex may develop. This Survey respondent, a teacher and mother, suspected her husband's pain over her affairs as the major cause of their relationship difficulties: "My husband and I have been having less sex in the last four months than we used to. Although we are both forty-eight, I don't consider age a factor in my case, although it might be in his. I think the reason for the lessening of frequency is ultimately due to my past affairs and my husband's experience of being extremely hurt. . . . Lack of sex and lack of my husband's interest are *major problems*!! Because I do enjoy sex. And not to have sexual relations with an available partner is most disappointing and frustrating. Our relationship is suffering."

Affairs are too complicated, too difficult, and not worth it: ♀ It takes too much energy and focus away from working on an intimate, happy marriage; ♀ They never really work. Or, as one woman put it: ♀ I've had a hard enough time dealing with sex in just *one* relationship.

Others wrote about **how affairs would affect them**: ♀ Cheating would change *me!*; ♀ I like myself too much to do that; ♀ I have to live with myself.

Would You Have an Affair in the Future?

Fewer than 10 percent of 2,108 respondents agreed that they would be open to having an affair in the future. Most women, and most men, too, do not approve of affairs and do not think they will have one. Just as few people go into marriage thinking they will get divorced, so, too, few people enter into a monogamous relationship thinking they will ever engage in sex with anyone other than that partner. Yet just as many people who never thought they would divorce actually do, our data clearly indicate that some women who don't approve of affairs and don't think they will ever have one— actually do. As **Vera (1940)** put it, "Yes, I had affairs many times. I never thought I'd do it, but I did." The woman whose struggles with infertility were described in this chapter is another who had an affair despite strong beliefs about monogamy.

Relationships are complex and difficult, and most go through periods of disappointment. Although having an affair is probably never the only way out of a frustrating situation, stresses and frustrations within a relationship together with an attraction outward can sorely test the strongest of convictions. Sometimes, the crisis of an affair will ultimately strengthen a relationship, but the breach of trust caused by an affair tends to be a very difficult wound to heal. Sometimes there is a moving on and everyone is better off, but often this is not the outcome.

The havoc wreaked by an affair can be very difficult to repair completely. The partner who did not have the affair may find it nearly impossible in the future to fully trust the one who did. Children who are aware of a parent's affair often experience the knowledge as a tremendous burden and also may develop an inclination to have affairs themselves later in their adult lives. Furthermore, a couple who begin their relationship as an affair while each still has another primary partner may have problems with fully trusting each other not to have affairs as solutions to difficulties within the relationship they have formed.

What Does This Mean to You?

Now, if you wish, pick up your notebook and express the thoughts and feelings you're having about affairs or sex outside of, or in addition to committed relationships. Here are some questions you might want to consider after you've done that.

- Where do your values fall on the continuum between monogamy and consensual nonmonogamy?

- Have you ever had an affair? Or contemplated one? If you have, what were your reasons for doing so?

- Did either of your parents have an affair? If so, how has that affected you?

- Is an affair ever justified? If so, under what conditions?

- If you are recalling experiences that you now regret, consider the circumstances, the roles of others, and how you saw your options at the time. Then, sit quietly with your eyes closed and imagine what you could now gently and lovingly tell your younger self that would be healing and would lead to greater self-acceptance

Part 4

Erotic Pleasures

8

Solo Eroticism: Masturbation and Fantasy

How does masturbation fit into your life now? That is one of the questions I asked the women I interviewed. **Lucille (1921),** who was divorced from her second husband and has had "no real sex partner" for about ten years, told me, "I like the intimacy of sex if you're with a man who you really like. I think it can be an absolutely wonderful experience with someone who reciprocates. Now that I'm seventy-one, I don't think a lot about it much anymore, but I still masturbate now and then—about once a week or so ... always to orgasm."

I'm amazed at how many women younger than Lucille—even women now in their forties or fifties—are surprised when I tell them that women Lucille's age and older continue to masturbate. Yet three out of five of the Survey respondents who were age fifty or older (61 percent) had masturbated at least once in the previous month.

We may be inclined to believe that *certainly women in my mother's generation wouldn't do that,* but women have been masturbating in middle and late adulthood—and admitting to it—for ages. This table, which describes the sexual behaviors of unmarried college women is adapted from material in Katharine Bement Davis'

Factors in the Sex Life of Twenty-two Hundred Women, published in 1929. These data were collected in 1921-1923! Only four of the women represented in this table were younger than twenty-five. The oldest woman—born around 1854—was of the same generation as my great-grandmothers, who were born between 1840 and 1857. Women of the average age represented in this table—37.1 years—were born around 1885, the generation of my grandmothers, who were born in 1879 and 1885.

Frequency of Masturbation

Age Group	N of ♀♀ = 928	Never Masturbated	No Longer Masturbate	Currently Masturbate
20-29	184	36%	36%	28%
30-39	434	34%	30%	36%
40-49	205	34%	29%	37%
50-59	82	39%	29%	32%
60-69	23	30%	61%	9%

How Many in the Survey Recently Masturbated?

In this century, the predominant cultural messages about masturbation have changed from a fairly strong proscription against it in the early decades to a strong permission, or even prescription, in the closing decades; but the practice is hardly universal. As a college student (1975) wrote in the margin of her Survey questionnaire in big sprawling capital letters, "*I DON'T DO IT!!*"

Of *all* the women in the Survey, about two out of three (66 percent) had masturbated at least once in the previous month. About three in four had masturbated at least once in the previous three months. The following table summarizes the experiences of the 1,724 Survey respondents who had masturbated in the previous month. Note that the percentages are based on the number of women who had masturbated in the previous month, not on all women in the Survey.

Number of Times Masturbated in Previous Month

Number of times	All ♀♀ N=1,734	% All ♀♀	♀♀ Age ≥ 50 N=336	% ♀♀ Age ≥ 50
1-5 times	1,271	73%	274	82%
6-10 times	295	17%	43	13%
11-20 times	141	8%	14	4%
21-40 times	33	2%	5	1%
60-90 times	2	<1%	0	–

These are the numbers. But how do women *experience* masturbation? How do you experience masturbation? **Alice (1938)** said she masturbates occasionally, "only when Ron is gone. For example, watching a steamy love story on TV might trigger that need. I used to think that was weird but I decided that it's not. I've never lived alone. Aside from Ron, there've always been kids here until last year. Time alone is different. There isn't somebody standing over you, there's nobody else to deal with in the house."

Some women told me that in addition to masturbating when alone, they sometimes will stimulate themselves with their partners involved. **Pat (1945)** masturbates when she has intercourse and doesn't come to orgasm. "If I do it lying next to George, he'll usually stimulate my breasts or hold me," she said. For **Cindi (1952)**, "It's often when I'm home alone. The frequency varies with the time of the month, typically it's about twice a week in addition to lovemaking. Sometimes if I'm having an outbreak of herpes or Mark's not interested, I will use the vibrator while he is in bed next to me, cuddling, doing whatever. That's nice, too."

Melanie (1970) masturbates about once a week: "usually because I get aroused by something I see in a movie or something I read. Or I'll just be sitting there fantasizing or, more often, thinking about my partner and what we do. That gets me all excited. I have a long-distance relationship, and my boyfriend encourages me to do it. He bought me a vibrator. I'd never even seen one before, but I was wildly curious. I was so embarrassed the first time he used it on me, I wouldn't even look at it. But I really liked it. Normally, I take all my clothes off and get in bed. I don't like absolute quiet, so I have the TV on with the volume low. Usually I start by touching my breasts ... running my hands down my stomach ... and then I'll use the vibrator on my clitoris, but not as a substitute penis. Occasionally, I use my hand, but that takes longer. My boyfriend keeps warning me—he's all scientific about this—*I've heard that once you do it too much with a vibrator, you can't get an orgasm the other way.*"

Vibrators

Is Melanie's boyfriend right? Can a vibrator make other paths to orgasm impossible? Because it can be so quick and effective in creating orgasm, a vibrator can be seductive. One could easily get in the habit of going for the quick rush and never go through a process of learning to pay attention to subtle sensations and shifts in arousal that could themselves be interesting and could create other paths to orgasm. That is not, however, the only way to include a vibrator in erotic pleasuring. A vibrator can be used to create some of those interesting subtle sensations and shifts in arousal.

For an expert's guide to the pleasure potential of vibrators, I recommend Betty Dodson's *Sex for One. The Joy of Selfloving* (1987). (See also www.bettydodson.com.) Dodson's book contains valuable information on how to use vibrators effectively and is filled with permission for those who experience guilt when contemplating self-pleasuring. Dodson says, "Instead of providing 'a quick rush,' on the contrary, the correct use of a vibrator will allow a woman to enjoy one- and two-hour sessions of self-loving with a series of orgasms" (personal communication 1999). With respect to women who have never or rarely experienced orgasm, Dodson notes: "If a woman has had little or no experience with childhood or adult masturbation, she has learned to say no to sexual feelings. For these women an electric vibrator provides strong, steady stimulation that can make up for the years of sensory deprivation" (1987, p. 93). A vibrator can be a wonderful solution, too, for women who begin having orgasmic difficulties after menopause and for anyone who wants to wake up and enhance a sex life that's become less exciting than it once was. Dodson told me that Melanie's boyfriend is inferring "that there is a 'right way' to orgasm." Her advice: "Use the vibrator all she wants. What he's really saying is he might no longer be the source of her orgasm. Many women have successfully incorporated vibrator use in partner sex with a secure male or female partner" (personal communication 1999).

Still, vibrators aren't for everyone. Some find a vibrator too mechanical or intense and prefer a hand and lubricated fingers—or something like a feather or a piece of silk or fur—when they want to build to a plateau of arousal and stay there, playing with subtle changes in sensations and energy. Differences in sexual experiences are like differences in music. A rock concert and a performance of a Mozart concerto are both music; both are enjoyed by many people. But they are dramatically different. We know that *too much* rock music that is *too loud* literally can damage and deafen the ears, making some of the subtle nuances of Mozart no longer perceptible. But this is not a necessary outcome of listening to rock; it is overdoing it—the problem is too much volume. And, at times, a vibrator is "played" in a Mozart style or a hand used for "rock and roll."

Sara (1949), whom we've met in other chapters (her abuse and early sexualization by her father were described in chapter 4), is into rock 'n' roll: "I was a late bloomer. I really didn't start masturbating until I was twenty-two. I had a new boyfriend, a very good lover, and the first night we made love, I had five orgasms. That had never happened to me before. And then he took me to an adult bookstore, and there I discovered vibrators. My sexuality just really blossomed after that. I got into using three hand-held vibrators, the seven-inch ones that in the magazine ads show the woman holding one to her face—I always thought that was funny. I have one in my asshole, one in my cunt, and one on my clitoris. With two inside your body, the reverberations bounce off each other so that the rhythm gets uneven. It's like: buh' buh-buh-buh-buh-buh, buh' buh-buh-buh-buh, buh' buh-buh-buh. And it's almost like somebody fucking you. 'Cause it's just a little off, to where it's very hot." Now, that's definitely rock 'n' roll!

Emily (1919) (whom we also met in chapter 4; she played on the bed with her father on Sunday mornings when she was a little girl) prefers Mozart: "Vibrators never worked for me. They numb me. My genitals are so sensitive that that rhythm was just far too fast." **Connie (1956)** prefers Mozart, too: "I have a vibrator, but it doesn't do anything for me. I prefer the finger, thank you very much."

Often getting a vibrator is an event, sometimes an event involving someone else. For Sara, in the narrative above, that someone else was a boyfriend. Others told of going vibrator shopping with a woman friend or of receiving a vibrator as a gift. **Teresa (1946)** said, "When I was still married a good friend and I secretly bought vibrators and encouraged one another to use them . . . my first experience with vibrators. That was really fun. I still use mine." A woman friend gave **Barb (1955)** a vibrator a few years ago: "I've used it a couple of times, but I don't need that to orgasm. As long as I have a man with an erection, I just don't feel I need the vibrator. I haven't tried any other toys."

There are other women who, like Barb, tried a vibrator and either didn't like it or didn't continue to use it. A woman friend gave **Madeline (1915)** a vibrator years ago. She explained, "I'm kind of a mothering person for her, and I think she's the daughter that I didn't have. She was always kidding me about not having sex. And so at one point she said, *I'm going to get you a vibrator.* And I said, *Be my guest! I guess I'll try it. I don't know.* Maybe I blushed. So she did. And I tried it and it was, *Ennhh.* But then I left it in the drawer and some time later when I got it out and tried to use it again, it had rusted or something and didn't work. So I threw it away."

Again we see that tension between wanting to explore some new aspect of sexuality and embarrassment or shame. Madeline is curious and willing to explore something new, but she also blushes and feels somewhat inhibited. So do Doris and Donna in the following examples. No matter our age, there may still be some of that sense that *someone is watching* or *someone is going to find out!* **Doris (1930)**, who hasn't used a vibrator, said, "I told this friend of mine: *I would like to get one of those, but I'm always afraid I'll die and my kids'll find it and say, 'Mother was a dirty old lady.'* And my friend said, *Well, if you're dead, what's the difference?* But I haven't had the nerve to. But I've thought of getting a vibrator. I think it would be great." **Donna (1949)** started experimenting with masturbating and tried a vibrator during a three-year celibate period: "The vibrator worked with a degree of success, I guess. But according to my morals it didn't seem like it was something I should do all the time and it wasn't necessary. Sex toys aren't a big part of my life."

Some women who have never tried vibrators or sex toys aren't planning to start. **Maria (1965)** said, "I'm not into foreign objects like vibrators. I like the warmth of the body, the feel of the skin." **Alicia (1967)** thought about a vibrator after a friend told her last year, *"You should use one of these things; they're a great invention."* She described her reticence: "Maybe it's a combination of I didn't want anybody to find it if I had it; I didn't want to buy it; I didn't want to order it from mail order; and also I just didn't really feel like I needed one."

Deborah (1949) found her way to a different outcome—to greater self-acceptance for her practice of masturbating with a vibrator, a practice she still continues, both alone and in the presence of her partner. Her parents had a massage chair with a hand vibrator attachment: "I was at their house when I was twenty or so and wondering what it would feel like to try masturbating with it. I was really surprised to discover I could have orgasms very quickly. I liked it, but I felt guilty about it, even dirty. Then I experimented to see if I could come again. I did ... my first ever multiple orgasms. My thinking began to change and the guilt began to fade. *Oh, the hell with guilt, I thought, this feels great! I don't care. Who decides masturbation can be bad if it feels this good?* I didn't stay hung up or feeling guilty long."

The emotion of guilt is often a message from one's inner self to consider: *I am breaking (or about to break) a rule. Where did this rule come from? At the place I am now in my life, is it still appropriate for* me *to follow this rule?* In a way Deborah did this. Sometimes we can use this question-and-answer process to fool ourselves into doing something that's not in our best interest. At other times, the process allows us to break out of old patterns that no longer fit our age and circumstances; this is what seemed to happen for Deborah.

Why Do Women Masturbate?

The Survey included a list of reasons a woman might masturbate; each respondent marked all answers that applied to her. The results are in the following table, where they are ranked from the most often to the least often selected. (Note that the percentages are based on the 1,866 women who had masturbated in the previous three months, not on all women who participated in the Survey. Of all the 2,226 women who responded to this question, 16 percent had *not* intentionally stimulated their genitals when alone in the previous three months; of those who were age fifty or older, 24 percent had *not* done so.)

In the last three months, I intentionally stimulated my genitals when alone ...	All ♀♀ N=1,866	% All	♀♀ Age ≥ 50 N=337	% Age ≥ 50
Because self-stimulation feels good	1582	85%	284	84%
Because I felt a physical urge to do so	1,531	82%	286	85%
To have one or more orgasms	1,195	64%	237	70%
Because a partner wasn't available right then	894	48%	155	46%
To relax	737	39%	113	34%

To help me sleep	595	32%	102	30%
To comfort myself	567	30%	99	29%
Because I was lonely	299	16%	50	15%
To feel more finished/relieve frustration after partner sex	283	15%	45	13%
Because I was bored	200	11%	21	6%
To relieve menstrual cramps	177	9%	8	2%
I have *not* intentionally stimulated my genitals when alone in the last three months	360		109	

In response to our invitation to write in their "Other" reasons not on our list, women offered many more reasons for masturbating in the previous three months. We might describe some of the reasons from women age fifty and older as a version of *use it or lose it.* "Because I'm getting old and I want to keep the engine running," said one respondent (1930). Others mentioned a husband not interested, masturbating to help with breathing during a spell of light asthma, procrastination with respect to something else, and choosing not to have a sexual partner at this time, but still feeling strongly sexual. A woman born in 1917 masturbates "because I am slow to arouse and intercourse isn't always satisfying."

"Other" reasons given by women younger than age fifty included "to engage in sexual fantasy and have orgasm." One likes to "sit outside and pretend I'm being watched." Another masturbates to keep awake when she gets tired while driving. Women of all ages mentioned that reading sometimes leads to masturbation: "I'm reading a great sexuality book, *Pleasures: Women Write Erotica* [Barbach 1984]," wrote one. Some among the youngest women in the Survey said that they masturbate "as a study break," "out of curiosity," because "it's good exercise," and as "foreplay." A young woman who wrote "I'm a *dancer, stripper,*" masturbates "because it gets me feeling sexy for work and I make better tips."

Many women wrote comments in response to the reasons listed in the Survey:

1. **Because self-stimulation feels good:** ♀ It's fun; ♀ It's so intense; ♀ I love myself; ♀ For self-love and affirmation; ♀ To

affirm the beauty of my body; ♀ Why not? Masturbation is part of my sexuality.

2. **Because I felt a physical urge to do so:** ♀ I feel addicted to it; ♀ I masturbate when I am tense or horny—it is a physical release; ♀ I was horny!; ♀ I felt compelled to; ♀ I *mentally* felt the urge to do so; ♀ I just felt like it.

3. **To have one or more orgasms:** ♀ We have great sex and a lot of it, but I get frustrated that orgasm doesn't always come; I know what spot works; ♀ I don't have orgasms with my partner; ♀ To work with my partner after intercourse or during so I can achieve orgasm; ♀ I have never had orgasm with my current partner during intercourse; ♀ I can only orgasm using a vibrator, and masturbate quickly and frequently.

Masturbation is also a way to learn about orgasm and one's sexual responsiveness; both of these women were born in 1973 and so were among the youngest *Survey* respondents: ♀ Because I'm trying to become good enough at it to achieve orgasm; ♀ To learn about my body and what feels best. One woman lamented, however, ♀ Masturbation doesn't usually end in orgasm for me!!

4. **Because a partner wasn't available right then; because I was lonely:** ♀ I have no partner at this point; ♀ I wanted sex and couldn't get it; ♀ My boyfriend encourages it when he's gone; I fantasize about my boyfriend or ex-husband performing oral sex with me; ♀ Because my husband hasn't been making love to me frequently; ♀ Masturbation gives me an opportunity to "keep the home fires burning" but I often miss my partner so much afterwards that it spoils the pleasure; ♀ To relieve physical longing for someone I'm attracted to; ♀ Because my partner and I sleep different hours due to our work schedules; ♀ Because my partner's frequency preference doesn't match my own.

Some women masturbate even when a partner is available: ♀ . . . to avoid sex with my partner; ♀ . . . because I'm too tired for "partner" sex.

5. **To relax; to help me sleep; to comfort myself; because I was bored:** ♀ I was frustrated and upset about something; ♀ I had too much to drink; ♀ I was depressed; ♀ To relieve migraine headaches and relieve anxiety; ♀ To avoid thinking; ♀ Pro-

crastination!; ♀ Because I had a stomachache and head- ache, gas; ♀ Because of itching (I had a vaginal condition).

Not all women find masturbation relaxing or comforting. Some of their comments went like this: ♀ I suffered a lot of internal judgment about it before I was married, but not since; ♀ I may start out to comfort myself but it is soon the opposite, an upset; ♀ Afterwards I feel unsatisfied, unfulfilled, empty; ♀ I really haven't experienced total satisfaction with masturbation; I'm just now beginning to experiment; ♀ I am consumed with thoughts of sex while I'm doing it, then feel guilty later; ♀ During masturbation I feel turned on and "hot and bothered," kinky. After, I feel relieved, relaxed, but also empty and almost pathetic.

6. **To feel more finished/relieve frustration after partner sex:** ♀ My husband is impotent; ♀ Sex is no longer fulfilling with my partner, but we're trying to work it out; ♀ I came home from a date with a fellow that sexually stimulated me.

7. **To relieve menstrual cramps:** ♀ To bring on a period; ♀ At ovulation and menstruation because of heightened sensitivity; ♀ Because I have a physical urge before or right after menstruation. Not all women find masturbation helpful for menstrual cramps. One noted: ♀ Actually, masturbation *gives* me *heavier* menstrual cramps.

Orgasms in Masturbation

Do women reach orgasm more easily by themselves than with a partner? This is what some sexologists claim. There is a way in which this makes sense. Orgasm can be more complicated to create with a partner than by yourself, because being with a partner involves the complexities of couple interaction and what may be the different needs and desires of two people. When you are alone, stimulating yourself, it is easy to make subtle changes in stimulation. Your hand is not going to get its feelings hurt or think you are criticizing it when you want it to change what it is doing and try something else. Neither is your hand or vibrator likely to finish before you want it to. As **Penny (1946)**, who has only once had an orgasm in partner sex, describes her experience, "I have no trouble having orgasm with a vibrator. I've never gotten that kind of satisfaction with a man. I can even have multiple orgasms with the vibrator. With the vibrator, I don't feel I have to do anything to make it happen. I just find its place and that's it; it happens very quickly, usually in a minute or two."

One hundred and sixty women, 4 percent of *all* Survey respondents, said that they reach orgasm alone but not with a partner. Other women find, however, that interaction with a compatible, involved partner provides more varied and richer stimulation to orgasm than their own hand or a vibrator. There are body scents and tastes, visual impressions, mutual sounds, and shared emotions and images. There are also the rhythms created by the giving and receiving of touch, and the mutual movement and building of sexual energy. Obviously, these mutuality factors are not present when creating the release of orgasm alone. One woman noted that for her it's "more enjoyable" with a partner, "even though reaching orgasm isn't any easier!"

Other respondents wrote that the ease with which they reach orgasm depends on the partner: ♀ Now, I reach orgasm more easily by myself. My second husband has impotence. With my first husband, orgasm was easy, natural; I was married to him for twenty-four years; ♀ If it's *a* partner, it's easier by myself; if it's *my present* partner, it's definitely not. Seventy percent of the Survey respondents agreed that they generally have or had more enjoyable orgasms with their most satisfying sexual partner than by themselves.

Masturbation Fantasies

What is the nature of your solo sexual fantasies? Over half of the women who stimulate themselves for pleasure when alone say that they *usually* fantasize when they masturbate. But the use and the themes of masturbation fantasies are aspects of women's sexuality in which I found tremendous variety. **Cindi (1952)** seeks fantasy material and finds fantasies crucial. She said, "I usually get out the fantasies book and take it into the bedroom, plug the vibrator in. It's pretty quick, five to ten minutes. For me, fantasies are crucial to orgasm in masturbation." In contrast, **Lori (1969)** said, "During masturbation, I concentrate a lot on exactly what I'm feeling. I spend a lot of time trying to get to know myself. And sometimes there's a fantasy about my partner watching or my partner masturbating me. Ethereal kind of."

There are many themes in masturbation fantasies. They may, for example, be hot or naughty and involve strangers or unspecified partners. **Anna (1949)** says that "One of my typical masturbation fantasies is *the kinky waitress*, servicing a table of men, getting involved with somebody on the table, wearing a sleazy outfit. Most of my fantasies are about hot, lusty strangers rather than about anybody I know." **Ronni's (1955)** fantasies have often been "about some man coming in and taking me, not in a violent sense but in an aroused, passionate *I-want-you* sense."

Some are better described as images of a current partner than as fantasies that contain a story line. **Deborah (1949)** observes, "It's interesting to me that whenever I masturbate, I fantasize about the two of us, not someone else." And **Tracy (1971)** notes, "I don't know if I'd call them fantasies. When I masturbate, I tend to think of the person that I'm with, sort of imagining him with me."

Some fantasies are about someone who is known but who is not an actual partner. **Lou Ann (1944)** says, "When I'm masturbating I usually have fantasies of intercourse or other sexual play with particular people. They could be people I've been with or other people. But I haven't conjured up Mr. Right, so it's actual people."

Another common fantasy theme is having sex with someone real who is helpful—and perhaps forbidden—a doctor, teacher, attorney, repairman, auto mechanic, and the like. For **Susan (1958)**, it's her therapist: "When I stimulate myself, I actually have a fantasy about my therapist quite a bit, because he's fairly young and just really intelligent and handsome. And it's hard, because he's younger than my husband. He's like early forties. You know, it's that transference thing where you just fall in love with your therapist. That's about the only male fantasy I have."

And many, many fantasies are about behavior we can't imagine that we would ever really do or that doesn't even make sense in real life. **Barb (1955)** has fantasies she "wouldn't necessarily even want to carry out." She explained: "I have fantasies sometimes about making love with two or three men. Intellectually, I think that's disgusting. I would feel used, like they're just taking advantage of me. But that's a potentially exciting fantasy. I've had fantasies about dogs doing me, licking, although I'd never do anything like that, and I'm terribly allergic to animals. But dogs look like they know how to use their tongues ... and giraffes with their fifteen-inch tongues; I thought about that the last time I went to the zoo. Another masturbation fantasy is being with young men, like seventeen, eighteen. Intellectually I don't want to teach anybody so that goes back to *I wouldn't do that*. Plus, I think it would be not right, unfair, to initiate a young man that way; they have to find their own way; but sometimes I think about the virility of young men. I mean a guy gets hard like *that*! And you can just touch them and *Boing!* they come. That's pretty exciting."

Fantasy images also can be elicited as a way of letting ourselves experience something that we wouldn't usually let ourselves do. **Doris (1930)** uses her fantasies as a way to let herself be sexually aroused and out of control: "During self-stimulation my fantasies are with a man at the rear, not anal penetration, but where I'm not seeing him. I don't have to cope with this person in front of me that I might have to look at or him seeing how I'm reacting. I'm a very controlled person. And I think that sex means out of control. It's hard for me to be out of control. I've let myself go out of control in masturbation, but not with a partner."

Through fantasy, Doris has found access to a part of her sexual self that she enjoys but which isn't yet accessible when she is with a partner. For **Gloria (1944)** attempting to use fantasy has an opposite effect—another example of the great variability in the sexualities of women. If she *tries* to have a fantasy, she becomes so self-conscious that she neither enjoys what is happening nor is she able to lose herself to being out of control: "If I consciously try to engage in fantasy, it just doesn't work for me. But sometimes when I least expect it, I have an erotic fantasy. But it doesn't lead to anything because I'm so conscious of it. I fondle myself but I just don't enjoy it. I need a partner! Actually, I wish I knew how to stimulate myself. I guess I'm not patient enough. I even tried a vibrator a few times. It felt good but I didn't reach orgasm."

Variations

How variable are your masturbation fantasies? Some women not only have differences with respect to each other, they also have quite varied experiences themselves from time to time when they masturbate. **Janet (1955)** said, "Without fantasies, masturbation wouldn't be any fun." She described a range of fantasy images that included her new relationship with a man, ". . . sex with women . . . sex with more than one person, men and women combined." Also, "just plain old daytime sexual fantasies usually having to do with some guy who has just walked by," and, occasionally in the past, "angry ones . . . quasi-rape situations where I was being forced and being thrown down and being told what to do."

Karen (1957) used to use a lot of fantasy images to masturbate. She had developed a "repertoire of standard fantasy images that would expedite orgasm based on the *Penthouse* letters she read: "It's like this little recipe box of standard images . . . standard themes . . . like images of women having sex with animals, first sexual experiences. One is sort of a first sexual experience for teenagers where there is a father and stepmother and they decide to talk about sex with their teenagers, sort of with the guise of wanting to give their kids information on how to give pleasure, and then they end up demonstrating, and then they end up with the teenagers sort of getting into sex . . . the boys with the stepmother. So in this scenario there is some crossing of taboos, but not totally."

Using Erotica with a Partner

Another aspect of fantasy is the use of erotica or videos with a partner. Only a few of the interviewed women specifically mentioned using erotica to enhance self-pleasuring. For **Cindi (1952)** it was "some of the fantasies in Nancy Friday's books, *My Secret Garden* and *Forbidden Flowers* [1973, 1975]." **Marcy (1967)** has books on erotica, most written by women, "like by Anais Nin, and *Pleasures* [Barbach 1984] and *Herotica* [Bright and Blank 1991]." **Andrea (1972)** usually masturbates only when she's reading: "I read a lot of books. And the way I read books it's like a movie right in my head. So I'm going through sexual scenes, and it's just like watching a movie in a theater where you're watching two people have sort of sex. During the school year this happens rarely. I try not to read then because I tend to not be able to put the book down. So then it's mostly just those little teeny flashes, where something somebody says triggers some quick image."

The fantasy dimension of our sexuality is also expressed with great variability in partner sex. You will find a discussion and examples of fantasies while with a partner in chapter 13.

We indulge in pleasurable self-stimulation for a multitude of reasons. Some of us masturbate because self-stimulation feels good, we feel an urge to do so, to have orgasms, or because no partner is available. Masturbation can be relaxing, a way to self-comfort, and help us sleep. For some of us, it is a readily available antidote for loneliness and boredom and a solution to frustration when a partner finishes before we want to; for others, it can lead to loneliness or frustration; and, as one woman told us, it's a way "to keep the engine running" as we get older and want to *use it, not lose it.*

What Does This Mean to You?

Now, if you wish, pick up your notebook and express the thoughts and feelings you're having about your fantasies and masturbation. Here are some questions you might want to consider after you've done that.

- Are you satisfied with the role of masturbation in your life? If not, what changes would you like to make? What are some first steps toward implementing those changes?

- Are you satisfied with the role of fantasy in your life? If not, what changes would you like to make? How might you begin?

- If you are recalling experiences that you now regret, consider the circumstances, the roles of others, and how you saw your options at the time. Then, sit quietly with your eyes closed and imagine what you could now gently and lovingly tell your younger self that would be healing and lead to greater self-acceptance.

9

Sexual Satisfaction and Partnered Sex

What qualities make sex pleasurable and satisfying for you? Have you at some time in your life had at least one partner with whom you've had what you considered to be really fantastic sex? Most of the women responding to the Survey—about 80 percent—said that they had such a partner. But what is fantastic sex? What makes great sex special?

Satisfying Sex and Associated Feelings

Recall for a moment your own most satisfying sexual experience with a partner. (If you have not yet had satisfying partner sex, imagine what you think it would be like.) What are five feelings in addition to "satisfied" you felt—or imagine you might feel—during great sex—or right afterwards? Does your list include any of these words: *loved, passionate, happy, wonderful, aroused, erotic, pleasured, ecstasy, sensual,* and *loving*? These were the ten words selected most often by the Survey respondents from the list of fifty-seven choices we provided. The next six words were *excited, desirable, playful, peaceful, romantic,* and *desired*. Most amazing, however, was the variability in the combinations of descriptive words women selected from the list. Every word was marked at least twice, and the most selected word on the list, *loved*, though it was selected most frequently, still was marked by fewer than half of those who answered the question.

With respect to feelings experienced most often during and immediately after sex with a current or most recent partner, some words changed across age groups. For example, *excited* dropped from 70 percent of women ages 20 to 29 to 53 percent of women aged 60 to 69, and *merged* increased from 26 percent at ages 20 to 29 to 41 percent for women between the ages of 60 to 69.

These differences are indications that how we experience and express our sexuality changes as we move through our lives. In our sixties, even if we replace some of the hormones we no longer produce ourselves, we don't have the strong hormonal support for lush arousal and sexual excitement most women have in their twenties. A woman in her sixties, however, who has a loving sexual partner, is more likely to be in a stable ongoing relationship in which she has had more time and opportunities than a younger woman to explore and become skilled in the transpersonal and perhaps spiritual aspects of sexual expression.

Women who did not experience sex with their current or most recent partner as pleasurable and satisfying were likely to have included some of the following cluster of feelings we found associated with sexual dissatisfaction: *bored, dissatisfied, disappointed, lonely, sad*, and *frustrated*. The contrasting cluster associated with satisfaction was *passionate, sensual, excited,* and *sexy*.

Satisfying Sex in Ongoing Relationships

If you have ever had *satisfying* sex with a partner within an ongoing relationship, consider the most recent period in your life when that was true for you. If you have never had satisfying partner sex, imagine now what that would be like.

What follows is a question from the Survey. As you answer it, you probably will find that some of the items on the list do not match your experience. For example, if your most satisfying sex was with a woman, *being aware that I might become pregnant*—among others— would not apply to you. Consider the items that apply to your own experience and disregard the rest. In the Survey, women who had never have had *satisfying* sex with a partner did not answer this question. However, if you have never had satisfying partner sex, go ahead and answer it as you imagine what satisfying sex would be like.

Factors affecting sexual satisfaction within a relationship. In this relationship that I am considering or imagining, the following were **usually** or **always** present in my **most satisfying experiences** with my partner (Mark all that apply):

Before Sex

_____ Feeling close to my partner before sex

_____ Arguing before having sex

_____ Having an alcoholic drink before sex

_____ Using marijuana or another recreational drug before (or during) sex

Partner and Situation

_____ Feeling loved

_____ Feeling safe in the relationship

_____ Knowing we could take as much time as we wanted

_____ Knowing there was no risk of getting or transmitting a disease

_____ Knowing there was no risk of getting pregnant

_____ Being aware that I might become pregnant

_____ Knowing my partner would give me the physical stimulation I needed

Behaviors and Feelings During Sex

_____ Talking with my partner during sex about what we were doing

_____ Talking about or acting out a shared drama or fantasy

_____ Focusing on a stimulating fantasy of my own

_____ Feeling really attuned with my partner during sex

_____ No pressure from my partner for me to have an orgasm

_____ No pressure from myself to have an orgasm

_____ My partner was accepting of my desires, preferences, and responses

_____ My partner got and maintained an erection

_____ My partner did not ejaculate quickly

Stimulation

_____ Extended stimulation of other kinds before intercourse

_____ Breast stimulation

_____ Manual stimulation of my genitals

_____ Oral stimulation of my genitals

_____ Using a vibrator

_____ Using a dildo

_____ Anal stimulation

_____ Having intercourse

_____ Steady, reliable stimulation that continued through orgasm

Outcomes

_____ One or more orgasms

_____ Simultaneous orgasm with my partner

_____ Knowing that I gave my partner a wonderful experience

_____ Emotional closeness after sexual activity

Other

_____ (Please specify): _____

Age of most satisfying sexual experiences with a partner. What was your age (or were your ages) in the period of your life you have been considering as you answered the above question?

Closeness, Love, Acceptance, and Safety

The Survey demonstrated what many of us already intuitively know:

- Most women associate sexual satisfaction in an ongoing relationship with closeness, love, acceptance, and safety.

- For most women, sexual satisfaction is an emotional experience closely linked to feeling attuned and connected with a sensitive partner.

Overall, the top three items associated with satisfying sex by the women in the Survey were _feeling close to my partner before sex; emotional closeness after sexual activity;_ and _feeling loved._

Others in the top ten included *one or more orgasms; feeling safe in the relationship; knowing my partner is accepting of my desires, preferences, and responses;* and *knowing I gave my partner a wonderful experience.*

Also selected by a majority were *knowing that my partner will provide the physical stimulation I need* and *feeling really attuned with my partner during sex.*

Closeness, love, acceptance, and safety were mentioned frequently in the interviews as important dimensions of sexual satisfaction. **Emily (1919)** finds the best kind of sex in a love situation: "I'm not sure that men always understand that. Love creates an ongoing quality of closeness. Without love it's like *here today and gone tomorrow.*"

Victoria (1946) finds that, "There's a difference with maturity. It's more an expression of love and caring for the other person than sexual gratification. It's a mature coming together based on total commitment to each other. There's no underlying fear, it's total safety. I won't be left or abandoned. No matter how long it takes me to have an orgasm, he will be there. And he'll be there beyond the orgasm and the sex. It's so comfortable and good."

When **Barb (1955)** has sex, her first objective is to please her partner, "but," she said: "I need to know that he would please me. If he shows no interest in that, then that's probably the last time I'd be sleeping with him." **Susan (1958)** likes "all the passion and the hotness of sex to be there along with just how calm and steady and sweet it can be when it's combined with an emotional attachment in a committed relationship—being able to go from one to the other and have both at once." **Kirsten (1970)** likes "the feeling of being close to him, both of us having a good time. I just feel intensely in love at that point. He doesn't have to do anything especially. At the best times, both of you have a really good feeling afterward."

Satisfying Sex in Not-So-Satisfying Relationships

I don't want to leave the wrong impression. The Survey question addressed satisfying sex in an ongoing relationship but, sometimes, women's most satisfying sexual experiences don't occur in the most stable or satisfying relationships, and some women have had their most satisfying sex with partners with whom they didn't feel especially close.

Hilda (1915) described a man she was with for a number of years: "He was just insatiable. He could go for five times in a row! I would be worn out to a frazzle. I'd say, *No more!* and he'd say, *Oh yes.*

Yes you can. He was very handsome . . . had a body like a Greek god. It was just very exciting. But he was no good as a person. He was single, a lot younger than me; he drank a lot, didn't often want to work . . . *not marriage material.* But a great lover!"

In the Survey margins, women noted: ♀ I've had some of my best orgasms with the worst partners; ♀ The relationship had multiple problems but the sexual chemistry was present throughout, even after divorce. I still miss the sex occasionally, but not the relationship. Strange!; ♀ The best sex I've ever had was with a guy I didn't get along with very well. But for the two years we were together, the sex was *great!*

A college student (1970) wrote: "Before this relationship (that began three months ago), which is emotionally satisfying with a loving, soothing sexuality, I was in an intense, erotic love-like, pleasure-pain relationship for four years. They are very different. Sexually, the four year relationship was more intensely satisfying, but my current relationship is also satisfying. It is hard for me to let go of the pain-pleasure I became accustomed and attached to, but I believe that [the former relationship] was an unhealthy sexuality that I need to replace with a loving companion."

Sexual Activity and Alcohol and Drugs

When the conditions are right, alcohol and some drugs can enhance sexual pleasure. Alcohol is very tricky, because its effects depend on how much you drink. Just enough alcohol can release inhibitions and enhance pleasurable sensations, but a little too much may dampen your sexual responses or make you teary or angry; it can even put you right to sleep.

About 14 percent and 6 percent of survey participants reported that alcohol and recreational drugs, respectively, were usually or always part of their most satisfying sexual experiences; some others noted that these were involved *sometimes* or *occasionally*; a few respondents indicated that they had used one or both in the past, but did no longer. One respondent noted: *We quit using and sex went stale.*

If you've never or rarely had sex without alcohol or some other kind of drug, and then you give up the alcohol or drug, you are likely to find that you have to learn new ways to get into the feelings and altered state of having great sex. As **Anna (1949)** illustrates, it may seem as if you have to learn how to have sex all over again: "In college I did almost all my lovemaking stoned or with a few drinks. I miss the feeling, the mushy flow of lovemaking when you're slightly high on grass; I feel so much freer and looser when I'm stoned. Unfortunately my husband won't smoke; he's not that kind of person. It's been a real adjustment for me."

If you use alcohol and/or other recreational drugs during sex, you might want to think about whether using these mind-body altering chemicals enhances or detracts from your sexual experiences. If it detracts, consider what changes you would like to make and perhaps talk about them with your partner or someone else close to you.

Arguing Before Sex

Arguing before sex was the least selected item from the Survey list of possible components of satisfying sex. This may be because an argument can generate feelings of distance and insecurity rather than the feelings of closeness and safety many women associate with sexual satisfaction. As **Susan (1958)** reported, "Fighting doesn't make me interested in having sex like it does for some people. I like getting to a good place emotionally where we're not separate, where we're really together, there's a good flow and I feel open enough to have sex." However, *Arguing before sex* was usually a part of the most satisfying sexual experiences of 3 percent of the women who responded to this question.

Many people assume that being angry at your partner means you shouldn't or can't have sex, but that's not necessarily the case. Nevertheless, it's *not* a good idea to use sex time after time as a way to avoid discussing and resolving your problems. It can enhance your relationship to use sexual reconciliation as a way to create loving feelings through which you can listen to each other's point of view and discuss change. It is not *always* necessary to work out your issues first. Having sex can be a wonderful way to kiss and make up.

In fact, many of the same physical responses aroused by sex are aroused by anger (Kinsey, Pomeroy, Martin, et al., 1953). When there is reconciliation, an argument can lead to an intense sexual experience and the arousal of the argument can become converted into sexual passion. There is an interesting relationship between sexual feelings and anger. Sexual feelings are blocked by holding on to resentments and holding in anger; sexual feelings can be released by talking out resentments and asserting what you feel and want. Some couples do use friendly—or not so friendly—arguments to fuel their sexual arousal. One woman noted that for her: "Arguing before sex is actually fun."

Orgasm

For the women we surveyed, orgasm is important for sexual satisfaction, but it is not essential for all women. *Emotional closeness after sexual activity* was marked almost as often as the most frequently included item, *feeling close to my partner before sex.* And both were chosen more often than having one or more orgasms.

Although a majority did associate orgasm with their most satisfying experiences, nearly one in five did not. For 19 percent of the women describing sex with a partner in an ongoing relationship, one or more orgasms was not usually or always a component of their most satisfying sexual experiences. The qualities of satisfying sexual experiences with and without orgasm were described as follows:

Women fifty or older wrote: ♀ It's a very loving experience most of the time but I almost never quite get to an orgasm; ♀ I prefer to "ride the highs" rather than orgasm. I have fibroids that sometimes hurt when I contract in orgasm; ♀ I'm not as easily aroused as I used to be. I used to really get upset if I couldn't come to orgasm, and it became an unpleasant experience. At some point or another, I decided I'll do what feels good and if it doesn't feel good to orgasm, that's okay. So there are times I accept him and let him orgasm without really working for mine.

Two younger women reported: ♀ I *fake* one orgasm, even in *very* satisfying sex; ♀ I enjoy having an orgasm, but I don't see it as a goal of sex. . . . I used to focus on getting an orgasm and feel up-tight or resentful if I didn't. But gradually I realized that it's not worth getting uptight over. I don't really try. I either have one or I don't.

A woman of forty-nine who at forty-five had had a mastectomy and breast reconstruction and was currently taking the estrogen suppressor Tamoxifen for breast cancer wrote of the orgasms she *did* have regularly: "I was ill for a year during which time we developed our nonintercourse orgasms to an *art.* Often we don't have intercourse but bring each other to climax or at times watch each other masturbate . . . or one will just watch the other, although watching often stimulates the watcher to 'wake up.'"

Steady, Reliable Stimulation

One of the five orgasm items on the list, *steady, reliable stimulation that continued through orgasm,* was inspired by a study by Marc and Judith Meshorer published in 1986.

The Meshorers interviewed sixty women able to *consistently* reach orgasm through some means, which they defined as at least 75 percent of the times they had sex. One of the Meshorers' findings was that these women were unanimous in needing, in the final moments before orgasm, "steady, *reliable* stimulation, and a final, steady—occasionally increased—tactile rhythm and pressure." In our Survey, 1,653 women marked *steady, reliable stimulation through orgasm*, while 2,038 marked *one or more orgasms*, a difference of about 20 percent. *Steady, reliable stimulation through orgasm* seemed to be important but not unanimously needed by the women we surveyed. One woman further described her experience by adding: "steady, reliable stimulation that continued through orgasm *after orgasm after orgasm!*"

No Pressure

No pressure from my partner for me to have an orgasm and *no pressure from myself to have an orgasm* were each selected by about half of the respondents. Some explained: ♀ Both of us always reach orgasm; if it takes a while, the other person is patient; we are very attuned to what the other one likes; ♀ We've backed off on the pressure, and an orgasm usually happens—it's great now!; ♀ My partner (female) was wet, excited, soft. We felt complete and sated without orgasm; ♀ I don't feel the need to orgasm in order to have satisfying sex.

Katherine (1938), who has been married twenty-nine years, said: "I haven't had that many orgasms in my marriage. I think it's hard for some women to have an orgasm and I'm one of them. You have to have a man who's very patient. My husband can't sit still for five minutes. If we go out to eat and there're two people in line ahead of us, he won't wait. How's he going to wait for an orgasm?"

Many women did, however, experience *pressure from themselves* to reach orgasm: ♀ I always want to; ♀ I feel safe bringing my vibrator into our bed but I always express that my *real* desire is to have an "O" without it; ♀ If I start out not feeling turned on, then I worry so much about having an orgasm—performance pressure—that the orgasm isn't very pleasurable when it finally happens; ♀ There is definitely pressure.

Some women emphasized that *orgasm is very important* for their sexual satisfaction: ♀ Orgasm is very important. I don't like to have sex without orgasm. It's just like when a guy doesn't get satisfied. Very frustrating. Your body is all tensed up for that and then, boom, it's not there; ♀ Sex without orgasm doesn't feel like sex to me. Sometimes I think that the idea that sex is not just orgasm is something people who aren't having orgasms sell themselves; ♀ Right before my period I feel anxious and frustrated as if I'll never have an orgasm. Otherwise I am very satisfied and happy with my sex life.

And then, again, a woman may be satisfied with her orgasm but not with her partner: ♀ I usually have an orgasm but only through my own "mental" self-stimulation and imagination, so I am satisfied with the orgasm but not usually with my partner; we have been married for twelve years; ♀ I feel physically satisfied but frustrated and inadequate due to his unaroused state or seeming disinterest in sexual pleasure for *himself* and lack of expression of feelings.

It is clear that not all women believe that orgasm is the goal of sex or even that orgasm is necessary for sexual satisfaction. This may be surprising to some. Women who want orgasm every time and are frustrated when it doesn't happen may wonder at this. According to my Survey co-author, many men believe that orgasm is the best part of sex and the most important reason for engaging in it and, therefore, can't understand why a woman would want to have sex without wanting one. Yet nearly half of the participants in our survey who had had sex with a partner in the previous three months did not desire orgasm every single time they had sex with their partners. For many women, feeling connected, loving, and turned on is more satisfying than producing an orgasm with effort. (The meaning of *when having sex with my partner* in this question was ambiguous and interpreted variously to mean, for example, "*any* sexual contact, e.g., kissing" and "having *intercourse* with my partner.")

Feelings After Satisfying Sexual Activity

Women offered many spontaneous comments about how they felt or what happened after satisfying sexual activity: ♀ I have an increased consciousness of mutual love, increased gratitude for this woman being in my life, increased self-esteem, a sense of oneness with universal energy; ♀ We share appreciations; ♀ We experience spiritual closeness; ♀ We both sleep very well!; ♀ Playfulness always follows even if it's for only five minutes and then we're asleep; ♀ I experience a melding of body and spirit; I feel enriched; ♀ We talk.

One woman wrote: "I usually experience some *distancing* after intense sexual closeness and sexually satisfying activity." This is a fairly typical reaction to feeling very close in lovemaking. The capacity to reclaim your separate sense of self is an important aspect of being able to surrender to sexual union with another. Sometimes beginning to feel more separate after sex can be a sign of just how close you were able to be. I often say that *intimacy thrives on separateness.* An intimate couple constantly balances their mutual desires for love, merging, and companionship with their desires for independence, separateness, and autonomy.

Seventy-four percent of respondents said that *knowing that I gave my partner a wonderful experience* was a part of their most satisfying experiences, but some women wanted to modify slightly our choice of the word *wonderful*: ♀ A *good* experience; ♀ Knowing that my partner was pleased; ♀ I don't know about "wonderful"—very weighty word; ♀ . . . a *pleasant* experience; ♀ We'll settle for *good*.

Age and Sexual Satisfaction in an Ongoing Relationship

In response to the question about what period of their lives they were considering when they marked the items on the *factors in sexual satisfaction* list, 68 percent of the women answering said that their responses to this list of thirty-three items described satisfying sex in their current decade of life. As you might expect, the younger a woman was, the more likely her satisfaction was to be recent. For women in their twenties, 87 percent described their most satisfying sex as occurring in their twenties, *their current age*, whereas 63 percent of the women in their sixties described their most satisfying sexual experiences as having taken place in *some previous decade* of their lives. Some women had the good fortune of lifetime satisfaction; others described a much briefer period. A woman born in 1915 wrote: "I was married to this partner when I was forty-five to fifty-five—we divorced—then reunited at age seventy-eight; in my life, my sexual satisfaction was at its peak in my forties, fifties, and seventies."

Orientation and Sexual Satisfaction

Does sexual orientation make a difference in how women define sexual satisfaction? Whether women described themselves as heterosexual, lesbian, or bisexual, there were many similarities. *Feeling close to my partner before sex* was the number one item, and the other emotional and relationship factors were rated highly for all three groups. *Emotional closeness after sex, feeling loved, feeling safe,* and *knowing my partner was accepting of my desires, preferences, and responses* were near the top of the list. *Arguing before sex* was rarely selected.

The main differences associated with sexual orientation had to do with physical stimulation. Intercourse was, of course, associated with sexual satisfaction by many more of the *heterosexual women*; lesbians were far more likely than heterosexuals to associate anal stimulation and using vibrators and dildoes with erotic satisfaction. Overall, the Survey suggests that orientation makes only a small difference in the way women define sexual satisfaction and that this difference has to do primarily with what they do when engaging in sex.

Satisfaction with Frequency and Quality of Various Touching Activities

For those Survey participants who had engaged in sexual activity of any kind with a partner in the previous three months, 61 percent would have liked more affectionate nonsexual, nongenital touching, 68 percent would have liked more sexual/erotic contact that did not lead to sustained genital stimulation or intercourse, and 56 percent would have liked more sexual intercourse; virtually all of the rest of the Survey respondents thought the frequency of these activities was about right (only 2-4 percent would have liked less).

In her interview, **Cindi (1952)** said: "Nonsexual touching is important to me. I like to be held and petted and massaged. It's valuable as a way of keeping in touch with my partner. And it's something he values, too." **Lorraine (1957)** had this to say about the frequency of affectionate nonsexual touching in her relationship: "I would like to be massaged and to massage my husband but he's not interested in it. Which makes it very difficult for me. That's really a very sad missing link in my life."

In contrast, **Vera (1940)** doesn't regard touching as particularly important: "Touching isn't real important to me, but it is to the men I've had sex with. They like hugging and affection. I'm not really a hugger. I didn't have affection when I was growing up, so it doesn't occur to me. I like it when it's done to me, and I reciprocate, but I never think of it on my own."

With respect to the quality of the various activities, 58 percent *strongly agreed* or *agreed* that they were satisfied with the quality of affectionate nonsexual touching, 52 percent with the quality of erotic touching, and 63 percent with the quality of sustained genital contact or intercourse they'd had with a partner in the previous three months; 15 percent, 17 percent, and 11 percent respectively disagreed.

Satisfaction with Total Amount of Sexual Activity

With respect to the total amount of sexual activity (anything and everything sexual) in their current or most recent relationships, 26 percent said they wanted more than their partners, 32 percent said their partners wanted more, and 42 percent said that they and their partners wanted about the same amount.

Sara Socher's Research

Sara Socher of New York City analyzed the Survey data for her doctoral dissertation, looking for the factors that are most important to women's sexual satisfaction. In analyzing the data, she made some fascinating discoveries, which I have summarized in the following sections.

Sexual Affirmation and Sexual Satisfaction

Dr. Socher found that the strongest predictor of a woman's sexual satisfaction in both the previous three months and over her lifetime was a cluster of traits, a quality of the woman's sexuality that she called *sexual affirmation*. She describes *sexual affirmation* as "a combination of openness, assertiveness, and honest acceptance" of the woman's own sexual feelings and of the sexual feelings from her partner . . . "honest expression of likes and dislikes, self-acceptance . . . a mutually accepting interpersonal relationship" (Socher 1999).

The Survey statements that measure *sexual affirmation* include the following:

- I initiate sex whenever I want it.

- My current or most recent partner is or was comfortable with my initiating sexual activity.

- During sex, I'm comfortable telling my partner what I don't like or don't want.

- During sex, I'm comfortable telling my partner what I want and like.

- During sex, I communicate my desires as often as I want to.

- My partner gives me as much feedback about his or her sexual likes and dislikes as I want.

- My current or last partner is or was satisfied with how my body looks.

- I've been satisfied with my sex life with a partner in the last three months.

The Kundalini Woman

In her conclusions, Socher confirmed her assumption that defining a sexually satisfied woman solely in terms of her orgasms is not an accurate measure. She suggested that "for the woman who is sexually satisfied, with or without orgasm, an alternative to the term 'Orgasmic Woman' may be preferable" and she coined a new term, the *Kundalini Woman*, a description "borrowed from Tantra's culture, where reaching the creative power of sex is called 'Kundalini.'" This description is one that "represents a dynamic transition rather than a moment frozen in time; one that requires a level of comfort with one's own bio-psycho-social reality; one that permits (the woman and her partner) to seek the benefits of their sexuality in its full potential."

In summarizing her research, Socher concluded that a "Kundalini woman could be described as one who allows herself to experience (unrelated to procreative needs) the creative power of sex. This is a sensual person who is able to experience an intense physical and emotional pleasure while engaging in sexual activity (whether spasms occur or not); who allows loss of self into the feeling of lovemaking; and who reaches a higher level of self-acceptance as a result of this positive experience . . . a person who is accepting of and assertive about her sexual needs." She is a woman who might interpret a less satisfying experience as "an opportunity to grow . . . and a basis for corrective exploration" rather than as "devastating." She is likely to be comfortable with her own body and "in touch with her emotional and sexual needs."

Dr. Socher also noted that the ability to allow loss of self during lovemaking, although not measured in this study, seems to be an important component of sexual satisfaction. A *Kundalini Woman* loses herself while maintaining "a complete concern for her partner." She "may tend to be passionate but not compelled to experience her sexuality and may abstain rather than engage in a situation that is not appealing to her." Socher suggests that further research in this area could help us to "clarify the centuries-old Tantric claim that nonsexual self-realizing powers arise from sexual energy."

Sara Bridges' Research

Dr. Sara Bridges, now at Humboldt State University in California, also analyzed some of the Survey data for her doctoral dissertation; she, too, looked for the factors that are important to women's sexual satisfaction. Like Dr. Socher, she found that partner initiation and communication are very important in predicting sexual satisfaction.

Women who reported communicating their desires as often as they wanted during sex and women who said they were comfortable initiating sex with their partner tended to be more satisfied sexually than other Survey respondents. Dr. Bridges also found that physical affection and positive sexual attitudes in the woman's family of origin make it likelier that she will be sexually satisfied over her lifetime. Furthermore, she found that the women who masturbated most frequently were those most likely to be dissatisfied with sexual intercourse.

In summary, it is clear that, for most women in ongoing relationships, sexual satisfaction is closely linked to feeling attuned to and connected with their partners. When sex is satisfying, women feel loved and loving, passionate and aroused, happy and wonderful, sensual and erotic; they feel ecstatic, playful, peaceful, romantic, desirable, and desired. Although most women associate orgasm with their most satisfying experiences, satisfaction is associated even more strongly with assertiveness, communication, and feeling loved and close to one's partner before, during, and after sex.

What Does This Mean to You?

Now, if you wish, pick up your notebook and express the thoughts and feelings you're having about sexual satisfaction. Here are some questions you might want to consider after you've done that. If you have never had satisfying sex with a partner, imagine what that would be like and answer these questions from that perspective.

- What qualities make sex pleasurable and satisfying for you?

- If you've ever had what you considered to be really fantastic sex, what components of the sexual activity provided you with the greatest pleasure?

- Were your most satisfying sexual experiences with the best partner(s) for you overall?

- If you are recalling experiences that you now regret, consider the circumstances, the roles of others, and how you saw your options at the time. Then, sit quietly with your eyes closed and imagine what you could now gently and lovingly tell your younger self that would be healing and would lead to greater self-acceptance.

10

One Hundred+ Years of Women's Orgasms

There seems to be a reasonable basis for assuming that the human female's capacity for orgasm is to be viewed much more as a potentiality that may or may not be valued and developed by a given culture, or in the specific life history of an individual, than as an inherent part of her full humanity (Mead 1949).

The ideas many of us have about achieving orgasms and the kinds of orgasms we should be having underlie many of the problems I see in sex therapy. These ideas also influence us to fake orgasms. In this chapter my goal is to show you what we have been taught to think about orgasms and to present you with a liberating alternative.

Women probably have been thinking and talking about orgasm for centuries. When Dr. Clelia D. Mosher asked women about their sexuality—this was between 1892 and 1920—she asked them *Do you always have a venereal orgasm?* It would seem from the way she asked this question—*Do you always* . . . rather than *Do you ever. . . .*—that the college-educated women she was interviewing at the turn of the last century had, or expected to have, orgasms during sex.

In 1921-1923, Katharine Bement Davis and her colleagues asked 1,000 unmarried college-educated women about orgasms within the context of questions on masturbation. Their question was phrased: *How old were you when the orgasm was first induced?* Later, when discussing their findings, however, Davis noted that "the word 'orgasm' ... was unfamiliar to many" of their respondents.

Sexual Goals—Defining Sexual Success as Orgasm

I think it was the emphasis on clitoral and vaginal orgasms, which began with Sigmund Freud (1856-1939) and his followers, that firmly rooted the ideas I call the *manufacturing orgasms* sexual script into our collective consciousness.

Clitoral and Vaginal Orgasms

Few of us raised in this culture have escaped the influence of more than half a century of debate about *clitoral* and *vaginal orgasms*. The obsession with the two kinds of orgasm started with Freud. In *A General Introduction to Psychoanalysis*, published in English translation in 1920, he wrote:

> We know that the little girl feels injured on account of her lack of a large, visible penis, envies the boy his possession, and primarily from this motive desires to be a man. . . . During childhood, the clitoris of the girl is the equivalent of the penis; it is especially excitable, the zone where auto-erotic satisfaction is achieved. In the transition to womanhood it is most important that the sensations of the clitoris are completely transferred . . . to the entrance of the vagina. In cases of so-called sexual anesthesia of women the clitoris has obstinately retained its excitability (p. 274).

In 1927 he added that *"the abolition of clitoris sexuality is a necessary pre-condition for the development of femininity"* (p. 139).

Freud's opinions were repeated, quoted, and expanded upon in the marriage manuals and medical textbooks of the 1930s through the 1950s as if they were proven scientific fact. *Vaginal orgasms*, a woman's orgasms achieved by intercourse, were said to be the sign of marital maturity, and *simultaneous orgasms* achieved through intercourse were touted as the ultimate satisfaction in love-making. In his classic *Ideal Marriage, Its Physiology and Technique*, first published in 1926, Van de Velde wrote:

> ... in ideal communion the stimulation will generally be focused on and in the vagina. .... And this will be fully adequate for such a variety and intensity of sensation as will culminate in the orgasm.
>
> In the normal and perfect coitus, mutual orgasm must be almost simultaneous; the usual procedure is that the man's ejaculation begins and sets the woman's acme of sensation in train at once (1968 edition, p. 165).

And in *Love Without Fear*, a popular sex manual published first in 1947 and revised in 1957, Eustace Chesser advised his readers that "Both partners should, in coitus, concentrate their full attention on one thing: the attainment of simultaneous orgasm."

Manufacturing Orgasms

Van de Velde and Chesser, much read and influential in their time, specifically defined sexual success in terms of manufacturing orgasms to quite detailed specifications. They told their readers, many of whom were seeking to solve the mystery of how to do sex, that orgasm is the goal of sex. To be sexually successful in this *manufacturing orgasms* script, you *must* have an orgasm. The orgasm *must* occur in intercourse. And, according to these two prominent male physicians, the stakes are even higher: you and your partner *must* have not just any orgasms, but simultaneous orgasms.

Today, we recognize that these are just opinions, not truth. But isn't it interesting that all these books telling women how we are supposed to be sexually and how we should experience our orgasms were authored by men? There were some women writing marriage manuals in those days, too, but most were also based on Freud's ideas.

Women Who Have Vaginal and Simultaneous Orgasms

As each generation grows up and finds their way to understanding how they're supposed to have sex, they absorb the prevailing cultural messages and expectations of their time. **Emily (1919)**, who was influenced by the marriage manuals available in this era—

and who may even have read those cited above—described simultaneous orgasms as a regular part of her lovemaking: "I had read some books and they all promoted simultaneous orgasms and I had them with no problem in the first year of marriage. I had learned on my own how to build arousal. During intercourse I would tell him to stop for a few moments and let the feelings subside and then start again. And then again. I had tremendous orgasms by prolonging the event this way. I had discovered when I masturbated, that if I stopped right when I was starting to move that way and just let the buzzing and the feelings all calm down, and then I would go on, I would prolong the pleasure."

What Vera and Peg first learned about orgasms was that they were supposed to have *vaginal* ones. And they do have them. **Vera (1940)** explained: "I've never had an orgasm with oral sex. My orgasms are brought on by something inside that gets hit and I feel 'boom.' It doesn't come from the outside." **Peg (1948)** said: "I really like vaginal orgasms. I am one of the rare birds for whom intercourse doesn't necessarily have to be preceded with clitoral stimulation. I have clitoral orgasms also."

Women Who Don't Fit the Orgasmic Fashions of Their Times

But many women have experiences that do not fit the orgasmic fashions of their times. If they and their partners believe the socially imposed criteria about how they should respond, and then judge themselves by those criteria, they may think of themselves as sexually inadequate. That's what happened to this Survey respondent, a registered nurse born in **1940**: "A psychodynamic psychiatrist taught us medical-nursing students that clitoral stimulation to orgasm was immature. I felt inadequate and was unable to have intercourse orgasm (without manual stimulation, too) until my late thirties."

Freudian theorists and analysts, most of them male, labeled women who did not reach orgasm through vaginal penetration by a penis as *frigid, neurotic, infantile,* and *suffering from incomplete psychosexual development.* Long-term psychoanalysis was their treatment of choice for *frigid* women, although it often did little to improve sexual satisfaction. Another treatment, fortunately rare, for the so-called *problem* of clitoral sensitivity was to eliminate the clitoris entirely. Some physicians argued that removing the clitoris and its surrounding structures would keep this source of pleasure from interfering with the vagina's sensitivity (Barbach 1975).

How unfortunate that they didn't teach these women—and their partners—to be more skillful in their lovemaking! The problem, of course, was not vaginal sensitivity but that the Freudians were reducing the potentially wonderful variety of women's genital sensitivities and women's orgasms to just one "right" way. They were promoting their opinions about how sex and orgasms should be as proven fact.

A Liberating New Definition

My answer to the *manufacturing orgasms* script was to come up with a new *definition of sexual success* that does not define success in a sexual interlude in terms of physical functioning. Instead, I define success in terms of creating erotic pleasure with outcomes of intimacy, satisfaction, mutual pleasure, and self-esteem. This redefinition of success in sex has become the cornerstone of the *Intimacy-Based Sex Therapy* I do. I think of a couple as sexually successful when they *create mutual erotic pleasure, to whatever level and in whatever form they desire on any particular occasion, so that each ends up feeling good about herself or himself and the other, experiencing a good time and enhancing their relationship.*

I am frequently asked, *How do we achieve that?* Note how we so often associate the word "achieve" with sex! Observe that my definition includes the word "create," but not the word "achieve." Notice, too, that this definition doesn't say anything about having intercourse or how stimulation occurs, nor does it mention lubrication, achieving erections, lasting longer, achieving orgasms, or any other specific aspects of physical responsiveness. To create sexual episodes that fulfill this definition of sexual success for yourself, see chapter 13 for my Sexual Choreography guidelines.

More History

The Freudian psychological interpretations of sexuality influenced sex research throughout most of the twentieth century. But even in Freud's heyday, not everyone agreed with him. It wasn't long before sexual literature and research were addressing such questions as, *Are there distinctly different kinds of orgasms? If there are, is one kind more mature or better than another*? Kinsey, Pomeroy, Martin, et al. considered "clitoral versus vaginal" orgasms in their 1953 *Sexual Behavior in the Human Female*, and in *Human Sexual Response* (1966), Masters and Johnson asked: "Are clitoral and vaginal orgasms truly separate anatomic entities?"

From my perspective, the Freudians took a very narrow view of the glorious potential of a woman's sexual responsiveness. Focusing on one way of having sex as *the right way* or even considering a question like *Is it okay if there is clitoral stimulation during intercourse?* reduces sex from a dynamic, ever-changing interaction between two people to the rubbing of an erogenous zone or two to reach a goal by mechanical means.

In 1953, Kinsey and his colleagues described research in which gynecologists stroked areas of the vaginas, labia, and cervixes of more than 800 women with a Q-tip-like probe; these doctors also exerted pressure with a larger object. Since few of these women felt the touch when their inner vaginal walls were gently stroked or lightly touched and even fewer were conscious of a light stroke or pressure to the cervix, the Kinsey group concluded that vaginal sensation is limited to the outer third of the vagina, and "it is improbable that any area which is insensitive to tactile manipulation could be stimulated erotically" (Kinsey, Pomeroy, and Martin et al. 1953). They thought, therefore, that women shouldn't be expected to have vaginal orgasms.

This statement introduced an erroneous belief into our collective sexual mythology that still affects the way many people think about women's sexuality today: the idea that women's potential for vaginal/internal pleasure is quite limited. By the 1960s and 1970s, reactions against the Freudian dogma had swung the pendulum so far that some sex therapists, researchers, and feminists had replaced it with an equally dogmatic mythology that I call the "Clitoral Model" (Ellison 1979).

At its extreme, the Clitoral Model position can be stated like this: Women get little real stimulation from intercourse; orgasm is always caused by clitoral stimulation in some form. This was a dominant theme, for example, in the 1976 *Hite Report*. In the 1970s we were hearing women's voices, at last, even though some of these women were as dogmatic in their ideas as the Freudians had been. Although Katharine Davis was well known in the 1920s and 1930s (Bullough 1999, personal communication), her name and work had not remained in the public consciousness.

Masters and Johnson, who also greatly influenced our thinking, described sexual stimulation during intercourse as caused by the movement and tugging on the clitoral hood. They could not accept the idea that a woman might experience other kinds of movement and sensations from deep within her vagina (1966). They introduced a new medical diagnosis, *masturbatory orgasmic inadequacy*, for women who could have orgasms during sexual intercourse but could not have clitoral orgasms through partner or self-manipulation (1970).

Remember the discussion about *naming experiences* in chapter 2? When we label an experience, we impose values and judgments on it.

When Masters and Johnson introduced this label, they gave a new group of women, most of whom thought they were just fine the way they were, the message that they should consider themselves sexually "inadequate."

Experiencing orgasm in one way but not in another need not be a problem. As you will see, there is a nearly infinite variety in women's orgasmic experiences. What is a problem is feeling judged and inadequate because someone else is telling you what your experience should be—instead of validating the experiences you are having.

Whichever way the pendulum was swinging, there were dissenting views. Germaine Greer noted in 1971 that we had been infected by a *veritable clitoromania* and went on to say:

> It is nonsense to say that a woman feels nothing when a man is moving his penis in her vagina: the orgasm is qualitatively different when the vagina can undulate around the penis instead of vacancy. . . . Real satisfaction is not enshrined in a tiny cluster of nerves but in the sexual involvement of the whole person. . . . If we localize female response in the clitoris we . . . [substitute] genitality for sexuality (pp. 36-37).

In the male-centered Freudian image, the orgasm is produced by the thrusting penis. Greer gave us an image of woman-as-equal. The man is *moving* rather than *thrusting* his penis and the vagina is *undulating* around the penis. In Greer's construct, the woman is actively involved, rather than passively being done to.

The clitoral-vaginal orgasms issue was not exclusively heterosexual. In *The Joy of Lesbian Sex* (1977), for example, Emily Sisley and Bertha Harris wrote of how the term *frigidity* had "taken on the cultural meaning of being incapable of achieving vaginal orgasm with a penis" and said of the impact on lesbians of this way of thinking: "Lesbians, of course, suffered . . . from Freud's disqualification of the clitoris as a socially approved site of orgasm, and, even while the steam was pouring from their eyeballs from clitoral orgasm, believed . . . that 'mature womanhood' would be forever denied them until their vaginas could somehow make friends with a penis."

The Clitoris, Sexual Arousal, and Internal Sensations

The clitoris is unique in that, as far as I know, it is the only human organ devoted entirely to the generation of sexual pleasure. At least, that is our current understanding of its role. The clitoris is more than the visible external glans. It may have other functions of which we are unaware at this time. It may, for example, play a role in childbirth or other aspects of reproduction.

Many women report oral or manual stimulation of it as their most typical or preferable way to reach orgasm. Still, orgasm depends on a great deal more than where or what is stimulated. A woman's partner, mood, hormones, health, and the circumstances under which she is having sex are all important factors. A woman's experience of orgasm also varies according to her partner's skill as a lover, the nature of their relationship, her age, her sexual history, and more. As I will document, under certain conditions, stimulation of virtually any area of the human body, images from the mind alone, or experiencing the sexual energy of someone else, can all lead to orgasm.

The Kinsey researchers and the Clitoral Model proponents overlooked one very important element in the pleasure women can receive from intercourse or other internal stimulation. This is the importance of sexual arousal. A light touch from a probe such as a Q-tip in the vagina of an unaroused and perhaps nervous woman is not the same stimulation as a penis or dildo moving in the fully engorged vagina of a sexually aroused and actively participating woman. A thirty-year-old woman told me in 1979: "When I'm highly aroused by my partner and the situation, those intercourse movements are highly pleasurable. If I'm moderately aroused, the internal stimulation may feel good, but not nearly so good and intense as it does after we've been doing intercourse for a while and I'm really into it—or after we've done a lot of very arousing foreplay—for example, oral stimulation to orgasm or to the verge of orgasm" (Ellison 1984, p. 330).

One component of internal sensations during intercourse or vaginal containment of something other than a penis, such as a dildo, is compression of the spongy vaginal tissues. Another component may be movement of the cervix. Moving the cervix moves the uterus and the broad ligaments that support it. The uterus and these ligaments are covered with some of the most sensitive tissue in the body. This is the peritoneum, the membrane that encloses the abdominal organs. It has been suggested that stimulation of the peritoneum provides a broad base for sensation in the lower abdominal area (Clark 1970). Perhaps this kind of movement is the basis for some of the sensations **Terri (1971)** described: "I am orgasmic almost all the time in intercourse. It's more of an all-encompassing thing than a particular spot. When he goes in and out of me, that can be very stimulating. But if he's just inside me completely, that's stimulating as well. So it's not just the walls of my vagina or the complete inside, but I think it's all over."

The ligaments that support the uterus also play a role in the sexual pleasure—or sexual discomfort—of some women. Just as joggers stretch ankle ligaments before running to avoid pain or injury, some women seem to need their inner tissues stretched slowly so they can enjoy deep intercourse. Gradually applied pressure from, for example, a penis allows the tissues to relax slowly and stretch; subsequent movements can then produce deep sensations that are experienced as sensuous and pleasurable. Initial deep thrusts that are too fast or felt as jabbing may be experienced as painful.

Penis Size

Although in its aroused sponginess the vagina can receive penises of varying sizes, some women do report that penis size can make a difference in what they experience and in whether or not they have orgasms from intercourse. Women's bodies vary so much in size and shape, however, that what will be a pleasurable match for one woman may not suit another at all. Some men may be surprised that the women cited here do not consistently perceive bigger penises as better.

Some women did talk about what a full-filling penis means to them. **Emily (1919)** said: Penis size can make a difference for me. I feel more stimulation when there is more contact with the inner walls of my vagina. The entrance is where I feel most of the sensation, but the feeling of being filled is very satisfying to react with."

Susan (1958) described her experience of having a husband with a "pretty large" penis: "Sometimes it really feels nice because I feel filled up—and sometimes it hurts. We have to work with positioning so that it's not uncomfortable. But then, for me, there's this feeling of being filled up, and it feels nice. I haven't had that feeling with men who have smaller penises."

Susan was not the only woman to mention that *sometimes it hurts.* Other women noted that a man's penis can be too big. **Teresa's (1946)** former husband "was too big for oral sex and intercourse." She said she likes "a nice medium size, but size isn't the big be-all and end-all for me. Penis size is the least of my worries." And it took two years for **Bonnie (1966)** to come with her current partner inside of her, "because he's big and most of the time it would hurt."

Maggie (1965) had a boyfriend whose penis "was enormous and . . . bordering on painful," but she is adamant that "I do not enjoy sex as much with men with little penises. I think we're just trying to make men feel better by saying size isn't important." **Carole (1930)**, on the other hand, thinks that, while "there's an optimum size that is really nice . . . if a man who has a small penis is creative, he can make it very pleasing. Some of the men I was with did that."

It doesn't matter how big it is as long as you know what to do with it. We frequently hear this said about small penises, but it is true about large ones, too—and all of the sizes in between. **Michele (1972)** said she "was with one guy and he was huge. And even though he was big, it wasn't even good. I think it has a lot to do with what you know how to do. It's not just in and out, in and out. It's knowing when to do it hard or soft, or in circles, or whatever." She also observed that guys often think their penises are small when they aren't really: "My boyfriend has a medium-sized one, and he's like, *Oh it's small.* And I go, *Honey, I like it. There's nothing wrong with it.*" **Maria (1965)** was with a pleasing "partner who had a particularly small one." She said, "He was into bragging that it wasn't the size but what you did with it. And he was right. We had a lot of fun."

The G Spot and Female Ejaculation

In the 1980s, media and medical attention shifted again to women's internal responses with the rediscovery of what Beverly Whipple and her colleagues called the *G spot* and *female ejaculation.* The claim was made that women have an especially sensitive spot in their vaginas—the G spot—stimulation of which can lead to orgasm and even, for some women, ejaculation of a clear fluid. The G spot has been described as an erotic zone of erectile tissue on the anterior wall of the vagina along the urethra which engorges and swells in response to sexual stimulation (Grafenberg 1950; Ladas, Whipple, and Perry 1982).

After more than a decade of clitoral ascendancy, the G spot was promoted by those still interested in the clitoral-vaginal orgasm controversy as proof that vaginal stimulation was important after all—if only women would take the trouble to find this magic spot. It didn't take long before some women were frustrated because they couldn't find their G spot, or they didn't respond with orgasms or ejaculation when it was stimulated. Then there were new variations in sexual performance pressure. A woman, age thirty-two, wrote the following to the authors of *The G Spot* (Ladas, Whipple, and Perry 1982): "My husband used to ask whenever we made love, *Did you come, did you come?* . . . Now guess what he says? *Did you spurt, did you spurt?* . . . I don't ejaculate and I never have."

Do you recognize this as a new version of the *manufacturing orgasms* script? Now, in order to be successful in sex, you not only *must* have an orgasm, you also *must* ejaculate. But, of course, this is not so. It may even be that not all women have the physical capacity to "ejaculate" in this way.

Researchers tried to determine whether the G spot is a true anatomical structure or, as some suggested, not a particular *spot* at all but a variation for some women in how the spongy erectile tissue around the urethra engorges in response to sexual stimulation.

More interesting to me than the question whether the G spot really exists was to ask the women I interviewed: *Do you* experience *a sensitive spot or area in your vagina during sexual activity?* Some said, *No* or *No; my sensitive area is my clitoris.* **Emily (1919)** said, "I've never found anything in particular. My main sensitive areas are the clitoris and the outer and inner lips. But I've never actually looked for a spot." **Gloria (1944)** had experienced a spot many times before, but didn't know what it was until she read about it. She reported, "My orgasm is a lot more intense when there's a lot of contact with the clitoris or the G spot." For **Peg (1948)** the G spot is "terrific" and a trigger for orgasm in intercourse, particularly when the man is "on top."

In contrast, **Kathy (1949)** said, "There's a lot of talk about G spot orgasms but it's my least favorite orgasm. For one thing it involves an uncomfortable feeling of needing to urinate just before orgasm. And when the orgasm happens, there's a spurt of fluid and I don't like that; it feels like a loss of control. . . . Most of the time the stimulation's with fingers but one partner did it with his cock in me from behind. He has a large cock but it was soft. I think normally it would have passed by the G spot but because it was soft it was hitting the spot and his size was really massaging it well."

Not all women experience their *sensitive spot* in the same place. The G spot is described as on the front vaginal wall. **Marcy's (1967)** spot is somewhere else: "My sensitive spot is the back wall area. It's not like it brings me to an orgasmic state, but I'm always trying to push him in deeper. The penis has to be a certain size. It can't be too big or it just hurts, and if it's too small I can't feel it back there."

The Ejaculatory Phenomenon

Although some claim that stimulation of the G spot often leads to the forceful expulsion of fluid from the urethra at orgasm (Zaviacic and Whipple 1993), only a few of the women I interviewed had experienced any forceful spurting of fluid during and after their orgasms, and what they told me varied. For example, one woman for whom this happened fairly regularly said that it occurred "more with clitoral stimulation during intercourse than with G spot stimulation," whereas another woman for whom it also occurred regularly, said this was "generally with stimulation of the G spot area." She commented: "That was one of the things I had to go read about, because it seemed kind of weird." Another reported: "When I really have an orgasm, I literally squirt. I was shocked the first time it happened. I thought I had peed or something; it happens a lot in this relationship, but never with previous partners. I've had it happen with clitoral stimulation, but mainly with her finger inside of me." Other women reported a lot of wetness rather than a forceful spurting. One experienced "contractions and a lot of liquid, but," she said, "I don't spurt." Another said, "After I orgasm, I get very wet and sticky. It doesn't spurt, but it's just there, a lot of it."

Still More History

All through the 1970s and 1980s, the cultural and social pressures to *achieve* vaginal and simultaneous orgasms were replaced by subtle pressures to *achieve*, for example, total orgasms (Rosenberg 1973); multiple orgasms for both women and men (Hartman and Fithian 1984); G spot orgasms (Ladas, Whipple, and Perry 1982); extended sexual orgasms (Brauer and Brauer 1983); and the "Microcosmic Orbit" (Chia and Chia 1986). After a talk I gave for women medical students in 1990, one student told me, "My husband is really into Taoist sex and the 'microcosmic orbit.' He has read all of Chia's books and even taken some of his workshops. Frankly, this method is not easy and I feel a lot of pressure from him to make it work."

Reflect for a moment on how often we think or say "achieve orgasm" as if those two words go together. This is the *manufacturing orgasms* sexual script. Unless we pay attention, we tend to overlook how strongly the phrase implies that sex is work and orgasm is a performance goal. The idea that sex is about achieving orgasm is just that: an *idea* about how sex should be. It is a problematic script that has so permeated our culture that most of us take it for granted and believe it is true. But trying to "achieve" any particular physical response distracts from intimacy and pleasure. It is a setup for frustration, because it is a goal that most of us can't—and perhaps don't really want to—always meet.

Are vaginal versus clitoral orgasm issues and images still with us? Indeed they are. The messages about how orgasms are supposed to happen continue to be passed on from generation to generation. **Stephanie (1973)**, one of the youngest college students interviewed by Michaelle Davis, is still thinking in terms of *vaginal orgasms*. She said: "I'm not able to have an orgasm during intercourse. I usually have it during oral sex before intercourse—that's how we usually do it. My clitoris is the main source of my pleasure, that's why I like oral sex. I have an orgasm every time. The only sex problem I have is that I still can't orgasm vaginally. I'd like it if I could have vaginal orgasms. We're working on it."

And **Mary's (1972)** boyfriend asked her, in essence, *What's the use if I can't manufacture an orgasm for you?* She said: "I reach orgasm very, very easily. And that's just come with time. At first, it wasn't as easy or often, but now I reach orgasm at least once every time we make love. I can think of only one experience with my boyfriend when I didn't orgasm. I wasn't feeling well and I wasn't sure I really wanted sex. I enjoyed the experience, but I couldn't even get close to orgasm. He was very upset. He wanted to stop part way through because he's like *If you're not getting anything out of this, it's not worth it.* But I wanted to continue. It wasn't a big deal for me; I had a good time anyway." Mary was having an enjoyable and satisfying sexual experience. That particular time she didn't need or want to orgasm. She wasn't frustrated by her lack of orgasm. What frustrated them both was her boyfriend's belief that it was his job to give her one. Perhaps he also believed that if he didn't give her one, it meant that he was sexually inadequate.

Faking Orgasm

Have you ever faked orgasm? If you have, think about all of the reasons you had for doing that. If you have never faked orgasm, why not? Approximately 70 percent of the 2,311 women who provided Survey information about faking orgasm had done so at least once. About three-quarters of those who had ever faked had done so no more than fifty times, but some had done it a lot more than that. Nearly one in ten of those who had ever faked either entered a number between 150 and 10,000 times or wrote in another answer such as *countless*, or *a bazillion*. One woman drew an infinity sign as her answer.

What is it that motivates these women to fake orgasms? They offered a variety of reasons, and virtually all were based in a belief that the woman's orgasm makes a sexual episode *successful* or defines its ending—the *manufacturing orgasms* script for having sex.

Most of the women who have never faked orgasm, on the other hand, don't accept this script for their lovemaking. For them, orgasm is not the primary goal of sex. Some were rather matter of fact about not faking. **Ellen (1910)** said, "If I wasn't satisfied, I just said, you know ... *Forget it. There'll be another time.*" And **Maria (1965)** explained, "I've never been embarrassed to say that I haven't had an orgasm. I don't think it's a crime." Others were even more adamant. One Survey respondent born in 1916 wrote: "No faking in this house! If I didn't orgasm, I'd say *Better luck next time.*" And another, several generations younger, wrote: "I truly would not—I see this as an insult to myself and my partner."

Why Women Fake Orgasms

The belief that the woman's orgasm makes a sexual episode *successful* or defines its ending—reasonable or not—generates certain gender role expectations. There are interlocking female and male roles. The man, for example, is seen as in charge of orchestrating sex and satisfying the woman; the interlocking role for the woman is to be "satisfied" and thereby validate that he is a good lover. If she is not satisfied, what does that say about him? In my research, the women who had faked orgasm reported three main reasons that were not mutually exclusive.

1. To take care of what they perceive as their partners' needs or feelings. Many women think it is our job to protect the fragile male ego. **Deborah (1949)** explained: "He had to think he was a good lover, satisfying me. Basically faking was me taking care of the man. When I later learned my clitoris could be stimulated, I was too embarrassed to tell him at first. I sensed he'd feel inadequate if I told him that he had *not* been *giving* me an orgasm. So I took care of him at my expense and said nothing." Part of Deborah's motivation, she said, was feeling that she needed to please him so that "then he won't leave me and I'll have a boyfriend."

   Others, like **Liz (1951)**, said, "I've faked with men, but I've never had to with a woman. It's very important to men. They're put in a position by themselves and society where they think they have to perform, they're responsible for the orgasms. So I did it for them. I didn't want to hurt their feelings." Liz's partner, **Joanna (1957)**, added: "The same for me. A few times I said I hadn't come, but they'd get defensive when I asked for something. By that time their ego had shrunk and so had their [sound and hand motion indicating penis; laughter]. When I said *Well, you have a mouth, you have fingers, finish it,* they were really taken aback. It was easier to fake it than go through that hassle."

Some women, **Diana (1968)**, for example, have a blasé attitude about faking, assuming that's just what women do: "Yeah, hasn't everyone? You're so close but you can't climax, so you just say, *Oh, I came,* and then they feel better."

2. To shift attention away from the process of bringing her to orgasm. A woman's faked orgasm makes the question of whether she has orgasmed or not irrelevant and frees her of any pressure to have one. It may be, too, that she would like her partner to focus attention on something else, such as his or her own pleasure or their mutual caring and love.

   Penny (1946) described the man she was with for six years when she was in her early forties as *narcissistic* and *not a good lover:* "I faked orgasm with him all the time. I didn't do it in the beginning, I was trying really hard to be honest. I faked it to prevent him asking why I wasn't having an orgasm." A younger Survey respondent wrote: "I enjoy sex even without orgasm; I fake because my partner tries *too* hard to get me to orgasm and *that* turns me off." A few respondents mentioned that they have allowed partners to think they were having an orgasm without actually faking one. This, too, relieved them of pressure to actually have one. For example: "With my current partner, I didn't *fake* it, I just didn't say that I didn't come."

3. A desire to get sex over with. Over the years **Madeline (1915)** faked "probably half the time . . . because I wanted to get it over with and be through with it." **Carole (1930)**, now part-nered with a woman, said she had faked orgasm, "but not for a long time. Only with men. I faked a lot with my husband because I wanted it to be over with."

   Sometimes a woman may not feel the relationship is such that she can simply tell the truth. This was **Lou Ann's (1944)** experience: "I faked maybe a few times with each part-ner. Where I was tired and it felt like it wasn't going to hap-pen and it just wasn't worth the effort to keep trying. And the relationship wasn't such that I could say, *It's not going to happen, it's okay.*" **Beth (1961)** faked orgasms toward the end of her relationship with her ex-lover. She explained: "I didn't feel connected to her and I just wanted to hurry up the end-ing of our sexual contact."

Some women have faked orgasm throughout their entire sexually active lives. About one in four of those who currently fake orgasm fakes at least 50 percent of the times she has sex: ♀ Every time; probably 10,000 times; ♀ A million times! With all of my partners and 90 percent of the time with my current partner.

For a larger number of women, however, faking orgasms is something they did when younger but not presently. A great many more women faked in their past relationships than are faking in their current relationships. About two-thirds of those presently in relationships do not fake orgasm with their current partner, and over half of those who do fake orgasm do it only 10 percent of the time or less. The 36 percent of partnered women currently faking orgasm in our Survey is about the same as the 34 percent reported by Shere Hite (1976) in *The Hite Report* twenty-five years ago.

One Survey respondent faked almost always, before she got a vibrator. She wrote: "Without the vibrator, there's no orgasm. With it, orgasm is guaranteed." **Gloria (1944)** faked early on with her husband but then said, "Enough of this shit, if I keep faking there's no need to change anything." My research seems to have uncovered a trend: many women don't fake much beyond their twenties. **Barb (1955)**, for example, said that when she was "under twenty-five," it was "the thing to do." **Lorraine (1957)** faked orgasms before she was married, when she was eighteen or so. She explained: "I probably did it because that's what they expected. But in my marriage I realized I could have real orgasms and there's no need to fake them. I only faked them when I didn't know how to have them."

I only faked them when I didn't know how to have them. When they first become sexually active, many young women and their partners believe that to be successful at this new activity they should *achieve orgasm.* One way a woman can validate their mutual competence, if neither she nor her partner has learned yet to reliably create an orgasm for her, is to fake it. If she and her partner become more skillful lovers and more comfortable and open in their relationship as it matures, faking may no longer be turned to for this purpose. As **Cindi (1952)** said, " I faked when I was around twenty-six, but only until I got comfortable enough to tell my partner what I needed."

The quality of the relationship is an important factor in whether a woman feels comfortable enough to be vulnerable and open in her communication about orgasm. **Deborah (1949)**, mentioned above, was very hesitant to talk with her partner about what she needed once she learned to have orgasms. She said, "When I finally risked telling him that *my clitoris really needs some stimulation or I can't easily have an orgasm,* he tried it for little while and then asked me—irritated—*Well,* *just how long is it supposed to take?* When I told him, *Probably ten or twenty minutes,* he said, *Forget it! My hand's tired. You're just frigid. That's the problem."* His defensive, critical response validated Deborah's earlier fears that this was not a safe topic for discussion in that relationship.

Leslie (1971) described how faking orgasm fit into her sexual experiences in different situations and with different partners: "With my first boyfriend, I never faked an orgasm, because he knew I couldn't have orgasms. With my second boyfriend, we never communicated about sex or orgasms; I would fake it, because sex was so painful and so bad that I just wanted to get it over with. And then with one-night stands, I've usually faked, because it's either boring me or I just want to end it."

Clearly, faking serves many purposes for many women. It is a way they can appear to respond sexually in the way they believe they're supposed to when they first become sexually active. It allows them to give the appearance of having experience and knowledge about their bodies and responses until they—and their partners—actually acquire them. It is also a way that women can please or take care of their partners, shift the focus of a sexual episode away from orgasm, or end sexual activity when they wish to. Usually this is a relatively benign strategy for meeting these needs. Many of the women who regularly fake orgasm don't seem to experience faking as a problem.

However, faking orgasm has its costs. When a woman fakes an orgasm, her partner thinks she is pleased and is influenced to continue repeating exactly what he or she does that seems to be satisfying—but most likely is not. Another cost is the missing honest communication. And we saw with Deborah, whose boyfriend called her "frigid" when she asked him for clitoral stimulation, how difficult it can be with an uncooperative partner to end this pattern.

When the circumstances are right, not faking also can be an effective relationship strategy, as this Survey respondent explained: "With my first serious lover I was totally honest about not having orgasms with him but still liking sex with him. He was very playful and warm in response and eventually I had them with him all the time. I can't imagine *not* having them now."

If you regularly fake orgasms and it is a problem for you, consider this: A woman is not likely to continue faking orgasms, except perhaps through habit, if she and her partner can agree that their intention in sex is not *orgasm,* but *mutual erotic pleasure,* whether what they do together ends in orgasm or not. Consider talking with your partner about what you each want from sex. Remember, the goal of sex is to create pleasure together, feel good about yourselves and each other, and to have a good time, not to manufacture orgasms.

I do believe that a woman and her partners should seek to learn how to create not only mutual pleasure, but also orgasms for her—and even simultaneous orgasms, if that is what they wish. But realizing your potential for erotic and orgasmic pleasure is quite different from putting pressure on yourself to have a particular kind of physical response every time you have sex. There is infinite variety in women's orgasmic experiences.

What Does This Mean to You?

Now, if you wish, pick up your notebook and express the thoughts and feelings you're having about orgasms and the sexual scripts you follow. Here are some questions you might want to consider after you've done that.

- How has the *manufacturing orgasms* sexual script affected you?

- What role has faking orgasms played in your sexual experiences?

- If you engage in heterosexual sex, does the size of a man's penis make a difference to you? If so, in what ways?

- Is there anything about the sexual scripts you follow you would like to change?

- If you are recalling experiences that you now regret, consider the circumstances, the roles of others, and how you saw your options at the time. Then, sit quietly with your eyes closed and imagine what you could now gently and lovingly tell your younger self that would be healing and would lead to greater self-acceptance.

11

The Infinite Variety of Women's Orgasms

The Experience of Orgasm

Recently, a fifty-two-year-old woman came to see me for sex therapy because she couldn't have orgasms with her partner without using her vibrator. When I questioned her, however, she did tell me that without her vibrator she usually experienced a wave of relaxation and a feeling of completion after sex. I suggested that she was probably having orgasms, but orgasms so different from those she had with her vibrator that she wasn't recognizing them. After thinking about this, she agreed, quite relieved by the possibility that there could be variety in her orgasms.

So, what is an orgasm? As a *physical event,* an orgasm is a discharge or release of physical and energetic arousal. It is a process that returns your body to a less-aroused or nonaroused state. But to describe orgasm simply as a physical event is much too limiting. Orgasm is potentially a *multidimensional experience* that can involve all of your senses, your imagination, and your emotions; it can evoke a spiritual dimension, and even more.

How Women Experience Orgasm

What words or images would you use to describe your own experiences of orgasm? If you know that you've never experienced orgasm—or if you're not sure—what do you imagine having an orgasm is like? Some women find it impossible to describe their orgasms. Others find themselves in the realm of verbal creativity.

In the interviews, typical descriptions of the experience of orgasm include perceptions of a peaking of intensity, a release, relaxation, and pleasure. For example, **Madeline (1915)** said, "Gosh, I don't know how to explain that. Just that it was a peak clitoral sensation of some kind. It didn't last very long for me. I don't have a series of orgasms." **Doris (1930)** said, "How do you describe something wonderful like that? It's a release, like an explosion. I feel it in the vagina and then the relaxation spreads over my whole body." **Chris (1970)** described it this way: "It feels like thousands of feathers rubbing all over you. And water exploding out. And butterflies dancing on your inside." **Jessica (1970)** said, "It's an emotional and physical release, a draining almost."

Tracy (1971) thinks of orgasm as "a little spot that just starts and then grows. And it's like little creatures in there that get really excited and start jumping around. And it just spreads. Generally, I can feel it right down through my toes. The orgasm itself is like an explosion of all my senses. It's like a little light that just sort of peeks through a hole. And then it just sort of starts erupting through the hole until there's this bright, brilliant, shining light that just warms up my entire body."

There is no right way to have an orgasm. In having an orgasm, you do not have to notice any one thing in particular. You do not have to be aware of a specific physical response, such as vaginal contractions. You don't even have to enjoy it. Experiences of orgasm might range—even for one woman—from, for example, *explosive releases* to *gentle rushes of warmth* or *sensations of tingling*. And your experiences and descriptions are valid, even if they aren't in any way like someone else's.

Variety in Orgasmic Experience

Is there variety in your orgasmic experiences? This is a question I specifically asked each of the women I interviewed. While some said, *No*, others, like **Pat (1945)**, described considerable variability. Her orgasms vary from "very much a pumping sensation" to "whole body ... an overall general feeling"; from "just a feeling of well-being" to "a very soft, rhythmic kind of thing." They vary in intensity from "like a wave washing over me" to "real hard, intense"; sometimes she feels her face contort. Sometimes, she wonders if she's orgasming "because it's so generalized" and she feels "release afterwards" but doesn't "actually feel the pumping." On those occasions, "It's very soft . . . feels good, very pleasurable. It's an overall feeling of well-being . . . a sense of release."

Donna (1949) contrasted her orgasms: "Some are stronger, some are weaker; . . . longer . . . shorter; exhausting . . . enlightening. Some days I have an orgasm and I'm ready to get up and go out and work. Other days I'm ready to crash." **Pam (1968)** differentiates between "surface orgasms and the really deep orgasms where my entire womb just shakes. The surface orgasms usually bring a lot of laughter and I know a lot of that is just discomfort and a lot of it happens when I'm being sexual with someone I don't know very well; sometimes when I'm trying to make light of a very intense situation."

Variety in Pathways to Orgasm

Thinking of sex as *creating mutual erotic pleasure* in whatever form that might take means, of course, that whether or not you want to have an orgasm during sex and how you might reach it are choices for you to make—not requirements for successful lovemaking.

Yet, as we saw in chapter 10, there have been cultural and medical establishments telling us for more than 100 years that there are *right ways* for women to experience their sexuality and to have orgasms—with the inference that, if there are right ways, then there must be wrong ways. As we saw in the previous chapter, there have been an ever-changing series of fads and new events in the women's division of the Orgasm Olympics—from vaginal, clitoral, simultaneous, and multiple orgasms to the more recent notion of female ejaculation.

Clearly, women's experiences of orgasm do vary. They vary even for the same woman from time to time. And, clearly, many of us have learned to think of our orgasms in language that describes them as being either *vaginal* or *clitoral*. I did find, however, that when comparing orgasms, many women talk more about the variety in the ones they have than about strong preferences for one way of having them over another. For **Cindi (1952)**, "There's a wide range. I like that sort of all-body sensation that an orgasm during intercourse gives me: that sense of huge tension and then relaxation as an all-body thing. But orgasms with clitoral stimulation are good, too, because they are really intense. They're very centered on the clitoris and nice in their own way."

Even two partners like Liz and Joanna may have quite different paths to orgasm and differences in the kinds of stimulation they enjoy. **Liz (1951)** said, "The more intense the orgasm is, the more I feel spent and relaxed afterwards. For me, orgasm has varied with different partners. With Joanna they're usually physically intense and very satisfying. With some women I dated in the past, I wouldn't come at all or the orgasm would be marginal, without real intensity. Penetration doesn't really do it for me. I need oral stimulation. Sometimes I come real hard and my whole body is into it. Sometimes it's just genital. The strongest intensity is usually after I've been able to satisfy my partner; that turns me on more than anything. If she does me first, it doesn't seem to be as strong as when I get her off first. My back is real sensitive; a couple of times I've had orgasm just from back stimulation—without any genital stimulation at all—or sometimes just from lying on her." **Joanna (1957)** said, "I don't think any of my orgasms are the same. If Liz takes her time and starts with my breasts or neck I can have a little orgasm, but I usually need her to penetrate. I like oral and I enjoy deep penetration with her hands. Sometimes I get an aching feeling for penetration. It takes me longer with her mouth than with her hand. The strongest climaxes now are when she does both, oral and hand penetration. I used to have a sensitive area in my vagina, I think the cervix, but not since I had a hysterectomy."

Crying and Laughing with Orgasm

Slightly over half of the Survey respondents had cried at least once during orgasm or had had crying released by an orgasm, with some respondents writing that they had had this kind of emotional release *lots, many,* or *hundreds* of times. Fewer respondents (41 percent) had laughed during or immediately after orgasm. As with crying, for some women laughter had occurred *many, countless,* or *thousands* of times. One woman claimed *zillions!*

It is rare to see a movie or television scene in which a woman's orgasm is accompanied by either tears or laughter. In fact, I can't remember ever seeing one. This is unfortunate because media role models are an important source of validation that an experience we may have happens to other people, too. Many of us don't know that the emotional releases we have associated with our orgasms are experiences we have in common with many other women. (Note that anger is another emotion that can be released by orgasm.)

The women I interviewed often identified their orgasmic tears as an intimate welling up of deep feeling; rarely did they associate these tears with sadness. **Carole (1930)** has "cried a few times and laughed a few times too. Crying with orgasm is just an incredible physical release and usually without any sexual imagery." Among the older women I interviewed others related: ♀ I cry because I feel so grateful for the experiences I'm having; ♀ Sometimes I'd laugh because it was such a fun release. I remember saying, *Geeze it's so good to feel this good*, and then crying because it was just so intimate, because of the emotions and intensity; ♀ It's crying in a passionate sense, like when you really feel close and it's the first time you're in synch or emotionally into this love thing. Younger women related: ♀ When I'm really satisfied or feel a really intense feeling of love, I can't help it, I just start to cry; ♀ Once, in the middle of intercourse I just burst into tears, not sad tears; it was just so beautiful and so emotional at that moment; ♀ I don't cry but I laugh a lot and sometimes I talk without being aware of it; it's like I enter another consciousness; once in a while my boyfriend has to cover my mouth to keep my screams and laughs down.

For another group of women, crying was a reflection of frustration: ♀ I usually cry only when I'm unhappy or frustrated with the relationship; ♀ I cried because I was almost there when my partner stopped; ♀ I've cried maybe thirty times from positive overwhelming emotion, and also a few times when I was upset during intercourse and there was no orgasm.

When I talk with a woman whose sexual feelings have been blocked for some time, I advise her that when she starts having sex again, she may find herself having crying orgasms. When the release occurs, tears may flow. For some women this never happens, for some it happens only once, and for others, many times.

Multiple Orgasms

Some women, some of the time, have more than one orgasm when they have sex. As we have seen, for most women orgasmic responsiveness tends to develop over time. And, because orgasm in partnered sex evolves out of the erotic dance of two people, orgasmic responsiveness can be quite different in different partnerships or at different stages of a relationship. The potential is there, but different histories, different partners, and different interests in sexual variety and experimentation all contribute to whether a woman is regularly or easily multiply orgasmic.

Experiences of multiple orgasms are quite variable. One woman might have two orgasms several minutes apart, for example, or a cluster bunched closely together. Another woman—or the same woman at another time—might reach a high plateau of sexual tension in which subtle stimulation generates gentle waves of peaking sensations and letting go that continue until she or her partner decides to stop. For the women who have them, multiple orgasms may occur often or only rarely.

Janine (1921) said, "When I was younger, I would have a vaginal orgasm with my partner and then I'd find myself going into more spasms for several minutes with his penis still inside. I also remember having one orgasm and then shortly after reinserting and having another." For Victoria (1946), there is "sort of a pulsing that happens, ten minutes, five minutes. Contracting and letting go, contracting and letting go. It's like I have an orgasm and then it goes down and then I have another one. It just happens. . . . He's still inside me, but he's not [actively] stimulating me. It's like I'm pulsating around his penis (it's fairly large)." Sharon (1962) goes "from one to the other and there's no real stopping point." Mindy (1965) said, "I've had multiple orgasms with men before, but never with Jody. Sometimes with a man I'll have an orgasm with oral stimulation and then another with intercourse after that." Mary (1972) reported, "Sometimes when I have four or five orgasms, the first one is nice and the last ones are almost continuous. It builds until my fingers and toes tingle. I can feel it in my teeth and hair."

In one variation of multiple orgasms, the biggest and most fulfilling orgasm is the last one. As Gloria (1944) explained: "It's like a buildup. You have little ones, little ones, and then the big crescendo. That's when I see stars." Emily's (1919) pattern is different: "For many years I would have one of these huge orgasms and after that I was genitally supersensitive and didn't want any more stimulation. Now I often build up to a big orgasm and then seem to have a whole bunch of them after. My pelvis just releases and releases. It's so marvelous that I laugh a lot and occasionally I cry."

Pat (1945) also experiences the clitoral sensitivity that some women have after some of their orgasms: "Typically, there's kind of a building process where I'll have one when we first start and then build to two or three, even five, with often a minute or two between them. I'm just getting more and more stimulated and then after a while I get so sensitive, its just *Don't touch me. I'm finished.*" This sensitivity is an experience women have in common with some men: the glans of a man's penis may be hypersensitive after some of his orgasms, too.

One way some women stimulate orgasm after orgasm is with a vibrator. With a vibrator, Carole (1930) "can have millions of them, but they're not as full." When **Pam (1968)** broke up with her girl-friend, she got together with a couple of friends and they bought vibrators: "That was a big thing, a liberating thing. I now know what it's like to have twenty-five orgasms in a night. It's mostly clitoral."

Factors That Facilitate Multiple Orgasms

As you may recall, a woman's most satisfying sexual experiences tend to be associated with feeling close to her partner before sex, feeling loved, knowing that her partner will provide the physical stimulation she needs, feeling really attuned with her partner during sex, and knowing that her partner accepts her desires, preferences, and responses (see chapter 9). These are very like the conditions that Kathy finds necessary if she is to have multiple orgasms. **Kathy (1949)** has had multiple orgasms with both women and men:

> My vaginal orgasms are always multiple orgasms. A sense of warmth and well-being comes over me in a wave. In ten seconds to a minute, another wave starts taking over and it'll be a little higher and the feeling will be even warmer and stronger, starting at the vagina and moving up. Where a clitoral climax sets off an explosion in my mind, this is more an emotional experience. Each wave might get stronger, then it might ebb a little bit but the waves just come and come and come. And, at some point, I can't take another wave, I've got to stop. There's not really a peak as there is with the clitoral climax, it's just a point where I've had enough and can't take anymore. When I stop, I feel complete—in bliss.
>
> I can't do this with everyone. My partner has to be really into me, into doing what they're doing. It's not any particular kind of stroking—fast or slow—as much as that my partner's being attentive to what's feeling good . . . like a mutual trance. I have to feel comfortable and really bonded with my partner, at least for that time, and my partner is really paying attention to my needs and what's making me feel good. If it's a man, he'll slow down and then he'll speed up, or he'll pull his cock out so just the head's in there for a little bit and tease me, and then he will thrust hard. He'll vary what's he's doing as a way of showing that he's doing more than just fuck, fuck, fuck. For me to have these orgasm waves, there has to be recognition of my

whole being, my whole body; my partner needs to kiss me throughout, a lot of that kind of thing has to be going on.

In addition to demonstrating how important it can be to feel really connected with your partner, Kathy gives us other information on how some couples might go about creating multiple orgasms. She and her partner don't just start out and go straight for orgasm, rather they tease; they vary their movements and the rhythms of intercourse in ways that allow their arousal to build in waves. The stimulation is intense and less intense, intense and less intense. Kathy and her partner kiss throughout, and each is attentive to what feels good to the other. They are absorbed in what seems like a mutual trance.

Lorraine's (1957) few experiences of multiple orgasms remind us that there are still other factors to consider. A woman's experiences of orgasmic release are also related to her own relaxation and health: "I've only had multiple orgasms a few times. I'm a tense high-strung person . . . clench my teeth in my sleep . . . I don't relax easily. And I have to be very relaxed to have an orgasm. Once, years ago, I had such a good orgasm with my husband, and multiple orgasms, that I cried because I'd never felt so good. And I rarely cry. It was such good sex I wanted to bottle it and keep it for later. We'd been married ten years and it was amazing to me that this could happen at this point in my life. It happened from nothing I could attribute it to either. What was the formula? Often my back tenses up after orgasm due to an old injury. I remember that this time it didn't. I was still relaxed and even though I'd orgasmed, I still wanted more stimulation."

Reactions to multiple orgasms are mixed. Not all women who have them regard them as the be-all and end-all of sexual pleasure. **Helena (1943)** has them about a third of the time, but, she said: "Having just one orgasm . . . is as satisfying as any multiple orgasm experience I've had." **Barb (1955)** finds two orgasms in a lovemaking session over several hours "so energy depleting" that she "can't imagine wanting more." And, although **Lisa (1970)** has had "a couple of orgasms during sex a few times," she concluded: "Having multiple orgasms is not really important to me, because after I've had one I usually don't care to have another. I'm usually pretty content at that point."

Orgasms from Nongenital Stimulation

Not all orgasms—not even all multiple orgasms—arise through genital stimulation. **Chris (1970)** recalled: "The best multiple orgasm I've had was with a partner. I have a real strong erogenous zone on my neck and in my ear, and he was kissing me there. I've also had them with oral sex." Women experience orgasms in a variety of ways that don't involve their genital area (clitoris, vagina, G-spot, anus) as the primary focus of stimulation or even being stimulated at all. There are, for example, orgasms primarily from kissing, breast-focused orgasms, and even orgasms that take place without any physical touching at all.

Breast-Focused Orgasms

One familiar variation of orgasms arising without genital touching occurs through breast-focused stimulation. **Deborah (1949)** and her partner call the orgasms she sometimes has from breast stimulation "*tittie-gasms.*" **Joanna (1957)** reported that she has very sensitive breasts and sometimes has a mini-orgasm "when Liz is playing with them—tugging on them, biting, sucking my nipples. But it's not fully satisfying," she said, "I still need more."

Although orgasms resulting from breast stimulation can happen at anytime in life, they may happen spontaneously when teenagers engage in exploratory petting. **Ronni (1955)** told me of an orgasm she had when she was in junior high school: "We were doing some heavy petting—mainly breast stimulation, nothing genital—and at the time I didn't recognize it as an orgasm. He kept telling me to calm down because he didn't know what was happening."

Not all women like breast stimulation, at least with their current partners. **Peg (1948)** is one of those: "He's convinced that I should get really turned on if he sucks on my breasts. But it doesn't do anything for me. You have to be down by my vagina."

Other Variations

When the circumstances are right, any part of our bodies can be eroticized and become the focus of orgasm. **Bobbie (1946)** said, "I used to feel like something was wrong with me because there are certain spots of my body, like behind my knees, that I can have orgasms with. I have to be relaxed and not tired and I have to like and feel safe with my partner. It's been amazing to me to find all these special little spots."

Orgasms Without Any Physical Stimulation

Clearly sexual orgasm does not require stimulation of any particular area of a woman's body. In fact, no body part has to be directly stimulated at all. Many Survey respondents have experienced an orgasm solely from mental/emotional stimulation—without *any* sexual touching and/or have awakened from sleep while having an orgasm induced by dreaming.

Dream Orgasms

More than 1,000 (40 percent) of the Survey respondents have awakened from sleep while having an orgasm from dreaming at some time. On their questionnaires nine women spontaneously mentioned that they had awakened from sleep experiencing their first orgasms. Because we did not specifically ask about that, I don't know how many more women in the Survey may have had their first orgasms in that manner. Several women recalled dream orgasms when they were quite young; one woman said she had had one "at age four or five."

Among the women I interviewed, women of all ages had something to say about having orgasms as they were waking from sleep. **Janine (1921)** said, "Once I woke up and was startled that I was having an orgasm. I was dreaming of my psychotherapist. He was an old man and didn't turn me on except during the dream." **Carole (1930)** occasionally has "orgasms in meditation and in dreams" and remembered "a couple of times when I had orgasms when I was between the waking and dreaming state, when I was dreaming something sexual." **Penny (1946)** thinks "It's so weird" that she wakes up having an orgasm: "I can feel it flooding my body. It feels real explosive. It's happened several times. I'd like it to happen more, it's really kind of cool." The first time it happened for **Marcy (1967)** she was in high school: "God, it's really strange, like a wet dream. I'll wake up in the middle of the night and I think my body actually starts to move like I'm having sex, and I wonder if my partner can notice. Something like that happens once a month or so."

When a woman doesn't have a sexual partner—or the partner she has is temporarily unavailable—erotic dreams are one of the ways her sexual needs can be met. When I interviewed her, **Gloria (1944)** was attending graduate school in California and her partner was working on the East Coast. She told me: "I guess I'm very lucky in that I have this wonderful body. Whenever I'm too needy, I have an orgasm. About once a month I have an erotic dream and wake up having an orgasm without doing anything. My body is doing it for me."

Awakening from sleep experiencing an orgasm is by no means an uncommon experience for women. The 40 percent of respondents in our Survey who had had at least one dream orgasm is very close to the 39 percent that Kinsey reported in 1953. Five percent of the women in his survey had had their first orgasms from *nocturnal dreams* (Kinsey, Pomeroy, Martin, et al. 1953).

Waking Orgasms Without Physical Stimulation

When my colleague Gina Ogden, author of *Women Who Love Sex* (1994), interviewed fifty women self-identified as *easily reaching orgasm* for her doctoral work in 1980, she found that 64 percent of these women said they were *able to experience orgasm "spontaneously" without any physical touch at all*. Later she and Beverly Whipple, the research scientist of G spot fame, invited women who could *generate sexual satisfaction just by thinking about it* to their physiology lab. There, they validated these women's accounts by taking a variety of physiological measurements while the orgasms were happening. There is no question that those orgasms were real ones. (This work is reported in *Women Who Love Sex* in chapter 5, "Thinking Off and Other Thoughts on Sexual Imagination.")

In our Survey, nearly 600 women (22 percent) had experienced an orgasm from mental/emotional stimulation—such as a fantasy, recalling a past experience, or reading—without at the same time touching themselves or being touched sexually.

For one of the women I interviewed, spontaneous orgasm was a response to puberty. When I asked **Penny (1946)** the circumstances of her first orgasm, she told me that when she was in high school she "was just exploding with sexual feelings. It would be spontaneous. I wouldn't even need to use my hands. I wouldn't even be touching myself genitally." Another Survey respondent was "at a chamber music concert, listening to music, not being touched physically; this happened once."

Spontaneous orgasm experiences often involve sexual fantasy and/or a trance-like state. This happened a few times for **Lou Ann (1944)**: "I wasn't touching myself in any way. It seemed like I was in a heavy trance. The usual touching wasn't necessary because I could imagine the stimulation. I wasn't masturbating. I was sort of in a half-awake, half-asleep state and thinking *Should I masturbate now? No, I don't want to*, just sort of thinking about it. And before I knew it, without ever touching myself, I had an orgasm."

For **Deborah (1949)** "It happened only once. I was driving to get my hair done and thinking about the first time I was with the man I was having an affair with, how exciting and erotic it was. I had a spontaneous orgasm in the car just with the fantasy of remembering. I liked that, and I even smiled thinking about how far I'd come since the day that old boyfriend had called me frigid!" Deborah's in-car orgasm was pleasant and benign. **Gretchen's (1949)** was disastrous! She said: "I can have an orgasm mentally, without touching myself, even with my clothes on. There's always a fantasy with it. I once got into an accident because I was fantasizing that this wonderful man I had seen loved me and I couldn't stop myself from mentally causing an orgasm. I crashed into another car, and it cost me $1,000. It was a very expensive orgasm!"

Connie (1956) had a spontaneous orgasm when she was thinking of someone real and nearby: "The first time it happened I was away with this fellow . . . totally platonic at that point. We had separate rooms, and he didn't even know I had the hots for him. I was lying in bed trying to go to sleep. I was imagining his body, the way he smelled and tasted, having sex with him, what his penis looked like, what he looked like . . . and I was so worked up that I felt like my body was floating above the floor. I got myself into such a state just thinking about it that I had an orgasm. I can still do that. I will lie in bed in the morning and start thinking about this man I like now. I'll get myself worked into an absolute frenzy. But if I touch myself, it won't happen."

There is tremendous variety in these experiences. One dramatic account, quite different from others I heard, comes from **Mary Jo (1947)**. After she told me that she has orgasms without physical stimulation, I asked her to describe the circumstances: "It can be anything. It's like just being excited about life. Recently I was camping with my lover and I was sitting in the tent, just enthralled, and it was just wonderful to be there with him and by the ocean. I love being outside and the wind was blowing and it was one of those magic moments. He was outside of the tent and I was in it with my back kind of turned to him and it was like something came out of the earth and I just had this huge, full body spontaneous orgasm and I went *Wow!*"

Mary Jo has spent a lot of time doing meditative breathing practices and learning to focus her attention in various ways. She has studied Tantric sex, an Eastern tradition in which sex is conceptualized as a meditative union, and she has explored some of the transpersonal aspects of sexual union with another. At times she and a lover have sought to create moments of communion and quiet bliss rather than physical orgasm by using such methods as synchronized breathing, sustained eye contact, and motionless intercourse without orgasm. These are all approaches to sex that might be of use to other couples who wish to enhance their sexual communion.

Simultaneous Orgasms

In selecting the factors that are usually or always present in their most satisfying sexual experiences with a partner, 39 percent of women in our Survey reported simultaneous orgasms (see chapter 9). Although my male co-researcher was quite surprised by this frequency, I was not. Partner sex involves, to varying degrees, the interaction of the minds, bodies, and emotions of two individuals.

Examples of the amazing ability of our bodies and energies to harmonize with those of others are everywhere, from a mother nursing her baby, to a church choir singing complex harmonies, to a volleyball player smoothly setting up a play for her teammate. Research has shown that activities as simple as reading aloud together can bring breathing, heartbeat, and even brainwaves into synchrony (Leonard 1984). It does not surprise me, then, that when couples join their bodies in shared sexual arousal they may experience a deep nonverbal resonance that swells into simultaneous orgasm. I have talked to many women whose partners' orgasms trigger their own. Some, for example, have described having orgasms while orally stimulating a partner's genitals, even when not receiving other direct physical stimulation themselves.

Vera (1940) attributed her simultaneous orgasms to her stable relationship: "It's so great when you have orgasm at the same time. It's real important and it's hard to accomplish unless you're in a relationship. That's the neat part about the stable relationship, that you know each other well enough to have mutual orgasms." But, as we know, there are tremendous variations in women's experiences. **Cheryl (1937)** is not in a stable relationship, and she only recently, while in her fifties, had her first simultaneous orgasm: "The man I was with was kneeling between my legs with his fingers inside me, and I had my vibrator on my clit while he masturbated and came on my stomach. This was the first time I ever tried doing what the books recommend—*having orgasms with your eyes open.* Which is wonderful! It was very intense. The first time I forced myself to do it. I said, *Why am I doing this? It's so uncomfortable. It's so weird.* But now I have a connection with this man that I'll have all my life even though we're not really compatible in terms of being really into a romance."

Facilitating Orgasm

Think for a moment: If you're orgasmic, what—if anything—do you do to facilitate the release of your orgasms? In the Survey, 2,371 women marked one or more items as applying to them from a list of fourteen we provided. Here is our list with the most frequently checked items selected first and the least frequently selected last. Each woman who answered the following question marked all items that applied to her.

> In addition to getting specific physical stimulation, I often have done the following to help me reach orgasm during sex with a partner . . .

Activity	N of ♀♀ doing it	% N=2,371
Positioned my body to get the stimulation I needed	2,145	90%
Paid attention to my physical sensations	1,960	83%
Tightened and released my pelvic muscles	1,780	75%
Synchronized the rhythm of my movements to my partner's	1,778	75%
Asked or encouraged my partner to do what I needed	1,756	74%
Got myself in a sexy mood beforehand	1,686	71%
Focused on my partner's pleasure	1,612	68%
Felt/thought how much I love my partner	1,548	65%
Engaged in a fantasy of my own	1,331	56%
Engaged in eye contact with my partner	1,080	46%
Engaged in a fantasy shared with my partner	777	33%
Detached from thinking about anything	758	32%

Synchronized my breathing to my partner's breathing	543	23%
Thought or imagined that I might become pregnant	272	11%

How to Increase Erotic Pleasure and Enhance Your Orgasms

So many women, born between 1916 and 1974, wrote in additional information about how they reach orgasm that I can present you with a smorgasbord of suggestions for increasing erotic pleasure and enhancing your orgasmic potential. I have put the respondents' comments into four categories: focus of attention; physical stimulation and techniques; the setting and other sensory enhancements; and communication and interaction with your partner.

Focus of Attention

There are many places you can focus your attention during sex. A woman may facilitate orgasm by paying attention to her physical sensations and pleasure, focusing on her partner's pleasure, feeling and thinking how much she loves her partner, engaging in a fantasy, detaching from thinking about anything, thinking or imagining that she might become pregnant, and more.

1. **Paying attention to physical sensations.** ♀ I totally focused on the sensations and touched myself with my partner in me; ♀ I focus on my physical pleasure; ♀ I concentrate on how I feel stimulation-wise, not emotionally. I think it is psychological. If you know you *can* have one and don't worry about it and just feel, it happens.

2. **Focusing attention on a particular idea or image.** ♀ I remember that I have a limited amount of time left to live and that I want to live it fully; ♀ I think about the act itself; ♀ I focus on my breathing or my mantra; ♀ I thought of and spiritually agreed to "give it up," to meld, become one with his spirit. During sex I feel propelled into an "otherworldly" experience or state—alone and with him; ♀ Sometimes I really watch what's going on.

3. **Focusing on orgasm itself.** ♀ I focus on the clock chiming, set a goal—orgasm before the clock strikes; ♀ I told myself I was capable and deserving of an orgasm; ♀ Sometimes I tell my body to start having an orgasm and it works.

4. **Focusing attention on an image of your partner.** ♀ I engaged in fantasy about his pleasure; ♀ I thought how much my partner loved me!; ♀ I noticed and appreciated how gorgeous and sensuous she is; ♀ I manually stimulated my own clitoris during rear-entry position with my partner, and I fantasized my partner saying erotic and/or loving things to me; ♀ I touched and caressed my partner's body, watched my partner's body movement; I thought of how intense or close my partner and I are.

5. **Fantasizing being with someone else.** ♀ I fantasized about another partner; ♀ I thought of other people; ♀ I fantasized about a more satisfying partner.

6. **Fantasies and images with a variety of other themes.** ♀ I pretend I'm someone else, e.g., a prostitute; ♀ I fantasized that *I* was the male with another woman; ♀ I fantasized we are married; ♀ I remembered previously satisfying sex, used "sexy" language and moaning; ♀ I created and/or saw images in my mind—not fantasies, but images—like the Amazon River; ♀ I visualize male ejaculation; ♀ I imagined my clitoris was a penis; ♀ I speak to myself sometimes using swear words like "fucking."

    You and your partner might also think of your bodies as like musical instruments through which you can create erotic pleasure. When you are with an attentive lover who is sensitively *playing* your body, you might be playing his or hers, too, or just doing nothing but experiencing what is happening. The feelings are there, the sensations build, the intensity builds, you don't have to do anything but experience them. And, at some point, some kind of energetic waves get going—or there is an intense release—or something else happens. Sometimes your partner may come into synchrony with you and therefore know what you are feeling because he or she is feeling it, too. Usually, this experience requires a partner with whom you feel open and safe.

7. **Detaching from thinking about anything.** ♀ I don't worry about having an orgasm; I just have fun; ♀ I deliberately stop thinking about distracting things, like work, etc.; ♀ I let go and floated; ♀ I lay still and close my eyes to close out

other distractions; ♀ I get into total quiet and rhythmic sensational movement.

8. **Focusing on and accepting whatever feelings are taking place.** Emotional responses—even anger and frustration—can facilitate orgasm: ♀ I stimulate myself sometimes due to longing for male companionship, relationship, and sex. Sometimes in my loneliness and frustration I feel angry and I notice that I'm more easily aroused when I'm angry. This happens when I'm with a sex partner, too: say, he's been stimulating my clitoris with his finger and he can't seem to either find the *right spot* or stay in the *right spot* once he's gotten to it, and I've almost reached orgasm once or twice; I become impatient and angry with him and/or myself and that sudden surge of anger produces a surge of increased stimulation, sometimes bringing me to the longed-for orgasm.

9. **Imagining becoming pregnant.** One very specific image is a woman's thought or image that she might become pregnant. Although this image of fertility-in-the-sexual-moment was the least marked facilitator of orgasm, it still was circled by women ranging in age from nineteen to eighty-four, about one in ten of all the women who completed the Survey. A woman who had come to the end of her childbearing years wrote: "I used to imagine often that I might become pregnant," and a younger woman said: "I thought of this a couple of times in the last two months." This choice, on the other hand, definitely generated some strong reactions from those who did *not* facilitate orgasm by imagining that they might become pregnant: ♀ Good grief *No!*; ♀ *Never*; ♀ That would end the fun!; ♀ Surest way to prevent orgasm!! Eek!

Shift Your Attention from Performance to Pleasure

Sometimes right in the middle of having sex your attention may shift to: *How am I doing? Am I going to make it?* When that happens, you might consciously turn—or return—your attention to one of the images suggested here or to the question: *Am I enjoying what's happening right this moment?* If the answer is *Yes*, continue to pay attention to the pleasure you are feeling. If the answer is *No*, then consider: *What do I need to change—or ask my partner to change—so I can enjoy this? Or, do I want to stop?*

Physical Stimulation and Various Techniques

1. **Various specific kinds of stimulation** that helped them to reach orgasm during sex with a partner were described by women of all ages: ♀ Manual stimulation from my partner; ♀ Cunnilingus; ♀ Clitoral stimulation—always; ♀ I touched my nipples or his or other erotic areas: neck, inner thigh, hot tease spots, etc.; ♀ Touched breasts; ♀ Mutual body massage; ♀ Oral sex!; ♀ I imagine entering her while giving oral stimulation; ♀ We used videos, massage oil, oral stimulation; ♀ I kissed my partner; ♀ I held my partner as closely as I could.

2. **Stimulating yourself during sex with a partner** can enhance pleasure and is one way to get the clitoral stimulation that many women find necessary in order to reach orgasm: ♀ Self-stimulation during intercourse results in stronger orgasms; ♀ Essentially I wasn't orgasmic with a partner until I started to feel comfortable using my own hand; ♀ I masturbated to finish; ♀ I stimulated my clitoris or nipple; ♀ I stimulated myself with both my partner's hand and my hand together; ♀ I masturbated during oral sex (which my partner approved of); ♀ I masturbate while he is inside me.

   Another variation is **stimulating yourself as your partner watches:** ♀ I did what I needed while my husband watched; ♀ I masturbated in front of her to show her what I wanted.

   Judith (1940), though, finds that sometimes, during the deeper sensations of intercourse, she does not want the sensations of direct clitoral stimulation. She also demonstrates that the experience of orgasm can change over time: "I like clitoral stimulation and I like vaginal stimulation with intercourse. From a man I want one or the other, but not both at the same time. If he's using his hand, I do like having his finger in my vagina. But not the penis and hand at the same time. In the last two years, my orgasms have been changing. Clitoral orgasms were easy for me to have. Intercourse orgasms are new . . . developing. I feel them deeper inside of me, more in my whole body; and they last longer. Orgasms before didn't come up as high; they were shallower, less satisfying."

3. **Using a vibrator or sex toys** in their partnered sex was mentioned by women of all ages: ♀ We used a vibrator; ♀ . . . a

vibrator during intercourse; ♀ I can only have a full blown orgasm using a vibrator; ♀ . . . a dildo and a vibrator—sex toys!!

4. **Tightening and releasing different muscles than those of the pelvis** were mentioned by some women. (The Survey list included *tightened and released my pelvic muscles*.): ♀ I tighten my thigh muscles with my legs raised about a foot off the bed; ♀ I tense all the muscles of the body; ♀ I relaxed *and* tensed—both can work; ♀ I tightened and released my leg muscles; ♀ I tightened and released my buttocks; ♀ I rock my pelvis.

5. **Breathing and relaxation techniques:** ♀ I position a pillow under my hips, use Tantric exercises, use rebirthing breathing; ♀ I breathed deeply and meditated before sex; ♀ I engaged in relaxing physical exercise, yoga; or, sometimes, I've been physically challenged—e.g., by scuba diving, etc.; both relaxation and activities like scuba diving facilitate orgasm for me; ♀ I relaxed beforehand; ♀ I take a shower or bath alone first.

The Setting and Other Sensory Enhancements

The context in which a sexual episode occurs can facilitate arousal, pleasure, and orgasm. Some couples use music, special clothing, and other sensory enhancements; some have favorite settings: ♀ We take the phone off the hook, have a glass of wine; ♀ We smoked marijuana; ♀ I ask my partner to wear specific items of clothing when coming to my house; ♀ We use music, smells, etc.; ♀ We drink alcohol; ♀ I wear lingerie and have my husband wear sexy male stuff; ♀ Our mutual favorite is making love outdoors in the sunshine at a state park when we know we'll not be discovered; ♀ We use candles, music, massage each other; ♀ We've gotten stoned.

Communication and Interaction with Your Partner

Women also can facilitate orgasm by communicating and interacting with their partners in a variety of ways.

1. Some did this by **asking or encouraging a partner to do what she needed:** ♀ I encouraged him to ask me to do what he needed also; ♀ I told him at the beginning of our sexual life together; now he knows; ♀ I demanded what I needed; ♀ I guided my partner's hand to where I'd like to be touched.

2. **Focusing attention on her partner** was noted by other women as a way to facilitate or enhance their own orgasms: ♀ I touch and caress my partner; ♀ I stimulated my partner so that she could orgasm with me. Incredible!!; ♀ I've done what my partner desired, requested or enjoyed; ♀ I focused on his impending orgasm; ♀ I encouraged my partner with my hands; ♀ I'd be submissive; ♀ I encourage her to feel sexy; ♀ I engage in eye contact often, but only to *enhance* the experience of orgasm, *not* to help me *reach* it; ♀ I asked his desires; ♀ I watched my partner's response; ♀ I teased my partner throughout the day with sexy talk; ♀ I did things that were pleasurable to him; ♀ I make my partner happy.

3. **Talking or making sounds during sexual activity** was mentioned by women ranging in age from twenty to seventy: ♀ I express my pleasure; ♀ I say my partner's name; ♀ I say "I love you" over and over; ♀ I yell out to express my pleasure.

4. **Talking about sensations or feelings of the moment** was another orgasm facilitator: ♀ I verbalize my sensations to my partner; ♀ My partner talks to me about how he feels or what about my body is turning him on; ♀ We are open about asking each other about our needs; ♀ We talk about what we are feeling; ♀ I ask my partner to share erotic fantasies about us while engaged in sex.

5. **Using intimate talk to reestablish contact and build trust was also mentioned:** ♀ We talked before sex to build trust; ♀ We had a long intimate talk (not fantasizing) before we began touching; ♀ Foreplay included talking about how we care about each other. A woman who is in a long-distance relationship wrote: "We discuss how much time has gone by since we last engaged in intercourse together and discuss how enjoyable the experience is." And some exchanges are nonverbal: ♀ We always laugh!; ♀ We made noises.

6. **Talking dirty** is another variation: ♀ My partner and I become very excited when we "talk dirty" to each other; ♀ I talked dirty and had him talk dirty to me; ♀ We talked "nasty"; ♀ I like very specific "dirty" talk from my partner.

7. **Sharing images of erotica, pornography, and other arousal enhancers** with a partner was mentioned by women of all ages: ♀ I read other people's fantasies with my partner; ♀ We read from *Playboy*; ♀ We watched naked bodies of women—erotic scenes; ♀ We've used magazines, movies; masturbated; gone to new places; parked after years of marriage; ♀ We watch sexy videos, drink, get high; ♀ We role played; I caressed myself, masturbated in my partner's presence; we ate foods before sex that we found enticing, watched porno, took pictures of each other, etc.

Clearly, women have many different ways of finding their way to orgasmic release. There is no one right way; there are a multitude of ways. What we see demonstrated here again is the uniqueness of each sexual self. What arouses one woman—for instance, imagining becoming pregnant or sharing fantasies—can turn another totally off.

Women Who Are Not Experiencing Orgasm

Among our Survey respondents, thirty-eight women said they've never had an orgasm, and another ninety-five weren't sure. (Of 2,471 women, 95 percent had experienced orgasm at least once in their lives; of these, 160 women had reached orgasm alone, but not with a partner.)

Among those who had partnered sex in the last year, 25 percent experienced *difficulty in reaching orgasm* and 17 percent experienced *inability to have an orgasm* all or most of the times they had sex. Of the orgasmic women who had engaged in partnered sex in the preceding three months, 30 percent were not satisfied with the frequency of their orgasms with their partners.

Orgasm Difficulties of Older Women

For postmenopausal women who are not on hormone replacement, the absence of estrogen can radically diminish the potential ability of the vaginal tissues for engorgement; consequently, this makes it more difficult to create orgasm. In addition, certain medications may make orgasm practically impossible for *some* of the women (of any age) who take them. Many of the drugs prescribed for depression such as Anaframil, Prozac, Paxil, Zoloft, Trazadone, and Effexor may have severe inhibitory effects on orgasm for some; many of these also take away sexual desire. Antianxiety medications such as Xanax, Klonopin, Valium, and Ativan may inhibit orgasms, although paradoxically they enhance the orgasmic response of some women. We are not all the same. Heart medications, antihypertensive medications, and other relaxants can also inhibit orgasm and sexual desire. With respect to sexual responsiveness, BuSpar may be a better choice for treating anxiety than those drugs listed above; Wellbutrin may be a better choice for treating depression. If you are having sexual problems that may be due to taking medications, consult a physician knowledgeable about the sexual side effects of medications and ask whether other drugs—or no drugs at all—might be better for you (Crenshaw and Goldberg 1996; Goldstein 1996).

An older woman with a male partner is likely to be with a man whose arousal and erections are not what they once were; this factor, too, may make it more difficult for her to reach orgasm. Survey notes from women over seventy included the following: ♀ I'm embarrassed to admit the lack of orgasm; ♀ I do all of the above (suggestions on the list) but no results. Younger women on birth control pills also experience diminished orgasmic potential if their pills do not provide as much estrogen as their bodies need.

Imagery for Learning to Become Orgasmic

The following is an adaptation of guided imagery used by my teacher, Richard Olney, who developed Self-Acceptance Training.

You might want to record it, so that you can listen to the words when you are relaxed, with your eyes closed. Or you might want to listen to someone else slowly read the words aloud.

> Listen to my words. As you approach orgasm, don't let yourself go too fast. Hold on, let go, hold on, let go—like that. Don't let go any more than feels safe. It's like swimming—or walking down—or up—a staircase. It's not necessary to try. Your body is capable of so many things. These body signals can have a new and joyous meaning to you now.
>
> Stop worrying about having an orgasm. Instead, often imagine yourself experiencing orgasm. Don't go toward or into the orgasm all at one time. Go only in little tiny steps you can control—like going down a staircase toward a bottom door beyond which everything is bright and cheerful. Go down these steps pausing to feel comfortable—

pausing to know you are only going to go one little step more. And in no circumstances go beyond the step on which you feel comfortable. If the steps are one to ten, and if the level where you feel comfortable ends at five, go to four. If it ends at eight, go to seven. This way you won't go beyond the point where you feel secure and you can feel comfortable—and you can feel so secure and comfortable doing it that way that you can forget about yourself if you want to. At no point are you going to take a deep plunge. You'll move to your orgasm step by step as you choose to move.

Put these three things aside: panic, critical judgment, and self-consciousness. So, you don't have to hold yourself back from pleasure of any kind anymore. Every day it will be easier and easier—not to be overcome—but to choose to surrender yourself to pleasure. [Pause] Are you aware of the power you have—the power that only you have—to enter into this experience. Only you have the choice—I have only one power—to point it out to you. You can get to orgasm if you just don't give a darn.

We have seen that learning about the responsiveness of one's body and how to create an orgasm by oneself and with a partner is a process that takes place over time. We continue to learn, change, and adapt throughout our lives. We also have seen that erotic pleasure and orgasm with a partner depend on a great deal more than where or what is stimulated; they depend particularly upon the qualities of one's partner and relationship. With a compatible, involved partner, visual impressions, mutual sounds, shared emotions, the rhythms created by giving and receiving touch, and the mutual building and movement of sexual energy all may become at least as important to the release of orgasm as the physical stimulation of any particular part of a woman's body.

If you want to experience orgasm for the first time, more easily, or differently, you may find useful suggestions in the intergenerational smorgasbord of suggestions above. There, and in the narratives throughout this chapter and earlier ones, are many suggestions for enhancing erotic pleasure and realizing your orgasmic potential. You may want to focus your attention in new ways; experiment with variety in physical stimulation, including, perhaps, stimulating some area of your own body when you are with your partner; acquire a sex toy or other enhancers; have sex in new settings; and explore new behaviors with your partner.

There is a great variety in women's orgasmic experiences. Any absolute standard about orgasm—that a certain kind, or number, or way is better than another—simply denies the truth of the incredible and wonderful variety in the ways women do experience orgasm—or not—and the multitude of ways they enjoy sexual activity in all of its wondrous forms.

What Does This Mean to You?

Now, if you wish, pick up your notebook and express the thoughts and feelings you're having about your experiences of orgasm. Here are some questions you might want to consider after you've done that.

- Is there variety in your orgasmic experiences? If so, how would you describe the variations?

- Is there any way your orgasmic experiences could be enhanced? If so, how might that occur?

- Is there anything in this chapter you would like to incorporate into your own solo or partnered lovemaking? If so, what?

- If you are recalling experiences that you now regret, consider the circumstances, the roles of others, and how you saw your options at the time. Then, sit quietly with your eyes closed and imagine what you could now gently and lovingly tell your younger self that would be healing and would lead to greater self-acceptance.

12

Sexual Concerns and Problems of American Women

In media sex, everything goes smoothly and perfectly. Bodies are picture perfect, no one is too tired or hassled for sex, no one is distracted, no one has trouble getting aroused, and everyone has a wonderful, passionate time. Many of us—often without even being aware of it—take these portrayals of sex as how sex should be and we judge ourselves by them. We know that Hollywood movies and novel writers exaggerate, but still we secretly think that the real-life sex other people are having is, if not that dramatic and passionate, at least close. Even when we don't take these portrayals completely seriously, we may feel inadequate or think we're not *normal* when our bodies or our orgasms don't match those we read about or see in the movies.

We can't help being influenced by media sex, because up to recently, most of us have had so little with which to compare it. Few of us have had access to information about what *really* goes on in other people's bedrooms or what concerns them about their sexuality and sex lives.

What *Actually* Happens When Real People Have Sex?

What is typical in the sex lives of contemporary American women? Seeking to answer that question, my Survey co-author and I presented the following list of twenty-three sexual circumstances to those Survey respondents who'd had a sexual partner in the previous year. We asked them to tell us which of these experiences was true for them and how often. Here is an opportunity for you to consider these sexual circumstances in your own life.

Forms of Sexual Expression

These are some aspects of sexual expression you may have experienced in the past year. Think about how often each of the following took place in your experience: *not at all, rarely, sometimes, often,* or *all the time.*

You will probably find that some of the items on the list do not match your experience. If your partner is a woman, for example, the items about a male partner's responses will not apply to you. Consider the items that pertain only to your own experiences and disregard the rest.

If you wish to write in your answers, you can use RAR for *rarely,* ST for *sometimes,* OF for *often,* and ALL for *all of the time.* Leave those items you did not experience in the past year unmarked.

I have experienced the following in the last year:

_____ Difficulty finding a partner I wanted to be sexual with

_____ Lower sexual desire than I wanted to have

_____ Being too tired to have sex

_____ Being too busy to have sex

_____ Not feeling sexually satisfied

_____ My partner not as interested in sex as I was

_____ My partner less interested in closeness after sex than I

_____ My partner choosing inconvenient times for sex

During sex in the last year I have experienced:

_____ Difficulty getting excited/aroused

_____ Feeling distracted

_____ Inability to relax

_____ Involuntary vaginal spasm so that vaginal entry and/or intercourse was impossible or difficult

_____ Inadequate vaginal lubrication

_____ Pain during intercourse or other internal stimulation

_____ Fantasizing that I am having sex with someone other than my partner

_____ Difficulty in reaching orgasm

_____ Inability to have an orgasm

_____ Reaching orgasm too quickly

_____ My partner seeming distracted

_____ My partner wanting shorter foreplay than I wanted

_____ My partner having difficulty getting aroused

_____ My partner ejaculating too quickly

_____ My partner having difficulty getting and/or maintaining an erection

_____ Other (specify): _____

From now on, when I refer to this list, I will call it the *Overview List*.

The Experiences

These events on the *Overview List* are a part of life! If you experienced at least one of them *sometimes, often,* or *all the time,* you are not alone. Of the 2,295 Survey respondents with a previous year sex partner, 98.6 percent checked at least one. Almost everyone experiences one or more of these events at some time or another. If we omit *sometimes,* 72 percent of the Survey respondents had experienced at least one *often* or *all the time.*

Problems—or "Just How It Is"?

If you've experienced any of the items on the list, consider: Which of these do you think of as *"problems"*? Which do you think of as "just the way life is"?

Just How It Is

Many of us seem to accept the realities and imperfections of our sex lives—at least up to a point. Depending on the item, from 50 percent to virtually 90 percent of those who had had a particular experience concluded: *That's the way life is* rather than *This is a problem.* No one item was called a problem by more than half of the women who'd had it happen at all, whether *sometimes* or more frequently.

However, there were six circumstances that were more likely than the others to be considered problems, even if they were experienced only *sometimes.* I call these *The Big Six.* You'll find more about these events that are perceived as problems later in this chapter.

Most Important Sexual Concerns and Problems in the Past Year

The Survey demonstrated that women across a wide spectrum of educational and economic backgrounds and life circumstances have similar sexual concerns and problems, although some issues—particularly those related to fertility, physical responsiveness, and health—tend to vary with age. The table that follows categorizes the responses of the 1,637 women who reported a most important concern or problem. There were 547 others who reported having *no* important sexual problem or concern in the previous year.

Problem or Concern Category	N of ♀♀	% N = 1,637
Desire/frequency	555	34%
Physical responsiveness	469	28.5%
Lovemaking	261	16%
Finding a partner	123	7.5%
Relationship	71	4%
Fertility/reproduction	45	3%
STDs/safe sex	37	2%
Her own body/health	31	2%
Miscellaneous—abuse, nonmonogamy, orientation, other	45	3%

Think for a moment: What was your most important sexual problem or concern in the past year? If you were to rank this on a scale of one to seven, with seven as a serious problem, and one as a slight concern, where would your problem be on this scale?

Issues of Desire and Frequency: The American Way of Life?

Did you mark at least one of these on the *Overview List: being too tired to have sex, being too busy,* and *lower sexual desire than I wanted to have*? It may not surprise you that these were the three most marked items on the list. There is no doubt that these are typical experiences of today's American women.

Selected by 555 women, the Desire and Frequency category—those three items plus one not included on the *Overview List: the woman and her partner having different levels of sexual desire and interest*—also led the more specific list of Most Important Sexual Concerns and Problems. One out of three of the women with a most important concern or problem reported an issue from this category.

Too Tired/Too Busy

Although *being too tired to have sex* and *being too busy to have sex* were the items selected most often from the *Overview List,* they were not among the experiences *most likely* to be considered problems when they occurred. In fact, they were among those most likely to be considered as *just the way life is.*

Being too tired and/or too busy for sex at least *sometimes* is a part of the American way of life that many of us take pretty much for granted. Often both a woman and her partner are affected. Women in their forties and early fifties commented: ♀ We're too tired *and* too busy. We both have to work many weekends currently, not ideal at our age, but imperative if we want any kind of future security; ♀ Lack of sex is due to exhaustion on both our parts. We are coming to terms with the fact we're older, work two full-time jobs, and are actively involved in our three young children's lives.

Younger women mentioned parenting and attending school: ♀ Difficulty juggling—balancing—being a parent, a worker, time for myself, my relationship and my sexuality; ♀ Grad school overwhelmed me! Over the summer our sex *almost* returned to normal. Since I returned to school in September, we've been having less "success" again.

Sound familiar? In these comments we see clear examples of what I call *role fragmentation*: one woman filling many roles, any one of which might be a full-time job if she hired someone else to do it. And many of us come to these roles with high standards. We want to do them well. We want to be good at our career, homemaking, parenting, companionship, physical fitness, spiritual practices, love making, and more. Plus we want time to read a good novel, get our hair cut, and do our nails. Is all this humanly possible? Role fragmentation is a part of the American way of life. Where is the energy and attention to come from for sexual desire?

Suggestion. Think of your time and energy as limited resources and think about how you want to allot them to the roles you fill. Develop a *Time Budget*. List the hours of the day and block in the activities that have to fill them. Don't forget to budget time for fun and pleasure.

For greater *self-acceptance*, repeat this statement at least once a day, more if you're feeling overwhelmed: *I can't do it all; my best is good enough.*

Lower Sexual Desire Than I Wanted to Have

Having *lower desire than I wanted* was more likely to be considered a problem than being too tired or too busy. Some respondents, however, specifically voiced their acceptance of their low desire for sex or noted that the role of sexuality in their lives was changing. One woman, around age fifty, explained: ♀ I no longer feel my low desire is a "problem" or "something wrong with me" but a path to a new way of being sexual. My partner and I are experimenting with sex that is not goal (orgasm) oriented. We are currently having a moratorium from sex while looking for ways to be stimulated from within rather than externally.

Some women of reproductive age noted a link between diminished desire and taking birth control pills. Other respondents mentioned its link to grief and loss, and to anger and resentment. One noted: ♀ I'm too tired for sex and resentful about housework. I need a full time *maid*!

Absence of sexual desire affects women of all ages. A young woman in her twenties noted, for example: ♀ I don't really want sex. This example actually may not be about absence of desire, *per se*, but perhaps a lack of interest or consent. A woman may have sexual feelings but she may not see having sex as fitting into her life.

Sexual desire is a combination of sexual *interest*—the idea you would like to have sex—and some physical arousal or urgency—not necessarily genital. Sexual desire is hunger—or like hunger—but hunger that seeks sexual experience rather than food.

Sexual Interest

Sexual interest, on the other hand, does not always include lustful, romantic, or even specifically sexual or erotic thoughts. Sexual interest could be, for example, the idea, without any genital excitement: "I would like to have sex because we haven't made love for a while; if we have sex we'll feel closer and be nicer to each other." Although sexual interest may occur without sexual arousal or genital excitement, it also can lead to those feelings and generate desire. I often tell couples: *Interest is all you need to start*. You will find more about how interest can build to desire in chapter 13.

Some women of various ages described problems and concerns that perhaps reflected more a loss of interest than lack of desire: ♀ Both of us have lost interest in intercourse; ♀ My husband and I aren't close emotionally; therefore sex is rare; ♀ ... We've gradually changed our relationship over the past year to a more platonic one ... we've "moved on"; ♀ I haven't been wanting to be with my primary partner in a sexual way. I am bisexual; I have two male and one female partners.

Sexual Arousability

Sexual arousability is the potential to respond physically and mentally to sexual cues. Most of us experience our arousability as regular, ongoing, transitory awareness of sexual feelings, sexual thoughts, and/or sexual fantasies. Sexual arousability is hormonally based and, in a woman, is maintained by androgens, principally testosterone, which are manufactured in her adrenal glands and ovaries. These hormones are needed for the ability to generate spontaneous sexual imagery and, along with estrogen, for such physical changes of sexual arousal as vaginal engorgement to take place. They are essential precursors of sexual desire. Arousability can be affected by such factors as health, stress, the phases of our fertility cycles, menopause, medications, and other drugs, including birth control pills.

Over the years I have been consulted by women who were interested in having sex and yet were extremely frustrated because they had absolutely no sexual desire and couldn't seem to get turned on. I recall one woman who had thoroughly enjoyed sex in the past, yet could not recall any recent sexual imagery or fantasies. In my therapist's role of sexual detective, this was a sign to me that she might be missing the hormones she needs for arousability. In fact, in this instance, it did turn out that, as a result of a recent hysterectomy that had affected her ovaries, she was indeed no longer producing these hormones. Hormone replacement was very helpful for her.

262 — Women's Sexualities

When appropriate, I make referrals to a physician who is very knowledgeable about hormones and their biological precursors. She prefers to prescribe the more natural hormones and is experienced and highly skillful in the fine art of hormone balancing and replacement for both women and men. I am fortunate that she is nearby.

If you are considering hormone replacement, inform yourself about the importance of balancing the various hormones your body produces. Also investigate the difference between your various options. The frequently prescribed Premarin, for example, is extracted from pregnant mares' urine, and "isn't exactly the same as human estrogen" (Wright and Morgenthaler 1997). Provera is a progestogen or progestin, i.e., an *artificial* progesterone, not the progesterone that the human body makes; certain molecules have been changed. These changes may lead to side effects, possibly even serious ones, not caused by "natural" progesterone. The good news is that replacement hormones biochemically identical to those produced by women's bodies are available, although some medical professionals are just learning about them. These are the hormones often labeled as "natural," although they also are synthesized in a laboratory. "Natural" progesterone is now available as Prometrium®; "natural" estrogens are available by prescription from compounding pharmacies. For more information, I refer you to the Wright and Morgenthaler book cited here and the books of Gillian Ford (see the References).

A Sexual Detective Considers Low Sexual Desire

In my sex therapist roles of detective and problem solver, I recognize that a lower desire for sex than someone wants is not just one simple condition that is the same for all; low sexual desire can be arrived at by many different paths and often reflects a complex combination of factors. If you are currently experiencing less sexual desire than you want, consider the following factors:

- When and under what circumstances did you first notice you had lower sexual desire than you wanted?

- Is there anything related to your health that may be affecting your sexual desire?

- Do you eat well and regularly? Do you get enough sleep?

- Are you experiencing any health problems?

- Do you experience chronic pain? If so, when is it most intense? Least bothersome?

- What birth control pills, medications, vitamins, and/or herbal preparations do you take?

- Do you smoke cigarettes, drink alcohol, coffee, and/or use other recreational drugs? If so, how many (much)? How often? Under what circumstances?

- Do you eat sweets and/or drink soft drinks? If so, how many (much)?

- Are you depressed? If so, how often? Under what circumstances?

- Are you resentful or angry at your partner?

- Are you sometimes not truly consenting when you have sex with your partner?

- Are you concerned that you might become pregnant or are you trying to get pregnant?

- Are you concerned that you might acquire a sexually transmitted disease?

- Do you get enough time for yourself?

- Are you protecting your relationship in some way by not having sex?

- Is your partner a skillful/satisfying lover? Is there something you would like your partner to know about his/her lovemaking?

- Are you and your partner effective together at initiating sex? If not, what happens when you initiate? When your partner initiates? Why do you think you get off the track?

- Do you have a history of sexual abuse or trauma that you believe is affecting you now? In what ways?

- What pressures and demands do you have in your life outside of your relationship?

Usually the answers to these questions will deepen your understanding of your sexual desire and suggest changes that might begin to enhance it. Desire is likely to be optimum when you are in emotional harmony with your partner and are yourself physically, mentally, emotionally, and spiritually in balance.

You may be wondering why I ask about such things as soft drinks, sugar intake, cigarettes, and alcohol. Excessive use of any of these can lead to circulatory and hormonal effects that inhibit sexual desire; it also indicates that you are probably not at the moment physically in balance. Excessive use could also be an indication that you have other mental, emotional, and/or spiritual concerns. If you are experiencing sexual difficulties of any kind, it may be helpful, once you have completed this list, to discuss it with a psychotherapist or physician who specializes in sexual issues.

Desire Discrepancy

For each of us, sexual desire has a personal ebb and flow that varies in accord with our unique rhythms. Each sexual relationship also has its own ebb and flow of sexual desire that is specific to that partnership. A couple's individual rhythms may more or less synchronize, or there may be a discrepancy in which one partner seems to desire noticeably more or less sex than the other. Over 100 Survey women specifically indicated that their major problem or concern was that *they wanted more sex than their partners did.* Their partners either were avoiding sex or were not as interested as they were.

It is noteworthy that many of the comments in this section were from the over-forty age group. As men grow older, their bodies gradually tend to produce less testosterone, the hormone that predominantly supports their arousability. There is, however, some evidence that a man's testosterone production increases when he feels like "a winner," but that other hormones that are antagonistic to testosterone become elevated when he feels defeated (Hollis 1996). I find this possibility quite provocative. It suggests to me that having sources of recognition and self-esteem and a sense of purpose in retirement, or at anytime in one's life, can help to maintain sexual arousability and interest for both women and men.

One group of women, who ranged in age from about forty to sixty, described male partners who avoided sex, were less interested in closeness after sex, and had difficulty getting aroused; some men also had experienced delayed ejaculation. In general, these women felt quite strongly about their partners' unavailability for as much sex as they would like: ♀ I'm not feeling sexually satisfied because of *not* doing it. Lack of sex and lack of my husband's interest are *major problems!!;* ♀ My husband works too many hours—he's always tired.

There's not enough sex and not enough romance in our marriage. I need more kissing and hugs before sex; ♀ I'm extremely frustrated that my husband doesn't enjoy sex as much as I'd like him to and that he can "take it or leave it." Some younger women also had similar complaints.

Some women had implemented or were seeking a variety of solutions. Here are some examples: ♀ I tease, beg, cajole, play, excite, massage, etc., to get his attention and instigate more sex. Other solutions mentioned included writing her partner a letter, recognizing the cyclical nature of a female partner's diminished interest in sex, seeing a therapist, and getting another partner in addition to the one she had.

A few women for whom discrepancy in sexual desire was a major problem—or perhaps embedded in more extensive relationship problems—found a resolution in ending their relationships. Sometimes it is not clear which came first, relationship problems or the sexual problem: ♀ My partner lost interest in all sex. We have divorced and I have had sex with three other partners in the last three months; ♀ My partner was not as interested in sex as I was—but it wasn't a problem. I just got upset and left him. It was bullshit and a control game.

Cultural myth tells us that it is men who want sex all the time and women who aren't all that interested. In the Survey, however, while more than 100 women reported their most important problem or concern as their partners *not as interested in sex* as they were, it was a much smaller number, ranging across the age spectrum, who said their problem or concern was *a partner with greater interest*. I should mention, however, that the Survey *Overview List* included *My partner not as interested in sex as I was* as one of the circumstances that could be checked off, while a woman would have had to write in that her partner was *more interested in sex than she.*

If a woman whose partner was not as interested in sex as she was were to see me for sex therapy, I would put on my sexual detective hat. If her partner were along, I would ask the partner: *Do you consent to engage in sexual activity with her?* If she were seeing me by herself, I would ask her to consider: *Does your partner consent to engage in sexual activity with you?*

If the answer were *Yes,* I would then put on my sexual choreographer hat and ask: *How can the two of you—given your problems and concerns as they are right now—create some kind of erotic experience that you both will enjoy, that will enhance your relationship, and will leave each of you feeling good about yourself and your partner?* Notice I didn't say "have sex" or " "have intercourse." I said "create some kind of erotic experience." I also would say this to someone with a problem related to physical responsiveness.

Problems Related to Physical Responsiveness

Of the reported *most important problems and concerns*, 28 percent had something to do with the physical responsiveness of the woman or her partner. Of the 457 responses in this category, 138 involved a partner's responsiveness and 329 her own. Of these, 186 had something to do with her orgasms, sometimes in combination with another problem or concern.

The Big Six

There are six items on the *Overview List* that were *not* the experiences of the greatest number of women, but they *were* the ones most likely to have been called *problems*, not just accepted as *the way life is*, by those who experienced them. I call these *The Big Six*.

What are they? *Every one of these six problems had to do with what went on during sexual activity.* Every one had something to do with attention or physical responsiveness—the woman's or her partner's—during sex. Three had to do with her partner's involvement and three with her own. Compared to the other items on the *Overview List,* a woman was more likely to experience it as a problem if her partner

- had difficulty getting and/or maintaining an erection,

- had difficulty getting aroused, or

- seemed distracted during sex.

The woman was also likely to experience it as a problem if she herself

- reached orgasm too quickly,

- experienced pain during intercourse or other internal stimulation, or

- experienced involuntary vaginal spasm so that vaginal entry and/or intercourse was impossible or difficult

Are any of these problems on your list? If so, did you put it in the *problem* category or as *just how life is*?

There were five other items that also were called problems and not just accepted as "the way life is" by many of the women who experienced them. Remarkably, these issues also were involved with what went on during sexual activity. They included the woman's own difficulty getting excited/aroused during sex, inability to relax during sex, insufficient vaginal lubrication, and inability to orgasm, plus one other experience that could well be related to the woman's own difficulties with arousal and orgasm: her partner ejaculating too quickly.

Obviously, many of us can accept being too tired and/or too busy for sex, or even not desiring to do it very often. We're much less likely to say *That's just how it is* when we don't get relaxed and caught up in sex or don't fully enjoy engaging in it. When we and/or our partners regularly don't seem able to physically, mentally, and emotionally join in the dance of sex, we are likely to experience that as a problem.

A Male Partner's Difficulties with Arousal and Erections

A man's erectile difficulties may have many underlying physical causes. These can include diabetes, problems with circulation, high blood pressure, alcohol intake, smoking, various medications and other drugs, and some surgeries. The penis becomes firm when three chambers that run the length of the penis fill with blood and the blood's outflow channel closes off to hold it in. Basically, erectile difficulties occur if the blood doesn't get into the chambers or if the outflow channel doesn't close and hold the blood there to maintain the erection.

One important psychological factor that often underlies erectile difficulties occurs when the man experiences a certain amount of pressure to perform, originating either from within himself or—real or imagined—from his partner. Performance pressure also can be a factor when a man with erectile difficulties seems distracted during sex. As one woman put it, *He pays more attention to his penis than he does to me!*

This Survey was conducted before the introduction of Viagra into the sexual lives of the American public. In my experience as a therapist, Viagra has been very helpful for some couples. It does concern me, however, when a man is given Viagra without any discussion of the importance of his partner's consent, receptivity, and pleasure. Those who prescribe Viagra often seem to forget that producing an erection should be an enhancement to creating *mutual* erotic pleasure; the erection is not an end in itself.

It isn't only older women who have partners with erectile difficulties. This next group of women were ages eighteen to twenty-one when the Survey was done: ♀ My partner has difficulty getting aroused and getting erections. He has been taking an orgasm-inhibiting medication (Zoloft) for the past five months. I have dealt with this by giving his mental well-being a higher priority than good sex; ♀ My man can't keep his dick hard for shit; ♀ My partner wasn't very good in bed. He had what I consider to be erectile dysfunction, and our sexual relationship went nowhere fast. I'd never before had a man I couldn't turn on in a big way. After six months we broke up; ♀ My partner has difficulty with erections and I have difficulty in reaching orgasm.

I'd never before had a man I couldn't turn on in a big way. Women whose partners have erectile difficulties often convey this sense of frustration at their powerlessness to elicit a sexual response from their partners. Frequently, however, a man's erectile difficulties have underlying causes that no amount of sexual attractiveness can overcome.

Whenever a man has erectile difficulties I ask about medications. I ask women about medications, too. Medications for blood pressure, heart conditions, anxiety, depression, allergies—in fact almost any medications—can affect erections in men and vaginal engorgement in women. One woman described her most significant problem or concern as "side effects of medications decreasing my desire; I take a beta blocker for coronary heart disease." Unfortunately, the effects of these medications on women are not studied nearly as much as effects on men. When there is a medication involved, I often recommend that someone having engorgement or erectile difficulties talk to her/his physician about trying out a different brand or a related drug.

Emily (1919) told me of her acceptance that her husband of the last four years had difficulty getting strong erections: "But he's very good with oral. He wasn't at first, but I taught him what I want." **Lorraine (1957)**, on the other hand, described her frustration with her husband's difficulty with his erections and arousal: "When I say, 'I think you should see a doctor,' he gets completely upset and refuses, says he just needs time. I've done the reading and really tried to do things ... I've put on the short skirt and high heels; I do the trashy things that he likes ... just for sex play, to become aroused. There's only one position for sex where he can stay erect. It's really getting boring and tedious."

One benefit of the introduction and advertising of Viagra is that men like Lorraine's husband are much more willing to seek help for their erectile difficulties than was the case before Viagra was introduced.

Her Partner Ejaculating Too Quickly

When a man ejaculates quickly, it is often because he is not fully aroused rather than because he is too aroused. In men, ejaculation and having an orgasm are two separate responses. Often when a man ejaculates quickly, his genitals ejaculate, but he isn't fully aroused and he doesn't orgasm. Often, too, his attention and arousal are not in sync with those of his partner.

When a man consults me for what is often described as *premature ejaculation*, I work with him on paying attention to his body sensations and deeper breathing; developing the ability to take all the time he needs to become more fully aroused; and imagining expanding his arousal energy away from his genitals and out—to filling all the space available in his body. I tell him there is a point in becoming sexually aroused much like the "second wind" that runners may experience when running, where you are fully into the experience and your sensations, movements, and breathing suddenly feel integrated—at one. When that occurs, there is no need to be concerned about ejaculatory control; it just happens. And, again, if a medication is a factor, that too must be addressed.

Women whose partners ejaculated more quickly than they wanted reported difficulty reaching orgasm, anger, frustration, and feeling unsatisfied. A few wrote of addressing these difficulties by giving up on sex or leaving their partners. Often, the premature ejaculation is a sign of disconnection and other relationship difficulties. One respondent wrote: ♀ I have left the relationship (but for more reasons than that). On a different note, another respondent wrote: ♀ I get sore so I don't mind that he ejaculates quickly.

In her interview, **Gloria (1944)** described how it was in her relationship: "My ex-husband drank and that took its toll on both of us. It's hard to be in a loving mood when someone is reeking with alcohol. Between the marijuana and the alcohol, he couldn't always maintain an erection. He was quite amorous when he drank and smoked and he left me feeling unsatisfied. Also, throughout our marriage he had problems with premature ejaculation, so I had to learn I wasn't going to be satisfied the first time around, but I hung in there for the second time. It was often disappointing to me. There was this fantastic foreplay and then he'd enter and zoop, it was all over. I'd be left hanging. I told him I wasn't being satisfied and wanted to do something about it. I suggested counseling and he wouldn't have anything to do with it. In those days, men didn't do anything to satisfy women who hadn't been satisfied in intercourse."

Retarded or Absent Ejaculation

A male partner's *retarded or absent ejaculation* was not on our *Overview List* but it was among the problems and concerns that women mentioned. As with other aspects of physical responsiveness, delayed or absent ejaculation can be medication- or drug-related as well as indicative of distraction, performance anxiety, and breathing patterns that inhibit arousal.

A Note About Breathing

Focusing our attention on our breathing is such an important way to experience ourselves—our tensions, our emotions, sexual arousal, and spiritual states—that entire books have been written on the subject. How we breathe changes automatically as we experience different emotions or become sexually aroused, but we also can change how we feel or enhance sexual arousal by consciously changing how we breathe.

There is great variety in how different people build, spread, and contain the energy of sexual arousal in their bodies and then release this energy into orgasm. Most of us have some energetic holding patterns that to some extent inhibit our breathing, and therefore our sexual arousal process. These are the result of various psychological and physical influences in our personal histories. By becoming aware of how you breathe and engaging in exercises that release these holding patterns, you will enhance your capacity to become sexually aroused. *The Intimate Couple* by Jack Lee Rosenberg and Beverly Kitaen-Morse (1996) addresses these concepts and describes such exercises.

Antidepressants and Sexual Responsiveness

If you are having sexual responsiveness problems that *might* be related to an antidepressant, ask your physician if another antidepressant would be equally suitable or a better choice. One to consider is Wellbutrin (bupropion), which tends to be comparable to other antidepressants in relieving depression but also seems to facilitate orgasm and acts as a sexual stimulant for some of the women who take it. Like any medication, Wellbutrin isn't for everyone; it probably isn't the right drug for you if you suffer from a lot of anxiety or bulimia, for example, or if you feel sexually aroused constantly or have significant menstrual problems (Crenshaw and Goldberg 1996). The choice of what medication to take—if any—should be made in consultation with your physician.

Another question to consider is this: Is medication necessary at all? There are many ways other than medication to elevate mood. Here are some alternatives:

- Change your diet to enhance and regulate the mood-affecting neurochemicals in your brain.

- Change your exercise patterns. Both too little and too much exercise can be problematic. If you are getting too little exercise, there can be definite mood benefits from spending more time outdoors in natural light. Also walking, especially with an upbeat companion, can be a mood enhancer; so can gardening.

- Change your self-talk. Learn to observe and dwell on your strengths and the positive aspects of your life and relationships instead of on the negatives.

- Feed your psychological hungers. If you are depressed, it is very likely that some of your most basic psychological needs are not being met. By paying attention to these needs, you can make changes in your life and begin to fulfill them. Six of these psychological hungers include the needs for contact, stimulation, recognition, time structure, incident, and intimacy (Berne 1971). The numbered list below will give you a better idea of what it means to feed your psychological hungers.

1. Are you in *contact* with other people—family, friends, colleagues at work or in volunteer activities, etc.? Do you keep pet(s)?

2. Do you receive *stimulation*—physical, emotional, mental, spiritual? Are you touched? Do you listen to music? Read? Do you meditate or pray?

3. Do you receive *recognition*? Are you acknowledged? Greeted by name? Praised?

4. Do you have *time structure*—certain times to be up and dressed, a job to go to, scheduled activities?

5. Are there *incidents* in your life—events to look forward, to feel involved in when they happen, to enjoy, and to talk and think about afterwards?

6. Does *intimacy* have an active place in your life? Even if you have no sex partner, do you have someone with whom you can share touch and your intimate thoughts and feelings?

When needs—psychological hungers—are identified, creative efforts—sometimes with a therapist's support—can be taken to begin to fulfill them.

Other Aspects of Women's Physical Responsiveness

We rarely can reduce a problem with physical responsiveness to only one of its aspects. Inability to relax during sex, for example, may lead to and be a part of the difficulty in becoming aroused, which would be reflected as insufficient vaginal lubrication. Insufficient lubrication may be one of the underlying causes of pain during intercourse or other internal stimulation. Pain may lead to involuntary vaginal spasm to prevent painful vaginal entry. So, there can be a "domino" effect that can make it extremely difficult to pinpoint the precise cause of the difficulty with physical responsiveness.

Relaxation, Distraction, Arousal, and Vaginal Lubrication

Difficulties with relaxation, distraction, arousal, and vaginal lubrication (which is a reflection of engorgement) all may be related to a woman's own health, her partner's difficulties (e.g., her partner's inability to relax or to sustain arousal), to relationship issues, or to numerous other factors. In the next chapter, you will find a discussion of *transitions* in sexual experiences, which is one aspect of how individuals and couples can deal with relaxation, distraction, and some of the other issues presented here.

The inability to relax into sex affects women of all ages, and may be situational: ♀ My difficulties with relaxing and getting aroused improve when I have sex with my friend rather than my regular partner; ♀ Most of my sex in the past year was along the lines of "casual" sex; it's difficult to relax and let myself go; ♀ There's been some improvement in my inability to relax during sex since I got different birth control pills; ♀ I feel distracted during sex because I am busy; I'm looking forward to graduation.

A Relaxing Suggestion. When you and your partner need to get out of your heads and into your bodies, try starting with your feet. Sit together on the edge of the bathtub with your feet in warm water while you talk over your day. Or if you prefer being in the bedroom, put on some music and begin with foot rubs, followed by some leg caressing, and continue on up from there.

Vaginal Pain

Insufficient lubrication can lead to painful vaginal stimulation and intercourse, but not all vaginal pain during sex is due to insufficient lubrication. In my therapist detective mode I would ask: *What are the characteristics of the pain? Is it experienced as burning? Sharp? Sore? Aching or throbbing? Tenderness? Where is it located? When and how does it occur?*

Some Survey respondents described the characteristics of their sexual pain as follows: ♀ Pain during intercourse is a problem I'm still having after a hysterectomy a year ago; ♀ Pain during penetration—I have an obese husband; ♀ Pain related to endometriosis. One woman described how she was dealing with her pain during sex in this way: ♀ Asking him to pause or go really slow has helped with my pain during intercourse.

One pattern of pain involves the external genitals—both sets of vaginal lips, the clitoris, and the entrance to the vagina—which are collectively called the *vulva. Vulvodynia* is one of the medical words used to describe pain of this type; it also has been called *burning vulva syndrome.* Because symptoms can be quite subtle and may be cyclical, women with vaginal and vulval pain are much too often made to feel that their discomfort is primarily "psychosomatic" or all in their heads. With chronic burning, stinging, irritation, or rawness of the vulva, there may be few noticeable skin changes except, perhaps, irritation from rubbing or scratching. A medical practitioner can't see anything or figure out what's going on. Perhaps the symptoms are cyclical and don't even occur during some days of the month. The condition may not be immediately resolved, even with appropriate treatment. A woman can begin to feel, or be led by a medical professional to feel, that it must be her fault that she continues to have this problem. There even may be an implication that she is imagining it to avoid sex or for some other manipulative reason. Research, however, does not support this view. A carefully controlled study of women with intercourse pain did not demonstrate that they had more psychological problems or psychophysical complaints than a control group; the two groups also had similar attitudes toward sexuality. What the group with intercourse pain did have, however, was a greater number of the kinds of physical conditions that could be related to the pain they were describing (Binik, Meana, Khalife, et al. 1995).

Survey respondents described their experiences of this type of pain: ♀ Frequent yeast infection and burning; ♀ Bladder infections after intercourse; ♀ Inflamed Bartholin's gland; ♀ Chronic VVS (*vulvar vestibulitis syndrome*). For two months I have been taking Elavil for the pain. [Vestibulitis = inflammation of the vaginal opening]; ♀ Pain during intercourse. I had *vestibular adonitis* (gland inflammation) when I was twenty-six; ♀ A urethral syndrome I had was helped by urinating after intercourse; ♀ I experience irritation and swelling with intercourse and burning/irritation after intercourse; no latex or spermicide is involved.

In 1994 I heard Marilynne McKay, M.D., describe *vulvodynia*—chronic discomfort of the vulva—*as "a symptom with a variety of causes, not a diagnosis with a variety of treatments."* Dr. McKay, then an associate professor of dermatology and gynecology at Emory University in Atlanta, Georgia, distinguishes between four types of vulvodynia, each with its own causes and appropriate treatment. Women suffering from this condition may benefit from seeking out some of her medical journal articles, two of which you will find listed in the Reference section (McKay 1992; 1989).

Involuntary Vaginal Spasm

Although only six women marked *involuntary vaginal spasm so that vaginal entry and/or intercourse was impossible or difficult* as their *most important* problem or concern in the previous year, fifty-nine women said they had this experience either *often* or *all the time*, and that same number considered the experience a problem rather than *the way life is*. This experience is perhaps more common than many people realize; 10 percent of all respondents to this list of *sexual circumstances* question had experienced *involuntary vaginal spasm that made vaginal entry impossible or difficult* during sex at least *sometimes* during the previous year; 3 percent said this happened often or all the time.

A woman in her early seventies described a physical cause for which she had had corrective surgeries; for her, "vaginal jelly sometimes helps." Another respondent, in her late thirties, noted that she'd had pain during intercourse, but is now fine, so "perhaps vaginismus has reversed itself." A college student reported "vaginal spasm and insufficient lubrication" every time she had sex and wrote: ♀ Not being able to have intercourse because my opening is too small or because of improper lubrication has been a big problem and I don't know where to get help.

Some Sources of Help

If you have a sexual problem or concern, taking a college or university sexuality class might be helpful. Even if you don't take the class, a call to the instructor, who is likely to be able to recommend reading material or know of a therapist or medical practitioner from whom you can get sensitive help in your local community, might be useful. You also can call the American Association of Sex Educators, Counselors and Therapists, a national organization that certifies sex counselors and therapists, to get a referral from their national directory. Their number is 319-895-8407.

It is a good idea to first interview by phone someone you are considering seeing as a therapist. For vaginal spasming, for example, a therapist who focuses more on your autonomy, your right to say *No*, how *you* want to create erotic pleasure, and whether you are ready to welcome another person into your body would be a better choice than someone who wants to focus primarily on using dilators to open your vagina for intercourse, which is how some of the therapists and physicians who medically label vaginal spasm as *vaginismus* "treat" the condition.

Lovemaking Problems and Concerns

A partner-focused factor that inhibited some Survey respondents' arousal and orgasms was the partner's sexual technique. Again, there were similarities among women of all ages. Issues of sexual lovemaking technique included partners who wanted briefer foreplay than a woman wanted; didn't touch or kiss much; didn't like to perform oral sex; didn't make their needs known; weren't aggressive enough; didn't express their excitement more; and who were less interested in performing manual and oral stimulation than the woman wanted. One respondent wrote: "His inhibitions make me more inhibited."

Other issues had to do with the initiation and timing of sex: For example, ♀ My partner not initiating sex as often as I; ♀ My partner chooses inconvenient times. He is a night owl, I am more alert in the morning; he helps little with evening activities of dinner, children's homework, getting kids ready for bed, but expects my sexual receptivity regardless; ♀ My partner rejecting my advances; ♀ I felt too much distance, needed a closeness; sex is better and I want to do it more when we talk.

Other Aspects of Lovemaking

Some of the sexual concerns in this miscellaneous category included the weight placed on one woman by her overweight partner; a lack of confidence in lovemaking ability; excessive lubrication; passing gas at the time of orgasm; and a partner who climaxed and fell asleep while the respondent hadn't climaxed. For a lesbian, it was a partner "not wanting to receive (bottom) as much as I want to give (top)." Other women reported feeling too inhibited to express likes and dislikes; a partner not able to handle her being sexually aggressive; and needing pain for pleasure.

One aspect of lovemaking is one's decision about whether or not to engage in sex or sexual intercourse. This also was reported as a problem or concern by some. For example: ♀ I have a partner—not a sex partner. I have *not had* sexual intercourse. This does not mean I'm not involved in talking about it with my partner.

Suggestion. A good starting place for addressing almost any sexual problem or concern in a relationship is to start with the situation as it is and consider it in detail. That is your starting place. Then, think about how to proceed from there to create an outcome that will be enjoyable and leave each of you feeling good about yourself and the other.

Finding a Partner

The main problem or concern in the last year reported by 123 Survey respondents was *finding a partner with whom to be sexual.* Actually, there were even more women in the Survey population for whom finding a partner was a problem or concern, because women who had not had a partner in the past year did not answer the question about their most important sexual concerns and problems. Although difficulty finding a partner was mentioned by women of all ages, there is the reality for an older woman that the older she gets, the fewer *male* partners there will be available to her:

"Old age is a territory populated largely by women. Because women outlive men by an average of seven years, the ratio of women to men increases sharply among the elderly. For every 100 men sixty-five years of age and older, there are about 150 women. By the age of eighty-five, this ratio becomes about 100 to 250" (Butler 1996).

An older, once-divorced Survey respondent, whose last partnered sexual activity was fifteen years previous, wrote: "I think I would like to have a partner, but no one falls into the category of: 1) available; 2) interested in me; 3) attractive intellectually and physically. I have no physical impairment, I am active in several groups where it is not sedentary pursuits and I feel I could and would enjoy a fulfilling sexual life even at age sixty-six if Mr. Right came along." Another woman, over fifty, said of her recent good fortune: "Until I met my current partner ten months ago, I'd had no partner for two years since my divorce. I'm just realizing how fortunate I am!" A woman in her forties was interested in "finding the right woman to live with" and another in "finding a partner I want to be sexual with—but it's more about intimacy than sex. I need someone who cares for me, and don't really want to be sexual just for the sake of doing it." Others mentioned "finding a creative, stimulating, versatile sexual partner" and "just meeting someone—mutuality."

These were issues for women of all ages. A woman of about thirty wrote of wanting "a relationship with someone beyond sexual intercourse." In the past year she'd had "one-night stands." Some of the youngest women responding to the Survey wrote comments like this one: "I'm having a difficult time finding a woman who I am attracted to that is attracted to me" and "No one meets my standards."

Although the older a woman gets and the fewer close-in-age men there are, there are women who do find new male partners late in life. **Emily (1919)** remarried when she was almost seventy; another woman I interviewed, **Flo (1905)**, remarried in her eighties; both Emily and Flo married men close in age to themselves.

Some women who consider themselves heterosexual resolve the finding-a-partner dilemma by pairing up with another woman. I predict that with the "graying of America" more women will be making this choice. A woman in her fifties attached a note to her questionnaire describing this experience:

Alcohol allowed for sex to occur with another woman ... the only same-sex sexual relationship I've ever had. I've never felt any desire to have sexual contact with another female. Sexual fantasies are infrequent, but always with a male partner. I don't think of myself as lesbian or even bisexual, although I recognize that my behavior would be classified that way by others. This sexual relationship is loving and affirming but troublesome because we both feel that we would like to be, would probably prefer to be, in loving relationships with a man. Alcohol is never part of our relationship for years now. Sex is infrequent, but affirming. If we felt ourselves to be a "committed couple" it would probably be more frequent. We recognize that because the relationship is emotionally nurturing that it is unlikely that something better is likely to come along. Penetration by a male always sounds good. We both like men. We both would prefer to be part of a couple but are unlikely to give up something so nurturing to go seeking male contact, especially in light of the possibility of STDs including HIV and AIDS.

Other Relationship Issues

A great many of the problems and concerns already noted—differences in sexual desire and differences regarding sexual practices, for example—are relationship issues. The responses in this group are a miscellaneous assortment that did not readily fit into other categories. Included are issues of love and intimacy; the woman's dissatisfaction with her partner or the relationship; not desiring the partner she is with; coercion or pressure from her partner; and the ending of her relationship.

1. **Issues of love and intimacy**

    Women ranging across the age spectrum wrote of lack of love, not enough intimacy, and being with someone she wasn't "madly in love" with. Another woman was with someone she loves romantically but who loves her only as a friend; she noted: "confusion dominates the experience."

2. **Dissatisfaction with something about her partner or with the relationship**

    These concerns and problems included, for example, illness of a partner; a dilemma over whether to stay married to a partner who prefers to accept her lack of orgasm and satisfaction as her problem, not his, and refuses to talk about it; choosing a partner who hid his alcoholism that made him basically impotent; and feeling judged and resented for having a stronger sexual drive than a partner with erectile difficulties.

3. **Sexual boredom or not desiring the partner she is with**

Some of the responses in this category included desire for a former lover; boredom after fifteen years; and being with a partner who is kind but is not one with whom she feels connected. Other women described not finding a partner sexually desirable because he "is unwilling and uncomfortable with playing a dominant role" and "dissatisfaction with a current partner's oral hygiene, general physical condition and personal lack of hygiene." One woman reported that she was "getting bored" with a partner of five years with whom "sex is affectionate, but nonspontaneous, planned, a big project." She admitted that she has "a serious wandering eye" and was wondering if she should have an affair. She feared, however, that an affair "would just perpetuate the problem."

4. **Coercion or pressure to engage in sex**

An older respondent reported terminating a relationship due to "feeling coerced, feelings of 'fucking' rather than an expression of love." And a younger woman's problem was "My partner not taking *No* for *No*. He argues until he gets what he wants." Another reported: "My partner's a jerk when he's not sexually satisfied. He thinks he's 'entitled' to sex whenever he wants it. Sometimes if I'm only having sex so I don't have to deal with his mood swings I feel used, cheap, empty, and angry."

Suggestion. If I were able to sit down and talk with one of these women, I would suggest that when sex doesn't leave you feeling good about yourself and about your partner, it's time to do some serious thinking about the dynamics of your relationship and the rules (perhaps unstated) you are following. Then, make a decision about where to go from there.

5. **A relationship ending**

Among the responses in this category were a woman's recent loss of a partner for whom she cared deeply and another's loneliness after divorce. One woman described "depression resulting from breaking up" with a boyfriend and fearing that she would not love or be loved by future partners. She added, "This sadness affects all aspects of my life including my sexuality."

Fertility and Reproduction

Forty-five women wrote something about fertility or reproduction as their most important problem or concern of the past year. Fear of pregnancy was mentioned by women born from 1945-1974, sometimes accompanied by concerns about sexually transmitted diseases. Other fertility and reproductive issues included the inability to become pregnant, trying or wanting to become pregnant, being pregnant, having a new baby, and birth control.

The Reproductive Dimension of Sexuality

One of the most significant ways women differ from men is in how they experience the reproductive dimension of their sexualities. Women are cyclic in their fertility while men are not, at least not so dramatically. A woman's physical cycling is reflected in subtle, and sometimes striking, variations in her perceptions, moods, the images in her dreams, her sexual feelings, her receptivity to touch, and the tumescence and lushness of her body's tissues. Where she is in her fertility cycle also affects her mental clarity, her intuition, and her ability to critically evaluate the structure and quality of her life.

For the thirty to forty years between our first menstrual flow and our last, we women experience recurring fertility cycles that provide regular rhythmic evidence of the reproductive dimension of our sexual selves. This is a magnificent biological process. In the ovum a fertile woman releases each month, she carries the hereditary material that links her to those who have lived before her. A woman does not choose the ova she carries; these are her link with "the ancestral germ pool" (Shuttle and Redgrove 1990). But she can choose how she will use her uterus. She can, within the constraints of other influences, decide whether and when in her life to conceive and carry a child, and she usually can determine who its father will be.

Sex and Menstrual Cycling

It seemed to about two out of three of the Survey respondents that their sexual desire predictably varied or had varied due to their menstrual cycles. Fewer, about two out of five, thought that their sexual satisfaction varied predictably.

About one in five of the respondents had never engaged in sexual intercourse during their menstrual flow; about a third had done so rarely, a third had done so sometimes, and 13 percent had done so often. Fewer than half said that they had enjoyed sexual activity during their menstrual flow.

Fertility

A modern woman is likely to experience the fertility dimension of her sexuality quite differently than a woman of a century or two ago. In the 1700s and 1800s, a woman was much more likely to spend most of her reproductive years either pregnant or breast-feeding her babies than she is today. In earlier times, a woman might go through many pregnancies before having a child who survived infancy; she also was more likely to die in childbirth. Today's typical American woman, with her longer life, reliable and easily available contraceptives, and changed roles in society, will have several hundred recurring fertility cycles during her lifetime; an eighteenth- or nineteenth-century woman might have had only forty or so.

Ellen (1910) was the oldest daughter in a family with twelve children. Her mother was eighteen when she had her first child, forty when she had her last. Ellen said, "My youngest sister was born when I was a senior in college. I once asked my mom *Why don't you quit having babies, why do you keep on having them?* She said she tried everything. She just didn't know how. But, she did stop after the twelfth one. She chopped dad off at the pockets and said, *This is it. I've had it.* I realize now that, at that time, there were laws against doctors giving out information."

A Frequent Focus of Our Attention

In our fertile years, the possibility that we may become pregnant frequently occupies our attention. This possibility is likely to generate quite different concerns and feelings at various times in our lives. Many of us have felt, at different times, desirous of becoming pregnant, joyous, or alarmed that we have become pregnant, concerned that we might *not* become pregnant, and concerned or fearful that we might become or were pregnant. About 9 percent of the Survey respondents said that they had at sometime in their sexual lives had a problem because of inadequate availability of birth control, and 11 percent had had problems due to inadequate information about birth control. One Survey respondent reported difficulty adjusting to birth control pills as her most important sexual concern or problem: ♀ It took three different prescriptions for my body to accept them.

Difficulties Becoming Pregnant

The mature period for reproduction is generally thought of as lasting from approximately age twenty to forty, because these are the years of optimum hormonal functioning. An occasional woman will, however, conceive and bear a child before her first period or after what she thought was her last. In recent years we have seen an increase in the number of women choosing to bear children after age forty and, with new technologies, even beyond. A Survey respondent in her mid-forties attempting to become pregnant reported that taking Clomid (a fertility drug) for six months lowered her sexual desire and response; another woman, almost forty, was in the process of seeking an egg donor after two unsuccessful in vitro fertilization attempts. One forty-year-old woman summed up her major sexual issue in this manner: ♀ My major problem was not sexuality but rather infertility.

Every month a fertile woman's body demonstrates its readiness for a child. Sometimes, though, women who wish to conceive are misinformed about when that can occur. In a study of 192 pregnancies, conception occurred only when intercourse took place during a six-day period that ended on the estimated day of ovulation. The researchers concluded that the chances of sexual intercourse resulting in pregnancy ranged from one in ten when intercourse occurred on the fifth day before ovulation to one in three on the day of ovulation. If you want to become pregnant and don't have sexual intercourse until a home-test indicates ovulation has already occurred, you are waiting until your fertility window is almost closed. Sperm remain active for several days, whereas when ovulation occurs, the egg can be fertilized only for about twenty-four hours or perhaps even less.

If you're too tired and/or too busy to make love, your body also may be too tired and stressed out to ovulate regularly and/or to conceive. If you wish to become pregnant, here are my suggestions. Even if you are involved in medical interventions that will make it more difficult to do so, follow the spirit of my suggestions the best that you can.

Suggestions for aiding conception: During the five days before you think ovulation will take place, visit a lovely, relaxing setting for at least three days. Most couples need at least that much time to detach from work and the stresses of their everyday life and to become fully relaxed. Leave phones, e-mail, and all work at home. Walk in nature. Get plenty of rest—sleep in, take naps. Take the time you need to make love in a leisurely way. Talk about the mystique of participating in the creation of a child and imagine what it would be like to have a child in your life. If it's not practical to get away, stay home but create the same relaxing, leisurely conditions.

If it seems impossible to take three days from your life and devote that time to making love and creating a child, consider this question: Are you going to have time to nurture and enjoy this baby? It the answer is *No*, think about and discuss whether this is the right time to have a child, and what changes you might need to make so that you will be better prepared to welcome a child into your lives.

Becoming Pregnant

Several women reporting their sexual concerns and problems did become pregnant. Some, born between 1953-1956, reported becoming pregnant unexpectedly, lowered libido during pregnancy ("It was fine before that"), and a pregnancy that led to an abortion as their most important sexual concerns or problems of the previous year. One respondent reported happily that, after spending some of the year trying to get pregnant: "I'm pregnant now."

Consequences of Becoming Pregnant

Conceiving—becoming pregnant—can be a joyous occasion. Some Survey respondents described their happiness at becoming pregnant earlier in their lives: ♀ Happiness for me and my partner; ♀ . . . happiness the first time, surprise + happiness the second; ♀ Becoming pregnant resulted in a wonderful new chapter of experience and love for my husband and myself; ♀ The pregnancy was planned and enjoyable; we love our baby. One woman happily reported that her "partner, a woman, inseminated me with donor sperm."

A pregnancy can dramatically change the course of a woman's life. About 8 percent of all Survey respondents said that becoming pregnant had at some time in their lives resulted in their getting married sooner than they had planned. Four percent had married someone they had not previously planned to marry, and about 3 percent had married someone they never would have chosen to marry otherwise. Eight percent of all who responded had had a baby in a marriage before they felt ready to be a parent. About 4 percent had at some time had a pregnancy in which the biological father knew about the pregnancy but did not stay with her through it; 3 percent had had a pregnancy of which the biological father was unaware.

Abortion

Of the 4,478 pregnancies reported by the Survey respondents, 478, nearly 11 percent, ended in spontaneous abortions or miscarriages; 687, 15 percent, were ended by arranged abortions. One of the oldest women I interviewed, **Ellen (1910)**, told me of the abortion she had about a year and a half after she married. Her husband had been laid off from work and they'd gone to live with his mother. She said, "He didn't have any job and we just didn't have any money, and I just couldn't have a baby. So my husband inquired around, and I went to this little old, dark, dirty place and had an abortion. And I never regretted it. If people really can't afford to have children, if they can't afford to take care of them, having an abortion is not wrong."

Most women do not find the decision to have an abortion an easy one to make. **Cecile (1952)** said, for example, "I stayed pregnant for three months because I didn't know what to do. I was going to have it, I wasn't going to have it, I was going to have it, I wasn't going to have it. But I finally did have the abortion." As with other life decisions, we do the best we can with the resources we have and what we know at the time.

While most of the women I talked to did not regret the abortions they had, **Joan (1944)** felt differently about the abortion she had had at seventeen, when she was in high school: "I'm sorry now I had the abortion. I wish I could have had enough guts to go ahead and have the baby and give it up for adoption. But I wasn't mature enough to make a decision like that, and I was frightened." She went on to describe a process of empowerment and self-acceptance: "However, a lot of things came from that. I learned a lot about taking control of my life. I never took another chance as far as pregnancy was concerned, and I was much more cautious about other things. I took control. And later on, I was able to talk three women out of having an abortion, just by telling them my experience. Not by saying it's wrong or anything. And those three children are living. I am Pro Choice. I think you have to be, because our choices of all types are being taken away and undermined by whatever forces have power." I, too, am Pro Choice.

Pregnancies of the Survey Respondents

The table statistically tells the stories of the women who responded to the Survey. Of the 822 women in the table who had never been pregnant, 670 had never wanted to be pregnant. In my interviews, I heard of many pregnancies, some welcomed, some not; none of the college students interviewed by Michaelle Davis had ever been pregnant. Unfortunately, the space limitations of this book do not allow me to address the reproductive dimension of women's sexualities in the detail and depth I would like. Here, I merely touch

I have been pregnant _____ times. N = 2,458 ♀♀, with 1,636 ♀♀ reporting 4,478 pregnancies, 822 never pregnant

N of pregnancies	0	1	2	3	4	5	6	7	8	9	10	11	12	15	Total
N of ♀♀	822*	369	478	376	204	118	51	27	6	2	2	1	1	1	1,636
% of ♀♀	33%	15%	19%	15%	8%	5%	2%	1%	<1%	<1%	<1%	<1%	<1%	<1%	
Total pregnancies	0	369	956	1128	816	590	306	189	48	18	20	11	12	15	4,478
were planned	460	406	386	124	37	9	2	4	-	1	-	-	-	-	
were unplanned	218	569	326	168	83	37	16	8	4	1	-	1	1	-	
resulted in live births	239	308	541	256	67	22	11	4	-	1	1	-	-	-	
ended in spontaneous abortion or miscarriage	754	356	87	22	7	4	2	-	-	-	-	-	-	-	
ended in an arranged abortion	615	420	178	68	13	5	1	1	1	-	-	-	-	-	
(of my babies) were given up for adoption	1056	31	-	1	-	-	-	-	-	-	-	-	-	-	

* 822 with 0 pregnancies are not included in the 1,636 total.

the surface of this extremely important topic. The remainder of the data I have from the Survey and the many narratives I have from the interviews (including a series done by Dr. Susan Hennings, using my interview questions with mothers who had recently had babies) will be presented elsewhere.

Having a New Baby

Having their first child is one of the most transformative events in the relationship of an intimate couple. Several Survey respondents noted that their most significant sexual problem or concern in the previous year was having a new baby. Some wrote: ♀ My vagina has been healing and I'm getting back to "normal" after having the baby within the last year and readjusting both mentally and physically to intercourse, non-birth control pill methods of birth control, etc.; ♀ Having a newborn was very tiring. This improved somewhat when my daughter started sleeping all night; ♀ I was concerned that I wouldn't be sexy after the birth of my baby (now seven months old).

STDs/Safe Sex

Thirty-seven women across the age spectrum reported a most important problem or concern related to sexually transmitted diseases or to practicing safe sex. The oldest of this group and a younger woman each had had three partners in the previous three months and both were concerned about safe sex. Several mentioned their fear of getting AIDS. One respondent resolved her concern about STDs by "dumping" her nonmonogamous partner, another by "being more selective, taking relationships slower," a third woman "by avoiding alcohol," and a younger woman "by not having sex."

One woman had caught genital herpes from a previous partner and another spent four months afraid she had caught herpes. Another respondent had a partner who "messed around" on her and so she thought she "might have caught something."

In her interview, **Joan (1944)** told me of the problems she had with getting men her age to use condoms when she was once again single:

> There's a lot of resistance to condoms in men over forty. The men I dated after I left my husband in 1988 hadn't even thought about condoms in the thirty years or so since high school. They thought condoms were for other people . . . it's

enough that they have vasectomies. Another popular misconception is that men can't pick up the AIDS virus from women; I even believe it sometimes. I found it very difficult to get men my age interested in using condoms. They don't want to, and if you try to insist, they'll lose their erection right away. So it's either no condoms or no sex.

In the beginning, I just let that happen. I fooled myself, or was in denial enough, to think that as long as I knew them, they would be safe. But I got really frightened when I found out my primary partner was having sex with other women, also unprotected. I was greatly relieved when I tested negative to STDs. I determined to take a really firm stand, and I tried to talk to people beforehand. But in the end, when it was impossible to get them to use condoms because of their erections, I would go ahead and not use them. And I would be terrified again.

That was the past. For the last two years I've been with a very exciting, passionate, tender, beautiful man ... more chemistry than I've had with any other man in my whole life. When he wanted to make love with me, I wanted it very much. I invited him over and we had a long talk about sex ... the things I've been through, my fears about getting pregnant again, AIDS, all of it. We decided that we would make love and use a condom. And here's a man, again, who has maybe never used a condom because he had long-term relationships. So we tried to use a condom, and it made the erection go away. It just didn't work. And we got hotter and hotter. And this condom was getting in the way more and more. And I also was using a diaphragm. I was just so hot and bothered that I ... we finally just gave up and went ahead and had sex. So there it was again, more unprotected sex. I was just aghast! We both got tested for AIDS and we were negative. Now we're monogamous, and he got a vasectomy, so here I am, back in the best place you can be in, as far as that's concerned ... able to have sex without using condoms.

This issue affects women of all ages. The most important problem or concern of a woman a generation younger than Joan was her "partner using his inability to maintain erection as an excuse to practice unsafe sex."

Getting a condom out of its package and onto the male body can easily disrupt the feelings of closeness and sexual connection that have been building. Even when this is a part of mutual sex play, both partners may lose some arousal in the process. Once a condom is on, taking some time to reclaim arousal and feelings of connectedness before proceeding to intercourse may enhance pleasure for both partners.

Suggestions. One way a couple can get used to using condoms is to engage in erotic play that includes putting a condom on without either of them expecting the man to get or maintain an erection. They might decide, for example, that the first few times they are together they will use a condom but engage in *outercourse* rather than *intercourse*. A man also can practice using condoms during masturbation.

Body and Health Issues

The most important problems or concerns of thirty other women were related to their own bodies or health. This tended to be an older group. As one woman put it: "My issue is degenerating health, plus my partner having major prostate problems. Hello! Old age!" Women born in the 1920s and 1930s mentioned not having "enough energy and breath" due to severe emphysema, slowing down due to age, and the effects of "illness, surgery, recovery."

Menopause

For one age group, those born between 1939 and 1946 (ages forty-seven to fifty-five when the survey was done), the important problems and concerns were the changes due to menopause and peri-menopause. A homemaker and costume designer, forty-seven when she completed her Survey, was experiencing peri-menopausal distress. She said, "My partner has complained of my lowered desire. It embarrasses and baffles me. My doctor says I'm not yet in menopause."

We don't have to be "in menopause" to experience physical changes. Throughout adulthood, progressive, irreversible changes are continuously occurring in our ovaries where many of our hormones are produced. The physical transition from full reproductive potential to menopause, the advent of which is marked by the last menstrual period, begins for most women in our late thirties or early forties. Over the next ten years or so, our maximum blood levels of the ovarian hormones—the estrogens and progesterone—gradually decrease. These hormonal changes begin to be reflected in the rhythms and characteristics of our menstrual flows, and at certain times in our cycles we may begin to experience vaginal dryness, changes in sleep patterns, hot flushes, and variations in sexual response. Periods are likely to become less predictable and blood flow may become very heavy or decrease. Many women have some episodes of very heavy bleeding as they near menopause. This is because their ovaries continue to produce estrogen but do not go through the cycle phase in which progesterone is produced. For most women, taking natural progesterone for twelve or so days each month will remedy the extra heavy bleeding. Still, a woman who is bleeding heavily should check with her health professional to be sure there is no other underlying cause.

Menopause, the time when we leave behind the reproductive capabilities of our sexuality, need not be a barrier to an active and enjoyable sex life, but it can be a time of changes, some of them striking, in how sex is experienced. During this transition a woman experiences a gradual decline in the lush readiness of her body to participate in sexual intercourse and a shift away from the particular erotic images and sensations she experienced in her reproductive years.

Other Body/Health Problems and Concerns

Other problems and concerns relating to the Survey respondents' bodies and health included avoiding yeast or urinary infections and the physical and emotional adjustment of recuperating from various surgeries, for example, hysterectomy or bilateral breast biopsies ("I'm keeping myself in good physical shape and buying nice lingerie"). Two respondents mentioned feeling inhibited by the weight they had gained. One of these, 5'5" tall and weighing 129 pounds, wrote: "The ten pounds I've put on have made me less daring and adventurous," and a young college student's most important problem or concern was being "uncomfortable with my body."

Other Issues

Themes mentioned as most important problems or concerns by one percent or fewer of the women responding included issues of molestation and abuse, sexual orientation, and nonmonogamy. The issues of molestation and abuse and of nonmonogamy have been addressed in detail elsewhere (see chapters 4 and 7).

Sexual Orientation

One of the final Survey questions was about regrets. Specifically, it said *Looking back over my entire life, I regret the following about my sexual life*. Among the choices we provided were *I had sex with partners I should have turned down* and *I did not have sex with someone with whom I wish I had*. There was also a blank line for *Other*. The following comments are representative statements from women who regretted that they did not realize, accept, and act on their lesbianism earlier in their lives.

Women born in the 1940s said, *I regret that . . .* ♀ I didn't realize I was lesbian earlier. It might have created some problems but it would have alleviated some others. I didn't feel it was okay to enjoy my sexuality; ♀ . . . It was too many years before I was honest about my sexuality. I spent too many years trying to be heterosexual!; ♀ . . . That I didn't come out as a lesbian till past age forty; and ♀ . . . I was ashamed of being gay.

Women born in the 1950s regretted *that* ♀ . . . I married the wrong gender. I just came out as a lesbian this summer—I've been married twenty years—my husband is my best friend and supports me in this. I'm having a difficult transition—meeting other lesbians, the gender switch, etc. I'm at a very heightened sexual prime now and the sex I'm having with my husband is sporadic—to relieve sexual tension with another person—masturbating gets lonely. Also, we only have "doggie" style intercourse—no foreplay, kissing, etc. It kind of works. We've been doing this for over 10 years; ♀ It took so long to make the connection mentally that I'm a lesbian. It would have been nice to explore women sexually in my youth; and ♀ . . . I "discovered" women in my mid-twenties instead of my teens; I wish there had been more sexual information available then.

Women born in the 1960s put it this way: ♀ Coming to terms with my lesbianism was, at first, difficult and caused me considerable emotional pain in my early twenties; ♀ I slept with men for too many years; and ♀ I was asexual all my life. I didn't fit into "straight" society but didn't know I had any other options.

Two younger women, both born in 1970, said: ♀ I didn't sleep with a woman soon enough; ♀ I repressed my lesbianism and therefore had unsatisfying sexual experiences with men.

These few comments illustrate the trend for women born after the 1950s to act on their lesbianism at a younger age than those women born earlier.

Concluding Remarks

We are not alone in the aspects of our sexuality that concern us or give us problems. Somewhere out in the world there are many other women with issues and concerns similar to our own. Sexuality and the themes of sexual problems and concerns do vary somewhat predictably as we move through our lives. The multiplicity of examples we find here can give us a clearer perspective of where we've been, as well as where we are now, and, perhaps, where we are going.

It is obvious that much of the real sex in America is not like the sex in most movies. Much of real life sex, with its imperfections, its very genuine humanness, is quite different—but it also may be even better than the Hollywood version! When facing problems or concerns, part of the key to dealing with them is knowing when to say *That's how it is.*

Another key is knowing when to ask, *How, one step at a time, can I improve this?*

And, finally, asking this question: *Is it possible, given things just as they are, to create a satisfying experience that leaves me feeling good about myself and—if I have a partner—about my partner, too?*

You may find some answers to that question in the next chapter as we turn our attention to sexual choreography and the creation of erotic pleasure.

What Does This Mean to You?

Now, if you wish, pick up your notebook and express the thoughts and feelings you're having about the various topics covered in this chapter. Here are some questions you might want to consider after you've done that.

- What was your most significant sexual concern or problem in the past year?

- If it's resolved, how did you resolve it? If it's not, what would a first step be toward resolution?

- Is being too tired and/or too busy for sex a reality in your life? If so, is there any way you might change this?

- If you are recalling experiences that you now regret, consider the circumstances, the roles of others, and how you saw your options at the time. Then, sit quietly with your eyes closed and imagine what you could now gently and lovingly tell your younger self that would be healing and would lead to greater self-acceptance.

13

Sexual Choreography: Creating Pleasure in Partnered Sex

The Experience of Erotic Pleasure

Erotic pleasure is a composition made of many different kinds of sensations. We can experience scents, tastes, visual images, the varying qualities of the touches we give and receive, feelings emanating from within our muscles and internal organs, and the voluntary and involuntary sounds made by our partners and ourselves. Using our bodies and breath we can create and experience sexual energy, pleasure, erotic feelings and sensations, feelings of love, joy, and the experience of oneness with another.

During sexual activity, your attention may shift between your sensations, breathing, fantasies, mental impressions, and the variety of your emotional feelings. You can sense physical tension developing, expanding, and releasing; you may notice sexual energy intensifying, moving, and releasing. You also may be aware of memories, judgments, and performance expectations.

Here is what some Survey respondents said about their most satisfying sexual experiences: ♀ Lying close with him, I feel an "electric" sensation running between us which is warming and wonderful; ♀ It's a spiritual union; ♀ I sense and enjoy the warmth and smell of my partner's body; ♀ I feel dominated; ♀ I experience great satisfaction knowing how to stimulate my partner the way she wants it; ♀ Our bodies become one with each other; ♀ I have no expectations.

Creating Erotic Pleasure

An erotic experience is a process in which one thing leads to another. Descriptions of some aspects of this process follow, together with specific suggestions you can use to enhance your lovemaking.

Transitions

One key to great sex is the transition you and your partner make from separateness to togetherness. Most of us spend most of the time in our "not-doing-sex selves." Our bodies, our attention, our emotions are *not* in a "doing-sex" mode. A sexual experience begins with a shift of attention and consciousness. Something happens—or many things happen—one thing leads to another—and sexual arousal and erotic feelings begin to occur.

A transition into your "doing-sex self" can be practically instantaneous or take place gradually, over hours, or even days. It may be stimulated primarily through something outside of yourself or from hormonal shifts, physical changes, emotional longings, and sexual images within you.

In partnered sex, you and your partner each shift from your personal "not-doing-sex self" into your "doing-sex self" and also, with each other, shift from feeling separate to experiencing a sense of connection—togetherness. These personal and interpersonal transitions may seem to happen spontaneously or they may be made with effort.

As **Amanda (1970)** explains: "Sometimes you just start fooling around and you'll be just so excited, you'll just be like, *Okay, right now, right here.* But other times I've felt like, *No, I need foreplay, I need everything. I need to feel close to you before actually engaging in sex.* If it's a nice day, or if you've maybe gone out and done some exercise together, or something really special, maybe had dinner or romance, there's that sense of coming closer together. Conversation and flirtation definitely play into it, too."

Transition Activities

On your own you might "warm up" for sex by, for example, taking a bath or shower, stretching, and breathing deeply—or you could bathe or shower with your partner. Doing something as a couple that isn't specifically sexual can be an excellent way of starting to feel close. It might be a date or sharing a walk, a meal, exercise, or a TV program. It could even be weaving in sexual innuendoes and play as you clean the kitchen together. Such activities can give sexual interest and arousal the time to build into impassioned desire.

As these Survey respondents noted, playing, talking, laughing, and engaging in spiritual practices together can be great ways both to feel closer and to build arousal: ♀ We tussle a bit first, before becoming more quiet and cuddly; ♀ We engage in playful chatter; ♀ My companion takes on different names: Dick Long, Mason Dixon Hardcock VII, Vargas Fusco, Harry Dick Long, Danny Fusco, Vince Fusco, Tomachi Fukamoto, Amos Windcock; ♀ We form a conscious intention of *knowing we want to connect in heart, spirit, and body*; ♀ We talk to each other, creating a different psychic space to move into; ♀ We pray together before intercourse (believe it or not!). A satisfying spiritual oneness is naturally followed by a satisfying oneness.

Building Arousal Through Simmering and Teasing

Some couples, like those in the following examples, are adept at simmering, i.e., lighting a pilot light of arousal and keeping their arousal fueled—simmering—in anticipation of later sex: ♀ A word or a touch can let me look forward to sex. I like to anticipate, be looking forward to something, before you actually ever get there; ♀ I like flirting, verbal foreplay, innuendoes, and physical kissing on the neck over a period of time before we get to the bedroom; I can turn it on in the bedroom but it's just not as easy; ♀ My desire is highest when I know we'll be having sex eventually, but I have to wait. Like we'll be out, close to each other, getting more and more excited, like in the car just waiting to get home.

The ease with which we make sexual transitions and how we go about making them changes as we move through our lives. As we get older sex doesn't have to disappear, but it does change form with the changes in our age, partners, health, and the circumstances under which we are able to have sex. To illustrate these changes, the next three narratives begin with the youngest woman first; the oldest is last.

Michele (1972) is a college student who lives in a coed dorm: "Pretty much anything is a turn-on. It's pretty random. Yesterday, I was wearing these loose shorts and he hugged me, and put his hand up my shorts and he was rubbing my butt. And I'm like, *Oooh, let's go downstairs.* I get really turned on really fast. I could stay in bed twenty-four hours a day if my boyfriend would let me. He's twenty-one; I'm twenty. I guess we're just horny."

Ronni (1955) is married and living with her husband: "We know we're slowing down, yet it's important for us not to let sex go away or to go through long periods of time without sex. So we set up dates, like *Do you want to have a date tonight?* And that can be anything. We might dress up in nice clothes, even if we stay in the house all dressed up having a cocktail. We just set the time and place to do it. It might mean pulling out some erotica, it might mean lingerie, or playing strip poker. But we'll actively ask each other."

Emily (1919) has been with her current husband about five years: "I don't have the sexual drive I had in my forties and fifties. The way I like to have sex now is that it's preplanned, a time when we can be totally alone with no interruptions. We usually do getaways, go somewhere for a couple of nights or so. If you only go for one night, it's not enough time. I have a sack of goodies—candles, a fur mitt, feathers, all those nice things—and we give each other foreplay in a very loving way. It's very pleasurable."

Knowing We Can Take as Much Time as We Need

No matter how much time you actually have, you are likely to enjoy sex most when you feel that you have all the time you need to become focused into the sexual experience, and for your arousal to build. On one occasion that might be only a few moments in which a look or verbal suggestion triggers a sharp rush of sexual desire. Another time, it might be an hour during which there is a relaxed, unhurried buildup of sexual tension. On the other hand, sometimes the pressure of a time limit can make sex very exciting indeed. Quickies can be very arousing and a lot of fun. Typically, though, feeling rushed and pressured to hurry interferes with the physical and psychological changes involved in sexual arousal. In fact, if your partner's touches are too specifically genital or sexual before you feel ready, you are likely to pull away protectively, which will hinder rather than facilitate the unfolding of your arousal and your feelings of connection.

Imagine that you're having sex and feeling hurried or pressured; you're focusing on your genitals and *trying* to make something physical happen. Now, imagine instead that there is no hurry at all; you can *surrender* to feeling whatever is happening at the moment; all you have to do is *enjoy* what you're feeling; you can *let go* of control and *allow* sexual sensations to develop throughout your entire body. The sexual outcomes will be quite different.

Sexual Arousal

A woman's sexual arousal involves erectile tissues that are very similar in structure to the erectile tissues in a man's penis. During sexual arousal, these tissues fill with blood (often called *vasocongestion*) and the woman's body goes through an *internal* transformation in size and shape that, if we could watch it, would be as remarkable as the dynamic transformation of a man's penis from flaccid to erect.

Women's erectile tissues are of two types, one more firm and the other more elastic or spongy. The firmer tissues are in the clitoris. When a woman becomes sexually excited, her entire clitoris, including the part we don't see because it's inside, becomes engorged with blood, swells, and becomes firm. Unlike a man's penis, however, the typical clitoris does not become prominently erect and move *away* from the woman's body. In fact, as the rest of her vulva engorges and swells around it, the usually visible portion of a woman's clitoris may be pulled back and seem to disappear altogether. There is, of course, quite a bit of individual variability here, too. In this regard, Robert Rimmer, a novelist, once described the vulva as *the other lovely face of the female*, because, like human faces, no two are identical (1972).

The more elastic erectile tissues encircle the vaginal opening, lie within the skin of the vaginal lips, and also include the engorgable areas that are sometimes described as the *urethral sponge* and *perineal sponge*. If we think of the aroused vagina as a cave, the *urethral sponge* is the soft, spongy tissue that extends inward along its ceiling, where it surrounds the urethra. If this *sponge* is fully filled during sexual activity, it can then transmit sensations and protect the urethra from irritation. You can locate it by inserting a finger into your vagina and pressing up and forward toward your pubic bone. The *perineal sponge* is similar tissue in the perineum, the floor of this cave; it can be felt if you press downward. As these spongy tissues swell, they serve to tighten the vaginal entrance. As arousal heightens, other internal tissues, including the woman's uterus, also may become engorged and expand.

Some years ago, Dr. Eric Golanty and I coined the term *pelvic erotic complex* to describe the various aspects of the pelvic region that contribute to one's ability to create and experience erotic pleasure. When this *erotic complex*—which consists of the vulva, vagina, uterus, and all their associated skin, muscles, connective tissue, nerves, and blood vessels—is fully engorged and distended, a woman's whole internal shape changes.

Her uterus and expanded vagina become more accessible to the stimulation of an entering penis, finger, or whatever else is desired. In their aroused sponginess, these tissues can transmit sensations of pressure and compression as well as perceptions of friction. As a woman becomes highly aroused and her pelvic erotic complex literally becomes differently shaped, she can experience sensations not available to her when she is internally less expanded and spongy. Note that one function of the rhythmic pulsations of a woman's orgasms is to massage the accumulated fluids out of her erotic tissues, helping to return her body to its nonaroused shape.

Full-body arousal takes more time to develop than genitally focused surface excitement. To become fully aroused, your body needs to make physiological and neurological shifts that usually can't be rushed, but can be enjoyed and experienced as relaxation, sensual pleasure, and the building of sexual arousal. When the erotic complex is quite engorged and distended, a woman may experience an "ache" inside, as **Joanna (1957)** does: "I like oral and I enjoy deep penetration with her hands. Sometimes I get an *aching feeling* for penetration."

The potential richness and fullness of this more deeply aroused kind of experience is missed by couples who always rush to intercourse or direct their stimulation only toward orgasm. Individuals and couples can experiment to discover their own preferences and develop more variability in their lovemaking. One Survey respondent, an artist, has found that *"extensive* foreplay . . . leads to a more ongoing eroticism throughout the relationship . . . sensuous, loving . . . very 'spiritual' in an unusual way . . . and to a much deeper release at orgasm."

For **Alicia (1967)**, the best times take place: "when I'm not worried about anything that has to get done and we've got a good stretch of several hours and time afterwards to take a little nap and a shower." Realistically, however, everyday life may rarely provide circumstances in which an afternoon or evening can be devoted to sex. As **Katie (1955)** explained: "My best sexual experience would be one that would last, including foreplay and everything, an hour. Before we had a child (now two years old) . . . there would be a lot of foreplay: kissing, caressing, music . . . just everything nice and slow.

Everything now is so rushed for us. There's usually not enough time unless we're away." Another woman who was not able to take as much time as she wanted was a Survey respondent with sons, ages fifteen and twelve, who noted: "With kids? Ha!"

There's usually not enough time unless we're away, Katie says. This is one reason it's such an important part of relationship maintenance to schedule time away—away from kids, job, phone, whatever gets in the way—ideally, once a month, but at least once other every month or so.

Erotic Stimulation: Creating a Composition of Sensations

In giving touches and in being touched ourselves, we can feel variations in temperature, pressure, texture, shape, shading, tone, intensity, and location of the touch. In making love we can also vary the mood and the setting. The possibilities for varying these in erotic experiences are endless.

Habituation

For most people, *pleasure is enhanced by varying touch*. One reason for this is a physical effect called *habituation*, which is the numbing effect caused by steadily stimulating one area. Habituation occurs when nerve receptors become fully activated and are no longer able to transmit more sensations. This effect is very useful. It allows us, for example, to feel a shirt against our skin as we put it on, but it protects us from being continuously bombarded with sensations from the shirt until we take it off again.

Because of habituation, continual unvarying stimulation of one place, even the clitoris, is usually not the most effective way to generate arousal and create erotic pleasure. Sometimes short-term continual steady clitoral stimulation is exactly what a woman wants to enhance her arousal or to release her orgasm. But frequently the steady, ongoing rubbing of the clitoris by a woman or her partner, or the continual application of a vibrator or a stream of water to the clitoral area, can have a numbing effect. When that happens, arousal may seem to reach a plateau and go no further—or an orgasm may occur but be less intense than the woman desires.

However, because different locations on the body and different qualities of touch have their own nerve receptors, erotic touching can be imaginatively varied. Allowing the intensity of stimulation and arousal to build and diminish—or a tension between *Will we?* or *Won't we?* to develop—may take longer than rubbing one place continuously to reach orgasm, but it also may create more tissue engorgement and richer sensations of arousal.

Emily (1919) said she "loved to resist until I had no choice but to surrender. I would hold on to my pants and not let the man pull them off until there was no choice. Or I would resist the man until he physically had me pinned down, and then I would surrender, and that would be just great." **Janet (1955)** loves "to be touched in places that I can't reach, like my back" and she likes " kissing . . . stroking . . . hugging and fondling, lots of touching, lots of skin-to-skin contact . . . teasing . . . prolonging—even not taking your clothes off for a long time or taking them off piece by piece—like a strip-poker type of slowness." For **Maggie (1965)** it's "definitely about the games, the flirtation, the seduction . . . like verbal teasing or rubbing against me when I'm clothed."

Transition, Physical Responsiveness, and Satisfaction

Personal and interpersonal transitions are essential for creating mutual erotic pleasure. Skipping or not taking enough time for these aspects of the sexual process will diminish pleasure and physical arousal. Difficulties with insufficient vaginal lubrication, reaching orgasm, and, for heterosexual couples, erection or ejaculation, all indicate there may be underlying difficulties with distraction, relaxation, and arousal. Couples who are tense and concerned about physical responsiveness are typically feeling neither *close to their partners before sex*, the top-ranked factor of satisfying partner sex, nor really attuned with their partners during sex. They demonstrate how important it is to take all the time you need.

Take Care of Details

The transition into sex is more likely to proceed smoothly and effectively if distracting details have been taken care of ahead of time. These details might be related to, for example, privacy, contraception, disease protection, music, or even something you want to talk over with your partner. Sometimes, reducing distractions can be as simple as locking a door, unplugging a phone, getting a pillow, preparing a beverage, or opening a condom package.

When Partners Have Different Sexual Styles

In my sexual choreographer role I see many couples whose differences in sexual style interfere with creating feelings of connection. A couple may differ, for example, in what most effectively turns each one on. Sex will become more satisfying if they can find a bridge between their styles. Just as there are many styles of dancing—foxtrot, Western swing, rock, waltz, jitterbug, polka, to name just a few—there are many different sexual scripts and turn-ons. You can teach your partner your style or together you can experiment with and develop another style (or others). Together you can enhance your abilities to become sexually aroused and to arouse each other.

Sensual Styles

One way two individuals may be alike or differ is in their sensory languages. Most of us use one or two of our senses more than the others to organize our experience and think and talk about our world (Grinder and Bandler 1976). Some people think predominantly in words, others in pictures, others in more abstract spatial images.

You are likely to respond most readily to a sexual invitation that involves your most developed sense. If your predominate sensory language involves touch and body sensations, for example, a physical caress is likely to turn you on more effectively than words. Your partner, on the other hand, may turn on more readily to words or visual images. Some couples unknowingly offer each other invitations in language that is not primary to the recipient—it is as if one is speaking French but the other better understands Cantonese.

Most people can determine what their sensory styles are by paying attention to the language they use. Here are four different people showing sexual interest. Note their words:

1. It turns me on just to *look* at you.

2. *Listen*, they're playing our song. Oh, I wish I could take you to bed right now and *whisper* in your ear what I'd like to do with you.

3. When you *touch* me like that, I *melt* all over.

4. I get such a rush of desire for you every time I *smell* your perfume. The *taste* of this wine always reminds me the first time we made love. M-m-m, I would love to *lick* you all over.

And here are some representative examples from the interviews, accompanied by some turn-on suggestions for each style.

1. **Sight/visual**. For **Marcy (1967)**: "Eye contact is a big turn-on. Tim gets really turned on by watching how turned on I am, how I can get really wild when I'm really horny, really want him." And **Alicia (1967)** said, "I like it when he's dressed up. When he's wearing a nice suit jacket, for example. That's something he does without intention that turns me on. One thing that he does intentionally that turns me on is he just looks at me and smiles. He looks really shy, like a little boy. I know that look, and I can't resist. He doesn't even say anything, he just looks like this innocent little person looking at me and then looks at the bed."

    Turn-on suggestions: Eye contact. You might use clothing that conveys mystique, because it both covers and reveals; sexy costuming; mirrors. You could remove clothing as your partner watches, look at erotica, dim the lights, light candles.

2. **Sound/auditory.** For **Alice (1938)**: "Really gentle foreplay turns me on more than anything else. Words turn me on. Sometimes Ron will ask if I want him to tell me a story, and I fantasize with a romantic story. I need words, the voice saying things." **Maggie (1965)** always talks "a lot and I want my partner to talk a lot." That wasn't always true, however; she said, "When I was younger I was really uptight about making any sounds; now I like to make sounds and I get much more pleasure when my partner is being loud." **Fran (1965)** is "really into talking dirty in sex; that's a real turn-on. It freaks him out a little bit, but I think that that's really fun."

    Turn-on suggestions: Turn-ons might include music, talking, laughing, freely allowing involuntary sounds. You can directly ask: Do you want to *make love . . . fuck . . . go to bed . . . fool around . . .* or you can use suggestive words, double entendres, private language, changes in tone of voice, shared stories.

3. **Touch and muscle sensations/kinesthetic.** One thing that was a big turn-on for **Carole (1930)** was "the quality of someone's skin." She said: "I was very turned on by being with Black men—that silky, almost hairless kind of skin that is incredibly smooth." **Karen (1957)** described how, for a long time she had been aware that "sex has this place in my mind, in my head, almost like this vacuum, that sort of doesn't have

words and pictures. I can think of doing *it* without a word attached to the *it*, although it is real clear what the wordless thing is. If I brought some words to it, I would say: Sex is fun . . . warm . . . explosive, surprising sometimes. There's a real physical release. It's a place where I feel close . . . connected to my body . . . connected with my partner."

Turn-on suggestions: Brush against your partner in passing, make suggestive movements, move closer; sit or lie down next to your partner. You might touch, hug with full body contact (front to front or front to back), snuggle, kiss, lick, exchange massages, run your fingers through your partner's hair, touch genitals.

4. **Taste and scent/gustatory**. For **Connie (1956)**, "Each person smells different, tastes different. I'll never forget the way Rob smelled—better than any other man. To this day I can think about how he smelled and get turned on." **Terri (1971)** and her partner have "tried different things, like food, whipped cream, honey—just eating it off each other." **Michele (1972)** and her partner have "love oils and massage oils that you put on and lick off."

With respect to the smell of our intimate partners, researchers found that when seventy-five couples, using no perfume or deodorants, wore white cotton T-shirts to bed for a week and the T-shirts then were lined up on tables, a majority, using only their noses, were able to find the shirt worn by their partner (Boyd 1984).

Turn-on suggestions: Rub each other with scented oils, wear a perfume your partner likes, or burn incense during sex. You might also share special foods and drink.

Partners with Different Sensory Styles

If your strongest senses differ from your partner's, you may experience problems with sexual communication and pleasuring until, as a couple, you discover satisfying ways to bridge this difference. For example, talking makes **Pat (1945)** feel close to her partner before sex, but talking does not seem to be his primary turn-on: "I like to talk about us, about my own processing of things. We'll wake up on a Saturday morning and we'll share things. I'll talk to him and he'll talk to me. Like I've got a captive audience. Once those good feelings are there, I'll let him know, *How about sex?* Sometimes it's aggravating to him. Sometimes I don't think he wants to talk. He would just like to have sex. But for me, I need the good feelings, both from talking and touching. I really need the touching."

Sexual Choreography. Pat describes both sound and touch as her preferred turn-ons. We can draw on all of our senses for variety and can condition those that are not highly developed. If I were talking with Pat and her partner, I would listen to his language and ask about his turn-ons. I would then suggest that perhaps he would be less aggravated if she were to weave in more of his preferred turn-ons and suggest also that he touch her more and that she talk somewhat less.

Discovering Your Sensory Styles. If you and your partner have never before considered your sensory styles, pay attention to the way you invite each other to have sex. You might also each make a list of your favorite turn-ons, and observe which senses are reflected in the words you use. To facilitate most readily turning on and fully enjoying sex, be sure you each receive stimulation of your preferred senses.

Fantasy During Lovemaking

Another realm in which partners may find themselves either similar in style and expectations or quite different is that of sexual fantasy. Among the women we interviewed many did bring fantasy into the bedroom in some way, although there was tremendous variability in fantasy themes and in how fantasy fit into their lovemaking. Sometimes fantasies were kept private and sometimes they were shared. Potentially, fantasies can both boost arousal and unify experience.

Some couples use fantasies to facilitate their personal and interpersonal transitions into sex. **Victoria (1946)** sometimes throws herself "out of my head space and into a fantasy space" because "it's just not happening . . . if I'm preoccupied . . . not happy . . . I've gone to bed in a bad mood and Tod wants to make love. I do always want to make love but it's like I'm distracted, not right there, and I need to be brought out, into what's happening. A way to do this that really gets me excited and includes Tod is to ask him to talk to me about what he's doing, what he likes."

Not all fantasies have to be shared. Sometimes, though, one partner having a fantasy that excludes the other can disrupt a couple's sexual experiences. This happened for a couple I'll call Marilyn and Scott, who saw me for sex therapy. If Marilyn were telling her story, she might say: "For a long time I thought being raped in college was the reason I would suddenly feel anxious and separate during sex with Scott. Then, in therapy, we discovered that Scott had a habit of slipping into fantasies of his own during sex. His attention would shift, and I would abruptly feel not *with him*. I would get an anxious reaction to that, and then I would think something was wrong with me. I was blaming myself and feeling inadequate. I found out that I was actually responding to the withdrawal of Scott's attention. I was staying with him. But he wasn't staying with me!"

Low-Key Fantasies

Shared fantasies don't always have to be a big deal. In a low-key way, they can be a part of the play of sex, as **Roberta (1943)** described: "With somebody I'm having a relationship with, we'll talk about fantasies during sex. We can each pretend we're somebody else or something like that. It's not anything grandiose. My last partner also wanted to hear about my other relationships. We shared those kinds of things."

Pursuing Novelty

In contrast, some people actively pursue novelty and excitement in their sex lives by playing out their fantasies in a larger arena. In one sexual style, *a novel thrill or novel self-expression* seems more important in the sexual moment than whether sex is safe, comfortable, or—sometimes—even physically enjoyable.

Fantasy Themes

In this, and sections that follow, I'm incorporating theories from Dr. Donald Mosher's 1980 article, "Three Dimensions of Depth of Involvement in Human Sexual Response." The dimensions he discussed are *sexual role enactment; sexual trance;* and *engagement with the sex partner.* Although one dimension usually predominates, more than one may be experienced during a sexual episode.

Sexual Role Enactment

Mosher describes the primary emotional tone of the *sexual role enactment* dimension as the active pursuit "of the novel thrill or novel self-expression." When this sexual style predominates, it is more important to the participants that sex be exciting than that it be comfortable, satisfying, or enjoyable.

Marcy (1967) likes to pursue novelty. For example: "The other day Tim came into the interior design store where I work, and there was nobody there, and he looked so cute. I had on a real short skirt, and we had sex standing up. It's almost like when I am in charge that we have the most satisfying sex. Even if I don't orgasm, it's just so fun being able to control him, just being able to maneuver him and tell him *Right here, I want to do it—now!* It's so nice to almost be in control. He loves to be controlled."

In fantasy play the slightly forbidden can be exciting and more-or-less safe. **Lorraine (1957),** married fourteen years, said, "I like sex where you're not supposed to, like in Larry's folks' shower at their house . . . breaking preconceived ideas of what's okay and what's not."

Michele (1972), who lives in a college dorm, has a pattern of doing *"wild things"* with her boyfriend. She likes "thinking of things I can do that I haven't done before." She said that her fantasies "make us closer." She "tied him up . . . a dominant thing . . . I liked that . . . and he tied me up. We also played, *I can touch you, but you can't touch me.* We tried anal sex, and I didn't like that." When Michele is in her room, waiting for her boyfriend to come over, she fantasizes about "what I'm going to do to him . . . his expression . . . how I can get him going and how far he can take it before he can't take it anymore . . . It's *bad*; I feel *naughty.* Lately we've been really risqué."

Sex with a Story Line

Fantasies may contain plots that are elaborately scripted; some couples actually act them out with props and costumes. As **Sandra (1949)** explained: "I acted out a lot of fantasies with this one guy. One thing he liked to do is go in the park and make love in the middle of the day. He liked sex being staged and he liked costumes—like for me to sit there and masturbate in front of him on a balcony in a beautiful floppy sun dress with things unbuttoned. It was like I was acting out his fantasies. It made him really happy, and it was a lot of fun."

Joanna (1957) likes to act out a fantasy about "being dominated, tied up. But not in a painful way." She explained: "In my profession I have to take control of the situation, make the decisions. Sometimes I want to be dominated, to not have to be in control. I want somebody to take that away from me, to make those decisions for me." Joanna, and Marcy in the next example, use fantasy to counterbalance the reality of their everyday lives.

For **Marcy (1967),** "Sex is really fun more than anything else. No matter what else is going on, even if you don't feel attractive or you hate your job, it's there where you can really conquer. In sex, you can be beautiful and sexy . . . just play, have fun, laugh. It's fun to explore things as long as it's safe. You can experiment. You can play footsie under the table in a restaurant, or do something sexual on the beach under a blanket with people walking by, or go out dancing with the idea of making eye contact with somebody just to get excited so you can go home and fantasize about it. Sometimes I ask Tim to masturbate and I'll tell him to close his eyes and think about some really beautiful woman, and I'll tell him this whole fantasy about what he's doing with her. We both get excited."

Fantasies of Playing Out Fantasies

Not all fantasies are acted upon. Some women talked of fantasies they imagine they may play out someday but haven't yet. **Lorraine (1957)**, for example, said, "I've always thought of having sex on a rubber raft in the middle of a lake in some exotic place." **Melanie (1970)** and her partner have several fantasies they have tentative plans to act out: "One fantasy I want to do with him, and this is my idea, is to put him five or ten feet away from me, and tie his hands up so he can't move, and then masturbate in front of him, which he really wants me to."

Relationship as Container

Shared fantasy can be a way to contain desires that might unduly complicate a relationship if acted out in life. Some couples, for example, imagine what it would be like to include other partners. **Joan (1944)** told me, "We like to read erotic material or look at erotic pictures, and we do a lot of fantasy about other men. A favorite we play around with is the idea of seducing our chiropractor. And I have a dream of having sex with two men at once, either oral and vaginal or vaginal and anal, or all three. Now I know that to have that work out is almost an impossibility. A fantasy is fun and so much better. Sometimes I use toys and masturbate while we're having sex to pretend that there're two guys. It's a lot easier than actually getting involved with another guy. But if the right person comes along and it feels right, we'll do it."

Cecile (1952) and her husband use fantasy to contain her bisexuality safely within their relationship: "We were able to deal with my bisexuality in a safe way by him acting out this fantasy when we were making love ... like a high school sex class and he was the teacher and I was the model brought in for the class. And he would act out all of the characters ... the kids, which included girls. They would come up and do things to me ... he would be doing things on my body and acting out their voices. So that was a safe way for us."

Intimate Trance

So far, these fantasies have predominantly had story lines or been about the pursuit of novelty and excitement. Another sexual style, called by Mosher "the sexual trance" focuses instead on a more passive and relaxed mood with attention drawn inward into sensation and, eventually, orgasm. Mental imagery may be scriptless sensory images rather than stories. Emotionally, "receptive joy" (D. Mosher 1980) may predominate over passion, although at times the trance itself may be truly exciting. Sexual techniques may be less playful and emphasize repetitive, sensual pacing that draws the partners into an *intimate trance* (Ellison 1984).

Marsha (1940) told me, "I don't think I have real fantasies during sex; my attention is very much on the pleasure I'm experiencing. I'm focused. The best parts of sex for me are the exploration of touching, and the primitive and regressive nature of sexuality: the sucking, licking . . . mutuality . . . intercourse . . . the kissing, the touching, and the affection."

The Loving Relationship

One's attention during sex also may be predominantly absorbed into one's loving relationship with one's partner. This is the dimension Mosher described as "engagement with the sex partner." **Deborah (1949)** experiences sex as a loving merger, a momentary loss of self: "I love, when I'm coming, to be able to look in his eyes and say *I love you* and just feel lost, merged with this person for a brief moment in time. I think this only happens now because I've a real clear sense of my own boundaries and he has a real good sense of his, so we are able to merge together and become one for a time, knowing that afterwards we will separate and become once again our separate selves. It's like two lights coming together. I'm one light and he's another. There's a moment when I don't know where he leaves off and I begin and vice versa and we're merged and it has this real spiritual aspect to it. Participating in that experience is the most wonderful part of sex with love."

In contrast, **Lisa (1970)** starts out with her attention focused on being close with her partner, but as orgasm approaches, she needs to reclaim some of her separateness: "I get real sentimental at the beginning. There's a lot of, *Oh, wow. It's the same guy.* That just makes me feel happy and good. It's not doing as much *down there* as it is mentally . . . it's more romantic and it's not as sexual as the stuff that comes later. We kiss a lot at the beginning, and I'll touch his back . . .

skin touching is really sensual to me. Then there's a shift: I still know he's there, but it's a lot more my own thoughts. When I'm reaching orgasm, I'm really doing it for myself. I'm still liking him there and the touching and stuff, but I don't think I can achieve it if I'm just looking at him. I have to have other thoughts."

Mosher believes that deep involvement within the dimensions of *sexual role enactment* and *sexual trance* can occur with a range of partners, and in casual encounters. However, the deepest levels of involvement in the partner dimension—a peak experience of mystical union for example—require a "maximally acceptable partner" with whom one has a loving bond.

Sex Outdoors

There's something about sex outdoors that attracts women of all ages. Some report a sense of taking a risk. For others, it's just a wonderful setting for a sexual event. For **Pat (1945)**, it's "something we've been able to do on hikes and while camping. There's always that little bit of risk of being caught. I'm a bit of a risk-taker, but not so much that you're caught." Privacy is important to **Elena (1953)**, but she loves "to make love outdoors—certainly in the water, it could be a swimming pool or the ocean—or hiking." And with her partner, **Amanda (1970)** "acted out some of my fantasies—like having sex in the pond or just going to a beautiful place in the woods." Sex outdoors may involve any of the dimensions Mosher described and perhaps others as well.

Fantasy in Lieu of Involvement

When involvement with a partner is not a possibility or not a turn-on, some women use fantasy in its place. **Ruth (1943)** wasn't truly turned on to her first husband and would fantasize to get herself sexually aroused: "Sometimes it was about him," she said, "sometimes other people. That's what makes me know the marriage wasn't right. Because I don't do that anymore. With the man I'm married to now it's just always there. He's wonderful, so attentive, and I'm so turned on to him. So it's not what they do. It's what you feel."

Every relationship is different. Whether it is desirable that fantasies be shared and attention unified during sex has to be considered within the context of the individual partnership. Each of us can consider: *Does the way we include fantasy in our relationship—or not—enhance us individually and enhance our partnership?*

When Partners Have Different Images and Expectations

Some women were aware of having images of sex or wanting something different from sex than they perceived their partners as having or wanting. **Anna (1949)** told me: "Once or twice I had a fantasy during sex with my husband without telling him and feeling this little twinge of, *Should I be doing this?* My fantasies include what I think of as a little kinky stuff—leather outfits, strip-tease joints. He doesn't have to know I'm not thinking about him at the moment; maybe that's healthier because I'm not so focused on taking care of his needs instead of my own. My husband is a very gentle lover and very attentive in a kind, tender way. I don't know how I could tell him this, but there's a part of me that wishes he would grab me by the hair and be rougher. But it's not his style, that's not the kind of person he is. So I bring this stuff in with my fantasies."

Anna seemed to have found a solution that worked for her, at least for the time being. If a *difference* in style is causing a problem, however, that *difference* can be addressed. Here, too, differing styles do not have to be evaluated in terms of which is better, but only acknowledged as different. The solution lies in finding a bridge between the differences.

Sexual Choreography. One approach to resolving problems that involve one of you imagining sexual experiences in one style while the other wants something else is to share your sexual images and then experiment with creating new sexual scripts. Here are some suggestions for doing that:

- On occasion, have sex incorporating words and images you have both contributed, such as romantic poetry and sexy costuming.

- Take turns being in charge of scripting and taking care of arrangements for sexual dates.

- Seek out new images and experiment with ways of having sex that are entirely new to you both, such as, for example, Tantric sex.

Invitations and Sexual Initiation

To consistently create satisfying sexual experiences, you need to know how to invite your partner to join you in sexual encounters effectively and how to successfully accept, reject, and negotiate the invitations your partner makes. A truly consenting adult knows how to say *No* or *As soon as I finish what I'm doing* . . . as well as when and how to say *Yes*. Mutual consent is a requirement for a sensitive intimate connection. Without consent, sensual pleasure cannot develop fully. Consent means: *I agree to be here; I choose to be here; I'm doing this because I want to do this.*

One aspect of low sexual desire may be an absence of full consent. *I want to make my partner happy* we may say to explain why we go along with a partner's requests for sex at times when we don't really want to engage in sex ourselves. At face value, it seems a good intention to do this, and, in some relationships, going along with a partner's wishes succeeds in making both partners happier and the relationship enhanced. In relationships where it doesn't do this, however, a woman typically finds herself avoiding her partner eventually and not desiring sex very much at all.

Saying "No" to Sex

Just say "No" to sex is at times good advice, even in an intimate relationship. A lot of us feel guilty about saying *No*. We don't want to hurt our lover's feelings and we believe it is our responsibility to take care of our partner's needs. (Remember that old phrase: *It's your wifely duty*.) But taking care of a partner in this way may lead to overlooking an alternative: we can consider our own needs, too. We can consider mutual needs. With appropriate skills and a sensitive, cooperative partner, we can negotiate for outcomes that are *mutually* satisfying.

Let's consider Josie and Joe, a composite of many couples who have seen me for sex therapy: Josie never directly said *No* when Joe suggested sex, nor did she suggest some other activity she would prefer; but she would frequently participate only half-heartedly. When she did that, Joe assumed that she didn't really want to have sex with him. And, at those times, she didn't! He felt rejected and resentful. Joe had no way of knowing when Josie genuinely consented to sexual intimacy, and her passivity kept her from becoming totally turned on. She was rarely orgasmic when they did have sex. She claimed that this didn't bother her, but it did bother Joe, who assumed her nonresponsiveness meant that he was a less-than-adequate lover.

The partner who is unable to say *No* typically begins to avoid sex, and this was true of Josie. She began to counter Joe's invitations by going to bed early and falling asleep before he got there. For a while Joe had seemed to be after sex all the time, but gradually, as we would expect, he had begun to initiate sex less and less. By the time they saw me for sex therapy, they had not had sexual intercourse in several months. Both partners were resentful and concerned about their low sexual desire.

From my perspective, neither was to blame. If they had known better ways to deal with sexual initiation, they would have been doing them. When I work with couples, I don't look for who is at fault. I see two people who want to have satisfying sex, but have gotten into interlocking patterns or roles that keep that from happening. As sexual choreographer, I look at just how they are when we begin to talk as the starting place, and together we talk about ways in which they may be able to go from there to create the kinds of sexual experiences they want.

Consequences of Just Going Along

Even with the best of intentions, a person who frequently says *Yes* while actually meaning *No* and then thinks: *I really hate this, but I don't want to displease you*, sets up a situation that has negative consequences for both partners and for their relationship.

With respect to oneself: When you too frequently put your partner's wishes before your own, you feel estranged and resentful. If you almost always go along with sexual invitations you don't genuinely want to accept, like Josie, you probably will begin to tense up or pull away from your partner's touch, take measures to avoid or sidetrack his or her sexual invitations, or make other movements away from intimacy and the pleasures of deep sensual feelings. Your verbal *Yes* will be denied by a subtle—or sometimes not-so-subtle—physical *No*. This means that your sensual pleasure will be blocked. Your pleasure cannot develop fully because your are not surrendering to it.

From a partner's point of view: It is painful to perceive the person with whom you are having sex as not really with you, resentful, or only going through the motions. Usually, dealing with an honest *No* is a much less painful alternative. When your partner has sex with you half-heartedly or resentfully, you neither get your needs met nor are you set free by an honest *No* to meet your needs in a more satisfying way. You might prefer, for example, to read a book, go for a walk, or to masturbate instead of having sex with your partner who doesn't really want to have sex with you at that moment in time. Engaging in sex under such circumstances may, in fact, be depleting rather than fulfilling.

In therapy, Josie and Joe learned some specifics of sexual chore-ography—my definition of sexual success, the importance of taking time for *transitions*, and more pleasurable ways to touch, for example. They also learned how to more effectively make and respond to sex-ual invitations so that they could negotiate to *mutually consensual* sex-ual intimacy.

Consenting to Be Intimate: Effective Sexual Negotiation

There are many subtleties to sexual invitations. Intimacy cannot fully develop when the message, *I'm interested in sex and I would like you to join in a sexual experience with me* is either sent or perceived as, *I demand that we have sex, right now!*

Ideally, when you tender a sexual invitation, you accept your lover's autonomy and right to have feelings different from your own. You could honestly say to your lover, "You can say *No* to sex with me right now and I won't stop believing that you love and desire me." I say "ideally" because so many of us, no matter what our age, have triggers that set off a wave of hurt feelings if we interpret our part-ner's response as rejection.

No doesn't have to equal rejection, however. Although many of us have never thought about what our assumptions are, each of us has some assumptions about what our partner's requests mean. There are also rules underlying our relationships that influence us when we initiate sex, either verbally or nonverbally. A sexual invitation can open a negotiation in which you both know that you share similar underlying assumptions. These might be, for example:

- **That you will be completely honest in your responses to each other.** This assumption allows you to trust that neither of you will say *Yes* if you aren't really consenting. No one is *always* in the mood for sex. But you can't fully trust a *Yes* from a partner who will *never*, under any circumstances, say *No* or *I'd like to wait until later.* A clear, unambivalent *No* acknowledges your autonomy and sets you free to fill your needs in some other way.

- **That there are an infinite number of ways to create pleasure together, and when you decline to have sex you are not nec-essarily refusing to have intimate contact.** You are, *literally*, just declining to have sex or, perhaps, just declining to have sexual intercourse and/or orgasm. You can talk further about what is possible.

- **That in responding to a sexual invitation you will clearly state your interest level.** If you are not interested at the moment, you will, if you can, suggest other mutual activities in which you might be interested or provide information about when you might want to have sex or spend time together. For example, *I really feel like being alone this evening. Would you mind waiting until tomorrow night?* or *I don't think I want sex, but I would love to trade backrubs* or *As soon as I finish what I'm doing, I'll jump into the shower with you.*

Sexual invitations do have underlying meanings, even when they're abbreviated to a private sexual cue—a wink, a look, a movement, putting on perfume, a special touch, or a few words, for example. Each couple has their own "contract." An intimacy-based invitation might have an unspoken meaning something like this:

- I'm interested in sexual/sensual activity and I would like you to join me. Are you either in the mood or interested in getting that way?

- I acknowledge that you may not want the same level of physical intimacy as I do right now, and that sharing intimate feelings is more important than whether we have intercourse or orgasms.

- If I am more turned on than you are right now, my arousal level is not *better* than yours, it is only different. There is no need for you to rush to catch up. I can also ease back the intensity of my arousal so that it matches yours more closely. I recognize that our feelings about what we want to do may change as we proceed.

- My primary goal is to feel intimate with you and to create an experience that feels truly shared. I am making an effort to be aware of how you are feeling right now. I ask that you do the same for me, and if I do not perceive your mood or feelings correctly, I trust that you will tell me.

Sometimes we want to give gifts to those we love, which may include occasionally having sex when we aren't particularly interested. The key for evaluating how this plays out in your relationship is my definition of successful sex: Do you feel good about yourself and your partner afterwards? From my years of practice as a therapist, I do know that if you *always* go along with having sex against your own wishes, it will stop being a gift of love and begin to seem like an obligation. You will become resentful if you engage too often in activities, including sex, in which you genuinely don't want to be involved.

Mindy (1965) told me that one of the things she liked least about sex was: "being in a position where I don't necessarily feel the need for it, but perhaps she (my partner) does. And for me it's like, *Well, okay, I could take it or leave it.* Often in those times it's not that satisfying for me." **Tracy (1971)** spoke of how her attitude and awareness had evolved: "Now during sex my attention is definitely on mutual satisfaction. I was involved in a relationship where I think it was more for him. But that's over and done with. That was a learning experience."

A Sexual Detective Considers Nonverbal Responses

If you notice yourself tensing up or pulling away when your partner touches you, or if you are feeling conflict or discomfort about letting yourself relax into being with him or her, think about what your body is telling you. Such physical responses are signs that you're doing something you feel anxious about, don't want to do, or that wouldn't be in your best interest. If you told me you were involuntarily pulling away from your partner's touch, I would put on my sexual detective hat and try to determine the following:

- What is preventing you from connecting with your partner?

- What feelings and thoughts are blocking a relaxed sensual response?

- Do you need to say *No, not right now* or negotiate for something other than what your partner is requesting?

- Are you angry about something?

- Do you need more time for yourself instead of more closeness?

- Do you need more privacy for sex to be totally comfortable?

- Do you need to deal with birth control or protection against STDs?

- Are you feeling pressured or rushed?

- Are you afraid that if you allow *sensuous* feelings to develop, then your partner will try to be more *sexually* intimate than you want to be?

Sometimes, pulling away can be a response you learned long ago that has nothing to do with your present partner. The past may be interfering with your responses and pleasure in the present. Instead of an *active* response based on the present moment and your present partner, your response may be a *reactive* one—reactive to the situation and circumstances, but based in past experience. You may need to recognize that and learn to act creatively in the moment. For example, when you notice your reaction, you might think: *That was then, and this is now. Isn't it interesting how this keeps happening?* Then, take a deep breath and, as you let it out, think or say aloud *"I love you"* to your partner. This will help you to avoid self-judgment and to shift your attention back to your partner and to the present moment.

If you have such reactions, they may be more than you and your partner can resolve by yourselves. A knowledgeable therapist can help you to detach opportunities for pleasure and intimacy in the present from the mental images and body memories of earlier trauma. Remember, a stance of self-acceptance can begin with: *That's what I experienced. That's how it is. Where I am right now is my starting place as I go on to create the kind of life and experiences I want to have.*

All You Need to Start Is Interest

When you want to have sex, you do not have to wait for genital feelings or physical desire in order to begin creating a sexual experience. To start, interest and consent are all you need. It's enough to say, *It's been a while. It would be good for our relationship if we made love* and then begin making plans to make it happen, which might start with getting to bed early. Interest and mutual consent are steps one and two of the process. If you establish the right conditions arousal and pleasure will follow.

Put a Structure Around Your Spontaneity

You may be wondering: *But shouldn't sex be spontaneous?* Of course. But *spontaneous* can have many meanings. A dance performance in which every movement creates just the right emotional effect and seems fluid and without effort is ultimately a *spontaneous* artistic expression. The experience is real and satisfying, but the situation and mood were consciously created, and each dancer had personal responsibility for perfecting basic skills and learning movement patterns. When the dancers join together for the actual presentation, responses once learned with focused attention and effort seem effortless and always known; and emotionality and creative artistry guide their expression. Similarly you and your partner can develop your own erotic artistry.

Emily (1919) talked of a man she had lived with in the past: "He was the biggest turn-on for me sexually of any man I've ever been with. I just loved his body. But our schedules were so different, it became difficult to find time for sex. He suggested we schedule time for sex, which I first resisted because it wasn't spontaneous, but I went along and we scheduled three times a week, a commitment we kept for a long time. Spontaneity came out of what seemed like no spontaneity. I discovered that all my ticklish areas were also erogenous zones. When he kissed or touched them, they would be so erotic and ticklish at the same time that I would begin to laugh and get turned on. By the time we got to intercourse, my whole body was one big clit and I would have these marvelous orgasms with him. So I learned a lot from him."

Rather than expecting spontaneous physical desire to lead you to sex, you can, as Emily and her partner did, create a specified place and time, a setting—a structure around your spontaneity—and then surrender control and let one thing lead to another. You create the opportunity for a *feedback loop* to become established between the two of you in which subtle changes in breathing, muscle tensions, movements, gazing and being looked at, and even in tone of voice, feed back and forth between you. These kindle your arousal and change your moods. The dance goes back and forth, back and forth. Sometimes one may seem to be leading, sometimes the other. There may be anticipation, tension, knowing, and not knowing. *Will we or won't we?* And so it goes.

This is a process that takes two. If one of you has been sexually wounded or for any other reason the two of you are frequently unable to get into this feedback loop, perhaps consulting a therapist who specializes in sexual issues—a personal sexual choreographer— would be helpful.

Rituals for Relationship Maintenance and Enhancement

A couple can develop relationship habits—rituals—that increase the likelihood that intimate feelings and sex will regularly occur. For example:

1. **A date once a week** during which your intention is to create good feelings can be a very powerful aid in maintaining intimacy. It is important that during a date, no griping be allowed. If you get off the track, recall your desire to enjoy each other and do your best to create a positive mood.

   Special times together are crucial to the maintenance of intimacy. If you're a long-established couple, you may benefit from reclaiming some of the ways you used to have good times together. For example, these might be activities that involved shared interests in music, hiking, or reading aloud to each other. Typically, when a relationship is new, we plan many adventures and fun things to do. After we've been together awhile, we tend not to do so many fun things together and we may need to rekindle the habit.

   Dates don't have to be limited to a night out. If you can find a way to do it, a weekday affair—with each other, not someone else—can be very erotic and feel deliciously forbidden.

2. **A gripe session—or life maintenance session—once a week** is as important as setting aside time for a date dedicated to having a good time. If your date is the only time you have each other's undivided attention, you're going to want to talk about everything, including paying the bills and fixing the car. Problems and life maintenance issues are not the most effective topics for creating a pleasurable mood, so date times need to be balanced by opportunities to deal with decision making, life's little problems, and the conflicts in your relationship. If you can't end gripe sessions positively, you may need to read a book on fair fighting or work with a therapist.

3. **Coming from separateness to togetherness after a time apart is one of life's transitions.** A greeting ritual that immediately reclaims your coupleness when one partner is home and the other enters the house can be powerfully effective. A few minutes of contact and conversation can acknowledge your intimate bond and set the tone for all that follows. (Greeting rituals are powerful with children, too.)

4. **Evening walks before bedtime** are a good way to shed the day's tensions, step outside the roles of home, and end your day with a special time together as a couple or family.

5. **A goodnight ritual** is the realization of a shared intention to affirm your loving and caring for each other as the last thing

you do at night before falling asleep. Doing this allows you to end the day harmoniously and, I believe, to sleep more beneficially. Your goodnight ritual might be an expression of affection that takes only a minute or two or something more prolonged. When you're not going to bed at the same time, the one not yet ready to retire can join the other in the bedroom to talk and touch with mutually focused attention.

Weeknight Sex

An image you may find helpful in thinking about what your goodnight ritual might be is what I call "weeknight sex," which I contrast with the "fantasy/date sex" you might have on a weekend or on vacation when you are rested and have more time. Weeknight sex doesn't have to include either sexual desire or arousal and doesn't have to include either intercourse or orgasm, although it can. There are many ways in which you can express your affection through your sexuality—even when you're very tired.

Once you've begun to think of sex as creating mutual erotic pleasure rather than as manufacturing orgasms, sex is a continuum of possibilities. You may find, for example, that low-key genital—or even nongenital—stimulation can be surprisingly erotic and relaxing. Weeknight sex could be a minute or two of facing each other, legs wrapped around each other, cuddling, caressing, or scratching each other's backs and a brief *I love you*; or briefly holding or caressing genitals and breasts without the intention of peaking arousal or of orgasm; or lying in a "spoon" position and synchronizing breathing. It also might be one of you holding and caressing while the other brings herself or himself to orgasm; or it could include quietly joining together in intercourse, lying that way a few minutes, perhaps with a few gentle strokes, followed by *"Is that enough for you?"* "Yes. For you?" *"I love you. Good night."* The possibilities are infinite.

Genital stimulation and intercourse in this manner do not involve trying to build arousal in a way that would lead to tension and frustration if not released by orgasm. Weeknight sex might be, most of the time, a barely aroused expression of affection that involves your sexuality. It might be that, upon occasion, one of you, or both, would become quite aroused and want to continue, perhaps to orgasm. And, sometimes, you both may be surprised as one thing leads to another and you become caught up in an intensely passionate moment.

What Does This Mean to You?

Now, if you wish, pick up your notebook and express the thoughts and feelings you're having about your experiences with creating pleasure and satisfaction in the dance of sex. Here are some questions you might want to consider after you've done that.

- What are some ways in which you might enhance your erotic experiences?

- Do you and your partner have differences in your sexual styles that need a bridge between them? If so, how might you begin to create that bridge?

- Is there a fantasy you would like to tell your partner or act out with him or her?

- Can you recall ways you've had fun and created feelings of intimacy in the past that you haven't done for a long time? If so, are there any you would like to do again soon? Is there something you've never done, but would like to try?

- If you are recalling experiences that you now regret, consider the circumstances, the roles of others, and how you saw your options at the time. Then, sit quietly with your eyes closed and imagine what you could now gently and lovingly tell your younger self that would be healing and would lead to greater self-acceptance.

14

Sexual Self-Acceptance

Your Sexual Self

Who are you? How does your sexuality fit into who you are? In the Introduction to *Women's Sexualities* I invited you to consider these questions as the first step toward a deeper understanding of how you experience and express your sexuality. Think now about how your answers to these questions may have changed since you first read them there.

If you have been keeping a notebook or other record of your thoughts and feelings as you've been reading and reacting to this book, turn to it and review the steps you have taken on this journey of self-remembering. The journey is not over. Where you are now is the starting place for where you will go from here.

Self-Acceptance

Self-acceptance is the experiencing of oneself physically, intellectually, and emotionally in any present moment without the inhibition of simultaneous self-evaluation, self-criticism, or self-judgment.

—Richard Olney

Self-acceptance is a moment-to-moment possibility, not something anyone has all of the time. Furthermore, self-acceptance is not the absence of negative feelings. Self-acceptance is the acceptance of all of your various feelings as sources of information about your world and your experiences. Self-acceptance is present when you experience such feelings as anger, jealousy, fear, love, joy, or happiness fully when they occur and then let them go. Letting them go allows you be finished with that moment and ready to experience the next moment's emotions.

The founder of Self-Acceptance Training, the late Richard Olney, with whom I studied for about five years, believed only self-acceptance brings about peace of mind and transforms our self-destructive attitudes and behaviors into positive life-affirming ones.

Emotional Blocks to Self-Acceptance

There are some specific emotional blocks that can keep you from self-acceptance. Two of the largest blocks are these:

- Holding on to resentments and regrets rooted in the past, and

- Dwelling on fears and catastrophic expectations about what may happen in the future.

When any of these blocks consume your attention in the present moment, you cannot experience self-acceptance and inner peace. The stance of self-acceptance might be outlined something like this:

- Yes, that did happen; that's how it is.

- Yes, he did that, but that was then and this is now; it's time for me to move on.

- Yes, that may happen, but I've done what I can to be prepared if it does.

- If that happens, I'll deal with it then.

One woman who had never faked her orgasms told us in an earlier chapter, "If I wasn't satisfied, I just said, you know... *Forget it. There'll be another time.*" Her self-acceptance did not mean that she passively resigned herself to unsatisfying sex. It meant that she accepted what happened that time. *That's how it is. Forget it. There'll be another time.* Later, she might have taken action and told her partner some ideas she had about making sex more enjoyable for both of them.

Regrets

Looking back over your entire life, what do you regret about your sexual life? Here, from a list we presented, are what 2,560 Survey respondents said in response to that question:

- 50 percent regretted that they were too often not assertive enough about their needs;
- 49 percent that they had sex with partners they should have turned down;
- 43 percent that they had stayed too long in a relationship with the wrong partner;
- 38 percent said they had been too inhibited;
- 23 percent did not have sex with someone with whom they wish they had;
- 23 percent regretted that they got into sex when they were too young;
- 13 percent that they did not take more time to be celibate;
- 11 percent that they were celibate for too long; and
- 9 percent that they married the wrong person because of sex.

We all can examine our sexual histories and come up with something we regret. We've all had events in our lives that we might consider doing differently if we could live them over again. However, these experiences are woven into the fabric of the lives we've lived. They may be threads in the wisdom we have acquired. When you recognize the wisdom your unique history has given you, you are experiencing self-acceptance. You might even decide that, given an opportunity to live certain parts of it over again, you wouldn't change a thing. One way to share your wisdom is to tell your life story to others. The women who so generously contributed their life stories to this book have done that. Again, I thank them.

Forgiveness

The ability to forgive is one aspect of self-acceptance. Forgiveness—the act of forgiving—is not really about another person. Forgiveness is an act that *liberates you* from the image and deeds of that person so that you can get on with living your life and enjoying it. Forgiveness means you stop carrying someone who has mistreated you around with you. It means that you kick his or her image out of your bed. It means that you let go of old anger and resentments and free yourself to fully experience your pleasure in life now without being tethered to the past.

If you are holding on to regrets and anger—or any other emotion that is a reaction to an image you are carrying of something that occurred long ago—you are blocking your ability to experience pleasure and enjoy what is going on in your life now. The solution is to stop holding on to images from your past and let them go free. One way you might begin to do that is to sit quietly, close your eyes, and imagine the following:

> Imagine that you can blow up the person who harmed you as if he or she were a huge helium balloon. Blow all of your anger and resentments into that balloon until it becomes so gigantic that it could be entered in the Macy's Thanksgiving Day parade. Put any shape and features you want on your balloon. It's yours. Then, when you have your balloon exactly how you want it, open your hands, release the ropes and chains—and let it go! Let it go, taking all of your anger and resentments with it. Watch it go up and up—receding—growing smaller and smaller—until you can't see it anymore at all, because it has disappeared into the far reaches of the universe. Now move away from this place. Don't turn back. Go on with your life. Resolve to enjoy your life as much as you can from this moment forward. Notice how light you are, how free you feel.

Understanding

Forgiveness is one path to self-acceptance. Understanding is another. We may better understand some aspect of our lives if we can look at it from many angles and acquire new perspectives. Sometimes, it can help to sit quietly, recall an image of an experience you've had, and watch it as if it were a movie or the action on stage in a theater. You are the director out front. Various people, including your younger self, are taking part. Other players and external influences are in the wings, just offstage.

Consider the experiences of each person involved. What influences each actor? How do the participants interact? What are their personal histories? How were they influenced by earlier generations? What messages did they receive in their particular cultural niche?

Watch the players on the stage for a while, then begin to direct the action. Give the players new lines. Modify their roles. Allow them to say what needs to be said. Let them help and comfort each other. Bring some new, more satisfying, resolution to the drama.

We may hate what someone has done, but find that once we understand who and what shaped them into who they are, we no longer condemn them. For example, most of those who perpetrate child sexual abuse experienced horrific abuse themselves.

When we recognize this, we may hate their acts and the terrible consequences of what they have done, and at the same time we can feel compassion because their behavior is an aspect of the terrible consequences of abuse they suffered themselves.

Body Image Blocks to Self-Acceptance

Did you know that the height and weight of the average American woman is around 5'3-1/2", 146 pounds? Did you know that she wears between a size twelve and a size fourteen? The average-sized American woman has a curvy, rounded body that is mature, fertile or post-fertile, and therefore sexual. A *woman's* body communicates her maturity, confidence, wholesome life experiences, and acquired wisdom.

Compare a *woman's* body with the height and weight of the average female model. In 1980 this was 5'8", 117 pounds; in 1990 it had become 5'8" to 5'11", 110 to 115 pounds—taller and skinnier; and models continue to be much thinner than almost all of the attractive women you will meet in real life (Posavac, Posavac, and Posavac 1998). Many of the "women" with these unrealistic body proportions do not have enough body fat to support hormone regulation and regular menstrual cycling and fertility. The media's ideal "woman" has the body of a prepubescent, physically immature girl. She appears to have no maturity, confidence, wholesome life experiences, or acquired wisdom to convey to us.

According to the U.S. Department of Health and Welfare, well over half of normal-weight women say they want to be thinner. A majority of ten-year-old girls claim they're on a diet. What is wrong with this picture? A 1998 study (Posavac, Posavac, and Posavac) found that when most young women viewed images representing female attractiveness, their concerns about their weight increased. The authors of the study note that in their everyday lives women are exposed to quite a lot of these images. Fashion model images may be particularly likely to increase a woman's concerns with her weight because the media ideal is so extreme, and therefore more likely to be discrepant with the woman's own physical characteristics.

The women *least* likely to report more concern with their weight following exposure to media images were those who were generally satisfied with their bodies. The researchers suggest that women who are confident in skills and abilities—unrelated to physical attractiveness—are unlikely to be affected greatly by the media ideals of attractiveness; their confidence in other arenas renders their physical attractiveness relatively unimportant to them when they define their self-worth. They experience self-acceptance.

Survey Results

In response to a Survey question asking them to agree or disagree with the statement: *Overall, I'm satisfied with how my body looks*, 51 percent of the respondents indicated some degree of agreement, while 34 percent, about one in three, were dissatisfied.

Most of the women in our Survey realized that their partners accepted them as they are. Seventy-nine percent agreed with the statement *My current or last partner is/was satisfied with how my body looks*, while only 10 percent indicated some degree of disagreement. Consider this question: Is it more important to you that you match some external ideal, or that your partner likes you just the way you are?

Twenty-nine percent of the Survey respondents said that *their feelings about their bodies interfered with their sexual satisfaction* and 60 percent said their feelings did not interfere.

Terri (1971) explained: "When I don't feel good about the way I look, I really have a bad time with sex. I don't want to be touched, and I don't feel attractive. So it's hard for me to get in the mind-set of sex and pleasure and all of that. 'Cause I just feel like I should put big overalls on and sit there. It's really bad, actually, because I get turned on and off by it so quickly."

Eighteen percent of the respondents agreed with a Survey statement referring to health and body condition: *The physical condition of my body interferes with my sexual satisfaction;* 74 percent disagreed.

Many women, I think, are unaware of how attractive they really are. Often we focus dissatisfaction on some particular body part. *My nose is too big. My breasts are too small. My hips are enormous.* Others take in an overall impression. They see your body and clothing but they also experience your smile, the warmth you radiate, your friendly attitude, your interest in them.

We are immersed in a culture where the media do all they can to prevent us from accepting our physical bodies. The media, paid by advertisers to do so, perpetuate the myth that we need some kind of idealized body to attract a partner, be happy, or successfully participate in a relationship. Advertisers want us dissatisfied and buying their products to be more "attractive" as defined by the ideals they foist on us.

Kathy (1949) is an excellent example of someone who does not fit the media ideal and yet is seen by others as attractive and a desirable sexual partner. Kathy is physically disabled and spends her days in a power wheelchair. Her body is not that of a fashion model. When I interviewed her, she was in a committed but open relationship that allowed her to sometimes have sex with others and she regularly saw a second partner. I asked her for her thoughts on her success in having successful relationships. We all can learn something valuable from her reply:

> A lot of it is attitude. I've talked with other disabled women and some agree and some disagree with me. Some feel there's this real stigma if you're disabled, that people aren't going to be attracted to you. And I'll ask, *How much of that is because you don't feel like you're attractive?* I think it has a lot more to do with how you project yourself than with the fact that we're disabled. I think beauty really comes from the personality.
>
> I was once in a bar dancing (in my wheelchair) and having a good time and I wasn't there to pick anyone up. This guy asked me to dance and bought me drinks and he was trying to pick me up. He was a college football player and he wanted to take me home, but he was just so confused. He said, *I don't understand this, I'm really attracted to you.* I said, *Look, don't worry about it. I'm not going to go with you. Tomorrow morning you're going to wake up and say, "My, God. I cannot believe I was attracted to a disabled woman!" What's confusing you is that your body is everything to you. It's your ticket. And you can't imagine how horrible it would be to not have your body. And at the same time you're finding yourself very sexually attracted to me. And yet, my body doesn't work. And this is what's causing the confusion. You're just seeing me as a person.*
>
> I wasn't projecting myself as needy, I wasn't like trying to find a guy, I was just having a good time, and he saw that and he saw me and enjoyed what he saw. He liked my spirit, he liked my attitude and that's what he was attracted to. So I think it's important that people try to find those things they like about themselves and really explore and develop them.

For "disabled" in the above narrative we might substitute "too fat," have "... too big a nose," "... breasts that are too small," etc.

Most of us have some aspect of our physical body that concerns us. Useful statements of self-acceptance include: *I am not my nose. I am not my breasts. I am not my hips. I am not my disability.*

Another Look at What We Want Our Daughters to Know

In chapter 3 we considered six interrelated themes for the education of our daughters about sex and sexuality in this twenty-first century: 1) Value yourself; 2) Value that aspect of self that is your body; 3) Be aware that sex can be dangerous; 4) Sex is pleasurable; 5) Don't be pressured into sex that isn't right for you or that you don't want; and 6) Balance pleasure and responsibility. These are important ideas that apply to all of us. I summarize them again here as a reminder. For more detail, revisit chapter 3.

- **Value yourself.** Pay attention to what you want, your right to be treated well, and your entitlement to pleasure. Knowing and understanding what you think, feel, and want provides you with a foundation for satisfying relationships and informed sexual decision making.

- **Value that aspect of self that is your body.** It is through your body that you experience and express your sexuality. Value, protect, and honor it. And enjoy it. Although the media and advertisers try to tell you your body is not okay unless it looks a certain way, ultimately, you have to be happy with yourself. As **Chris (1970)** told us in chapter 3, your "body is absolutely fabulous the way it is, no matter what it is; . . . there's no perfect body." You have the power to honor, take care of, and enjoy your body. There are many moment-to-moment decisions that you are able to make. You can decide, for example, what you eat and what you don't eat, what substances you use to alter your moods, and whether or not to take medications. You can decide whether to engage in sex upon a particular occasion, and whether you will take precautions against pregnancy or sexually transmitted diseases.

- **Be aware that sex can be dangerous.** Protect yourself from physical and emotional harm, particularly when sexual activity is outside the safety net of a committed relationship.

- **Sex is also pleasurable.** Sex can be wonderful, either alone or with a partner, when circumstances fulfill your personal conditions for satisfying sex. Think about what your conditions are and actively fulfill them.

- **Don't be pressured into sex that isn't right for you or that you don't want.** In sexual situations, pay attention to your inner sense of what is right for you. Learn to trust your intuition.

- **Balance pleasure and responsibility.** Ultimately it is up to each of us individually to learn about how to fulfill our potential for pleasure and to protect ourselves from unwanted physical and emotional consequences of sex. The challenge is to achieve balance.

Sexual Self-Acceptance

You have your own unique way of experiencing and expressing your sexuality. It is up to you to create the relationship(s) and context(s) that work for you. You have your own unique way of being attractive that is much more than physical appearance. Other unique aspects someone might find attractive include your values, ethics, and ideas; the ways you express your emotions, laugh and have fun; your sexual and relationship skills; and your openness or not to spirituality and the transpersonal dimensions of sexual expression. We are all different. What will attract one person to you will not be interesting to someone else.

Make love in ways that please you. Put aside the *manufacturing orgasms* script. Open yourself to erotic possibilities, whether your experiences are solo or with a partner. Even if you do have a partner, sometimes have an erotic date with yourself; it can be a great pleasure.

Some Teachings of Richard Olney

Richard Olney had many sayings that those of us who knew him treasure. Among his statements to help promote self-acceptance were these gems:

- It's over, and that's the way it is.

- Everything that has a beginning has an ending.

- It is better to have a direction than to have a goal.

- I learn by going where I have to go.

- I do the best I can, and my best is good enough.

- There are three things I value: peace of mind, awareness of beauty, health.

- I'm alive. I'm real.

- Nothing ever stays the same. Everything changes.

- Well, we'll just have to see what happens, won't we.

- Here in the Hand of God I take my stand.

- Remember to breathe.

- Into Thy hands I commend my spirit.

- Take my hand and we'll walk together.

I hope some of these sayings will be as helpful to you as they have been for me.

Remember, your sexuality is a lifelong work-in-progress. Your journey of sexual self-acceptance has no specific end point. Where you are now is the starting place for where you will go. And where you go always will be another starting place. You find your way as you go. Enjoy!

References

Barbach, Lonnie Garfield, ed. 1984. *Pleasures: Women Write Erotica.* Garden City, New York: Doubleday.

———. 1975. *For Yourself: The Fulfillment of Female Sexuality.* New York: New American Library.

Berezin. 1972. Psychodynamic considerations of aging and the aged: an overview. *American Journal of Psychiatry,* 128:1483-91.

Berne, Eric. 1971. *Sex in Human Loving.* New York: Simon & Schuster.

Binik, Yitzchak M., Marta Meana, Samir Khalife, Sophie Bergeron, Deborah Cohen, and Danielle Hone. 1995. Painful intercourse: a controlled study. Paper presented to the Society for Sex Therapy and Research. March 10, 1995.

Blume, Judy. 1975. *Forever.* Scarsdale, New York: Bradbury Press.

Boyd, L. M. 1984. *San Francisco Chronicle,* "Grab Bag."

Brauer, Alan and Donna. 1983. **ESO: the New Promise of Pleasure for Couples in Love (*Extended Sexual Orgasm).* New York: Warner.

Bridges, Sara. 1999. *Predicting and Describing Sexual Satisfaction in Women: Physical Affection in Family of Origin, Sexual Initiation and Communication, and Masturbatory Practices.* Doctoral dissertation.

Bright, Susie, and Joanie Blank, eds. 1991. *Herotica 2: A Collection of Women's Erotic Fiction.* New York: Plume.

Bullough, Vern L. 1994. *Science in the Bedroom*. New York: Harper Collins Basic Books.

Butler, Robert N. 1996. On behalf of older women—another reason to protect Medicare and Medicaid. *New England Journal of Medicine*, 334:12, 794-796.

Chesser, Eustace. 1957. *Love Without Fear: A Plain Guide to Sex Technique for Every Married Adult*. New York: Rich and Cowan.

Chia, Mantak, and Manneewan Chia. 1986. *Healing Love Through the Tao: Cultivating Female Sexual Energy*. New York: Healing Tao Books.

Clark, Le Mon. 1970. Is there a difference between a clitoral and a vaginal orgasm? *Journal of Sex Research*, 6:25-28.

Comfort, Alex and Jane. 1979. *The Facts of Life and Love*. New York: Crown Publishers.

Crenshaw, Theresa, and James Goldberg. 1996. *Sexual Pharmacology. Drugs that Affect Sexual Function*. New York: Norton Professional Books.

Davis, Katharine Bement. 1929. *Factors in the Sex Life of Twenty-Two Hundred Women*. New York: Harper & Brothers Publishers.

DeAngelis, Tori. 1995. New threat associated with child abuse. *APA Monitor*, 26:4, 1, 38.

Dennett, Mary Ware. 1929. Sex enlightenment for civilized youth. In *Sex in Civilization*, V. F. Calverton and S. D. Schmalhausen, eds. Garden City, NY: Garden City Pub. Co. 97-108.

Dodson, Betty. 1974. *Liberating Masturbation: A Meditation on Self-Love*. (This later became *Sex for One: The Joy of Selfloving*. 1987. New York: Crown Publishing.)

Ellison, Carol Rinkleib. 1979. Beyond the clitoris: arousal and female sexuality. Paper presented to Society for the Scientific Study of Sex. San Diego, CA 9/29/79.

———. 1984. Harmful beliefs affecting the practice of sex therapy with women. *Psychotherapy*, 21(3):327-334.

Ford, Gillian. 1996. *Listening to Your Hormones*. Rocklin, CA: Prima Publishing.

———. 1992. *What's Wrong with My Hormones?* Newcastle, CA: Desmond Ford Pubs.

Freud, Sigmund. 1920. *A General Introduction to Psychoanalysis*. Authorized translation. New York: Boni & Liveright.

————. 1927. Some psychological consequences of the anatomical distinction between the sexes. *International Journal of Psycho-Analysis*, 8:139.

Friday, Nancy. 1973; *My Secret Garden: Women's Sexual Fantasies*. New York: Trident; Pocket Books.

————. 1975. *Forbidden Flowers: More Women's Sexual Fantasies*. New York: Pocket Books.

Goldstein, David P. 1996. *Effect of Psychotropic Drugs on Sexual Functioning*. Handout for presentation to the San Francisco Bay Area members of the Society for the Scientific Study of Sexuality and the American Association of Sex Educators, Counselors, and Therapists. December 6.

Grafenberg, Ernest. 1950. "The role of urethra in female orgasm." *The International Journal of Sexology*, 3(3):145-148. February.

Greer, Germaine. 1971. *The Female Eunuch*. New York: McGraw-Hill.

Grinder, John, and Richard Bandler. 1976. *The Structure of Magic II*. Palo Alto, CA: Science & Behavior Books.

Hartman, William, and Marilyn Fithian. 1984. *Any Man Can: Multiply Orgasmic Technique for Every Loving Man*. New York: St. Martin's Press.

Hindman, Jan. 1989. *Just Before Dawn*. Ontario, OR: AlexAndria Associates.

Hite, Shere. 1976. *The Hite Report*. New York: Dell.

Hollis, Karen. 1996. Getting Ready for Sex, Preparing for Battle: Pavlovian Conditioning Is More Than Drooling Dogs. Presentation to the American Psychological Association, Toronto, August 11, 1996.

Hunt, Morton. 1974. *Sexual Behavior in the 1970s*. Chicago: Playboy Press.

"J." 1969. *The Sensuous Woman: The First How-to Book for the Female Who Yearns to Be All Woman*. New York: Lyle Stuart.

Johnson, Eric. 1985. *People, Love, Sex, and Families: Answers to Questions That Preteens Ask*. New York: Walker & Co.

Johnson, Toni Cavanagh. 1999. *Understanding Your Child's Sexual Behavior: What's Natural and Healthy*. Oakland, CA: New Harbinger Publications.

Kaitz, Marsha, Pnina Lapidot, Ruth Bronner, and Arthur I. Eidelman. 1992. "Parturient women can recognize their infants by touch." *Developmental Psychology,* 28:1, 35-39.

Kinsey, A. C., W. B. Pomeroy, C. E. Martin, and P. H. Gebhard. 1953. *Sexual Behavior in the Human Female.* Philadelphia: W. B. Saunders.

Klein, Norma. *Breaking Up.* 1981. New York: Avon.

Ladas, Alice Kahn, Beverly Whipple, and John D. Perry. 1982. *The G Spot and Other Recent Discoveries About Human Sexuality.* New York: Holt, Rinehart & Winston.

Leonard, George. 1984. *The End of Sex.* New York: Bantam.

Lerner, Harriet Goldhor. 1985. *The Dance of Anger: A Woman's Guide to Changing the Patterns of Intimate Relationships.* New York: Harper & Row.

Lewin, Tamar. 1997. "Oral sex looks safe to teens. Norms changing in dangerous eras." *New York Times* article reprinted in the *San Francisco Chronicle,* p. A7. April 5, 1997.

Liedloff, Jean. 1977. *The Continuum Concept. Allowing Human Nature to Work Successfully.* Revised ed. Menlo Park, CA: Addison-Wesley.

Marcher, Lisbeth. 1991. Bodynamic character structures. Copenhagen, Denmark: BODYnamic Institute. (Course handout.)

Masters, William H., and Virginia Johnson. 1966. *Human Sexual Response.* Boston: Little, Brown & Co.

Masters, William H., and Virginia E. Johnson. 1970. *Human Sexual Inadequacy.* Boston: Little Brown.

Mazur, Ronald. 1973. *The New Intimacy: Open-ended Marriage and Alternative Lifestyles.* Boston: Beacon Press.

McKay, Marilynne. 1992. Vulvodynia: diagnostic patterns. *Dermatol. Clin,* 10:423-433.

———. 1989. Vulvodynia: a multifactorial problem. *Arch. Dermatol.* 125:256-262.

Mead, Margaret. 1949. *Male and Female: A Study of the Sexes in a Changing World.* New York: Dell Publishing Co. Laurel edition, 1968.

Meshorer, Marc, and Judith Meshorer. 1986. *Ultimate Pleasures: The Secrets of Easily Orgasmic Women.* New York: St. Martin's Press.

Metalious, Grace. 1956. *Peyton Place.* New York: J. Messner.

Miller, Alice. 1981, 1990. *The Drama of the Gifted Child.* New York: HarperCollins Basic Books.

Miller, Henry. 1961. *Tropic of Cancer.* New York: Grove Press.

Montagu, Ashley. 1986. *Touching: The Human Significance of the Skin.* Third Edition. New York: Harper & Row.

Mosher, Clelia Duel. 1980. *The Mosher Survey: Sexual Attitudes of 45 Victorian Women.* James Mahood and Kristine Wenburg, eds. New York: Arno Press.

Mosher, Donald. 1980. Three dimensions of depth of involvement in human sexual response. *The Journal of Sex Research, 16*(1): 1-42.

Ogden, Gina. 1994. *Women Who Love Sex.* New York: Simon & Schuster/Pocket Books.

O'Neill, Nena and George. 1972. *Open Marriage.* New York: Avon Books.

Perry, John D., and Beverly Whipple. 1981. Pelvic muscle strength of female ejaculators: Evidence in support of a new theory of orgasm. *Journal of Sex Research, 17:*22-39.

Posavac, Heidi D., Steven S. Posavac, and Emil J. Posavac. 1998. Exposure to media images of female attractiveness and concern with body weight among young women. *Sex Roles: A Journal of Research,* 38(3-4):187-199.

Rimmer, Robert. 1972. *Thursday, My Love.* New York: New American Library.

Rosenberg, Jack Lee, and Beverly Kitaen-Morse. 1996. *The Intimate Couple.* Atlanta: Turner Publishing, Inc.

Rosenberg, Jack Lee. 1973. *Total Orgasm.* New York: Random House.

Rubin, Lillian B. 1990. *Erotic Wars: What Happened to the Sexual Revolution?* New York: Farrar, Straus & Giroux.

Schuster, Mark, cited in Tamar Lewin, op. cit.

Shuttle, Penelope, and Peter Redgrove. 1988. *The Wise Wound: Myths, Realities and Meanings of Menstruation.* New York: Grove/ Atlantic.

Sisley, Emily L., and Bertha Harris. 1977. *The Joy of Lesbian Sex.* New York: Simon and Schuster.

Socher, Sara. 1999. *Correlates of Sexual Satisfaction in Women: A Dissertation Submitted to the Graduate Faculty in Social Welfare.* New York : The City University of New York.

Timmers, et al. 1976. Treating goal-directed intimacy. *Social Work,* 401-402.

Van de Velde, T. H. 1968. *Ideal Marriage, Its Physiology and Technique.* New York: Random House. (First publication 1926.)

Whipple, Beverly. 1997. How I became interested in sexology. In *How I Got Into Sex,* B. Bullough, V. L. Bullough, M. A. Fithian, W. E. Hatman, and R. S. Klein, eds. Amherst, New York: Prometheus Books.

Whipple, Beverly, E. Richards, M. Tepper, and B. R. Komisaruk. 1996. Sexual response in women with complete spinal cord injury. In *Women with Physical Disabilities: Achieving and Maintaining Health and Well-Being.* D. M. Krotoski and M. Turk, eds. Baltimore: Paul H. Brooks Publishing Co.

Whipple, Beverly. 1995. Research concerning sexual response in women. *Health Psychologist, 17*(3):16-18.

Whipple, Beverly, Gina Ogden, and Barry R. Komisaruk. 1992. Physiological correlates of imagery induced orgasm in women. *Archives of Sexual Behavior, 21*(2):121-133.

Whipple, Beverly, and Gina Ogden. 1989. *Safe Encounters: How Women Can Say Yes to Pleasure and No to Unsafe Sex.* New York: McGraw-Hill.

Wright, Jonathan V., and John Morganthaler. 1997. *Natural Hormone Replacement.* Petaluma, CA: Smart Publications.

Zaviacic, Milan, and Beverly Whipple. 1993. Update on the female prostate and the phenomenon of female ejaculation. *Journal of Sex Research,* 30:148-151.

Resources

The American Association of Sex Educators, Counselors, and Therapists (usually called AASECT), is a national organization that certifies sex counselors and therapists. To get a referral from their national directory, call 319-895-8407. Or you can write to P.O. Box 238, Mount Vernon, IA 52314-0238.

My Web site is www.WomensSexualities.com. There you will find other resources that will be updated periodically.

SEXSA Circles

In the Introduction I suggested that you might want to organize or join a women's Sexual Self-Acceptance (SEXSA) Circle in which to talk with other women about sex, sexuality, and each member's unique sexual development. SEXSA Circles can be peer groups or intergenerational. They might meet in members homes, campus dorms, or online.

One way to conduct SEXSA Circles is to organize each session around a chapter in *Women's Sexualities*. Circle members read the chapter before attending and the discussion focuses on the thoughts and feelings the chapter generates. Some topics, such as sexual development in childhood, sexual trauma, or sexual concerns and problems, could generate a series of discussions.

For some sessions, a circle might want to invite a guest facilitator with expertise on the topic to be discussed.

Some of the questions presented for your consideration at the end of each chapter can facilitate discussion. Here are some others. One question or topic might be all you would need for a session, or you might select several.

Chapter 1

- Each participant might introduce herself by talking about her answers to: Who are you? How does your sexuality fit into who you are?

- How are your answers to those questions different now from what they were ten years ago?

- Was there anything in this chapter that surprised you?

- How do you use the words *sex* and *sexuality?* Do they mean the same thing or are they different?

- Consider the variety in sexual comfort zones of the circle participants. Most people have comfort zones that are relatively narrow within the range of possibilities that exist. Is this true for circle members?

- What does *feeling* normal mean to each of you personally? Is that the same as being normal?

Chapter 2

- Was there anything in this chapter that surprised you?

- What are your first memories of yourselves as sexual? Some of you may have been too young at the time to know then that it was sexual.

- What do you remember of first naming your experiences of masturbation and orgasm? What were some of the effects of labeling your experiences?

- Compare early childhood experiences and then teenage experiences with shyness and embarrassment; shame and guilt; or finding your ways to self-acceptance.

- Discuss memories of puberty metamorphosis.

Chapter 3

- Was there anything in this chapter that surprised you?

- What kinds of messages—both verbal and nonverbal—did you get from your parents, or those who were like parents to you, about sex and sexuality?

- What kinds of messages do you think your parents got while they were growing up?

- What qualities of the relationship of your parents, or of those who were like parents to you, do you want for yourself? What qualities do you not want?

- Looking back, what were the most significant sources for you of sex information that was helpful or useful? Of information that was misleading or harmful?

- What would you like to see changed about how sex and sexuality are presented in the various media?

- What would you want your daughter to know about sex and sexuality? Your son?

- Would your children, if you have (had) them, say that in your relationship(s) you are (or were or would be) a positive model for them?

- Is there any aspect of your own sexual life that you now regret and would hope to spare your daughter(s) or other young women you influence from repeating?

Chapter 4

- Was there anything in this chapter that surprised you?

- Discuss the experiences of Emily and Sara described near the beginning of the chapter. What were your reactions to reading about their experiences? Emily assesses her experiences as a positive influence in her sexual development. Do you agree?

- Discuss the experiences Ruth describes at the end of the chapter. Is this situation in some way sexual abuse? If you think so—or if you don't—what are your reasons? How do you think Ruth may have been harmed? What may have been positive or empowering for her in these experiences? If you could interview the man involved, what do you think he might tell you of his experiences with Ruth?

- How do we decide if children's expressions of curiosity about sex and sexuality in their childhood play are appropriate?

- What experiences have group members had with that *edge* where curiosity, a little danger, excitement, and the slightly forbidden meet?

- Are there incidents group members recall in which—if they'd known the words and felt powerful enough to say them— they would have stopped a situation or changed course?
- If group members wish to discuss sexual experiences they've had to which they did not consent, proceed cautiously. If anyone has a history of serious trauma, invite a trained therapist to facilitate the discussion or to be available by phone in case a retraumatizing flashback occurs.

Chapter 5

- Was there anything in this chapter that surprised you?
- Discuss what you recall of attempting to solve the mystery of how to be attractive to boys—or to girls if that was your preference—when you were a preteen and teenager. Looking back now, what mistaken ideas did you have? Where did these mistaken ideas come from?
- What were some of your childhood questions and curiosities about penises?
- Talk about *at the edge* experiences in which you or others you know later wished you had known some way to say, *No. This isn't good for me.*
- How did (or will) group members decide where, when and with whom to have their *first times*?
- If you've had intercourse, what guidelines and sources of information and advice were helpful to you? What were harmful or misleading?
- Is there anything you wish someone had told you beforehand about deciding when, where, and with whom your first time would be?
- What guidelines would sexually experienced group members offer to young women making that decision today?
- What guidelines would you offer to women of any age deciding to have intercourse or woman-woman genital sex for the first time with a new partner?

Chapter 6

- Was there anything in this chapter that surprised you?
- How well should you know someone before you have sexual intercourse or other genital-genital sex?

- Under what conditions, if any, is "casual" sex okay?
- Do you feel the same way now about "casual" sex—do you have the same values—as you did when you were younger?

Chapter 7

- Was there anything in this chapter that surprised you?
- Discuss group members' experiences of consensual non-monogamy, if they've had them. Did they ever experience jealousy?
- Why do group members think people have affairs? Is an affair ever justified? If so, under what conditions?
- Discuss the impact on children of being aware of a parent's affair. What lingering consequences might there be in adulthood for a woman who was aware while she was growing up that a parent was having an affair?

Chapter 8

- Was there anything in this chapter that surprised you?
- Talk about how masturbation fits—or not—into your lives now.
- Share fantasies.
- Talk about ways to create and enhance pleasure.
- Talk about vibrators—whether you use them, how you use them, adventures in buying them, and so on.

Chapter 9

- Was there anything in this chapter that surprised you?
- Discuss the qualities that make sex pleasurable and satisfying for each of you.
- Have group members ever had satisfying sex in not-so-satisfying relationships?
- How satisfied are group members with the amount and quality of the affectionate nonsexual, nongenital touching in their relationships?
- With the amount and quality of sexual/erotic contact that doesn't lead to sustained genital stimulation or intercourse?
- With the amount and quality of intercourse or genital-genital contact?

- If there is dissatisfaction, what are some strategies for improving the situation?

Chapter 10

- Was there anything in this chapter that surprised you?

- How has the *manufacturing orgasms* sexual script affected each of you?

- Discuss my definition of sexual success. How might you apply it?

- Some other topics in this chapter you might want to discuss include penis size; clitoral and vaginal orgasms; experiences with the G spot and female ejaculation; and faking orgasms.

Chapter 11

- Was there anything in this chapter that surprised you?

- Talk about how group members experience orgasm and the variety in these experiences.

- Have group members experienced crying and/or laughing with orgasms? Multiple orgasms? Orgasms from nongenital stimulation? Orgasms without any direct physical stimulation? Dream orgasms? Simultaneous orgasms?

- Talk about the various ways group members facilitate their orgasms.

- Have someone read aloud the "Imagery for Learning to Become Orgasmic" while the other group members relax with closed eyes.

Chapter 12

- Was there anything in this chapter that surprised you?

- Do any group members find themselves often *too tired and too busy for sex*? Or with lower sexual desire than they want to have? If so, does this make sense given the many roles you fill and the lives you lead?

- What were the group members most important sexual problems and concerns in the past year?

- Have these been resolved? If not, brainstorm about first steps toward resolving them?

- Talk about the issues of the reproductive dimensions of your sexualities that are relevant for your age group.

Chapter 13

- Was there anything in this chapter that surprised you?

- Talk about the kinds of *transition activities* you enjoy and that are effective for you.

- Listen to group members' words and see if you can identify each individual's preferred sensual style; *i.e.*, does a group member's language seem to be based more on sight/visual cues, sound/auditory cues, touch and muscle sensations, and/or tastes and scents?

- Talk about the fantasy dimensions as described by Mosher: sexual role enactment; intimate trance; and focus on the partner and relationship. Do these descriptions apply to the group members' experiences.

- Discuss the underlying meanings in the sexual invitations you and your partners make.

- Talk about the rituals for relationship maintenance and enhancement you find effective in your relationships? Are there others you would like to adopt?

Chapter 14

- Was there anything in this chapter that surprised you?

- Talk about any regrets you have about your sexual lives up to now. Then talk about how *That was then. This is now. You go on from here.*

- Talk about how forgiveness and understanding have played roles in your lives.

- Talk about the sayings of Richard Olney. Can you come up with some new ones to add? If you do, please add them to the list on my website (www.WomensSexualities.com).

- If this is your last SEXSA Circle session, have some kind of closing ritual that you have planned ahead of time.

Index

A

Alice (1938) 158, 183, 302
Alicia (1967) 52, 59, 63, 68, 71, 186, 298, 302
Allison (1971) 43, 62
Amanda (1970) 72, 87, 150, 294, 309
Andrea (1972) 39, 107, 141, 194
Angela (1971) 31, 109, 141
Ann (1934) 38, 92, 122
Anna (1949) 70, 106, 125, 167, 191, 202, 310

B

Barb (1955) 63, 113, 125, 185, 192, 201, 228, 238
Barbara (1954) 19
Beth (1961) 37, 58, 67, 86, 109, 128, 227
Bobbie (1946) 239
Bonnie (1966) 41, 73, 92, 106, 129, 221

C

Carole (1930) 26, 71–72, 85, 121, 222, 227, 235–236, 240, 302
Cecile (1952) 30, 65, 70, 171, 173, 284, 307
Cheryl (1937) 66, 243
Chris (1970) 43, 69, 134, 232, 238, 328
Cindi (1952) 110, 124, 183, 191, 194, 208, 228, 233
Connie (1956) 26, 72, 104, 108, 185, 242, 303
Cynthia (1954) 47, 92, 127

D

Deanna (1971) 39, 128, 149
Deborah (1949) 44, 166, 186, 192, 226, 228, 239, 241, 308
Diana (1968) 59, 73, 85, 227
Donna (1949) 15, 35, 53, 150, 186, 233
Doris (1930) 71, 74, 88, 186, 192, 232

E

Eleanor (1912) 15
Elena (1953) 309
Ellen (1910) 25, 48, 226, 281, 284
Emily (1919) 42, 55, 60–61, 78, 160, 166, 185, 201, 215, 221, 223, 236, 268, 277, 296, 300, 317

F

Flo (1905) 277
Fran (1965) 69, 108, 302

G

Gloria (1944) 62, 73, 193, 223, 228, 236, 240, 269
Gretchen (1949) 242

H

Harriet (1938) 104
Helena (1943) 55, 238
Hilda (1915) 38, 120, 201

J

Janet (1955) 59, 193, 300
Janine (1921) 105, 121, 236, 240
Jennifer (1965) 69, 110
Jessica (1970) 19, 39, 104, 139–140, 232
Joan (1944) 27, 104, 108, 131, 284, 286, 307
Joanna (1957) 106, 226, 234, 239, 298, 306
Josephine (1913) 29, 63, 109, 129
Judith (1940) 60, 89, 116, 151, 248

K

Karen (1957) 15, 55, 71, 114, 193, 302
Katherine (1938) 18, 62, 84, 104, 205
Kathy (1949) 19, 37, 103, 223, 237, 327
Katie (1955) 69, 108, 298
Katy (1970) 15, 108, 141
Kirsten (1970) 39, 139, 201

L

Leslie (1971) 71, 114, 130, 152, 229
Lillian (1905) 18, 48, 60, 120
Linda (1940) 18
Lisa (1970) 54, 63, 134, 238, 308
Liz (1951) 75, 108, 226, 234
Lori (1969) 45, 107, 110, 130, 141, 191
Lorraine (1957) 91, 115, 208, 228, 238, 268, 306–307
Lou Ann (1944) 192, 227, 241
Luci (1959) 71
Lucille (1921) 15, 181

M

Madeline (1915) 44, 133, 186, 227, 232
Maggie (1965) 16, 30, 44, 73, 94, 171, 221, 300, 302
Marcy (1967) 37, 73, 194, 223, 240, 302, 305–306
Maria (1965) 153, 186, 222, 226
Marie (1965) 73
Marsha (1940) 41, 57, 308
Mary (1972) 225, 236
Mary Jo (1947) 15, 41, 111, 136, 158, 242
Marybeth (1972) 19, 64

Melanie (1970) 46, 75, 103, 183, 307
Michele (1972) 70, 103, 133, 149, 222, 296, 303, 306
Mindy (1965) 45, 148, 162, 236, 315
Monica (1940) 32

N

Nan (1917) 91

O

Olga (1971) 132

P

Pam (1968) 31, 34, 37, 75, 108, 110, 117, 138, 233, 237
Pat (1945) 104, 156, 183, 232, 236, 303, 309
Peg (1948) 31, 216, 223, 239
Penny (1946) 40, 66, 69, 103, 110, 190, 227, 240–241

R

Roberta (1943) 29, 157, 305

Ronni (1955) 52, 74, 109, 126, 150, 191, 239, 296
Ruth (1943) 25, 58, 98, 111, 309

S

Sandra (1949) 28, 306
Sara (1949) 25, 66, 80, 123, 137, 185
Sharon (1962) 25, 73, 236
Stephanie (1973) 225
Susan (1958) 16, 30, 70, 82, 192, 201, 203, 221

T

Teresa (1946) 35, 123, 185, 221
Terri (1971) 220, 303, 326
Tracy (1971) 192, 232, 315

V

Vera (1940) 176, 208, 216, 243
Vickie (1957) 15, 85
Victoria (1946) 32, 96, 201, 236, 304

Carol Rinkleib Ellison, Ph.D., is a psychologist in private practice, an assistant clinical professor with the Department of Psychiatry at the University of California San Francisco, and an adjunct faculty member at the Institute of Imaginal Studies in Petaluma, California. A fellow with the Society for the Scientific Study of Sexuality, Dr. Ellison is also an esteemed researcher and regular instructor of human sexuality courses for mental health professionals. She is the co-author of *Understanding Sexual Interaction* and *Understanding Human Sexuality*.

More New Harbinger Titles

SEX SMART

Demonstrates how childhood family dynamics shape our sexual selves and helps readers counteract troublesome emotional patterns.   *Item SESM $14.95*

UNDER HER WING

Dozens of women whose lives have been shaped by a mentor-protégé relationship share insights about developing mentoring relationships, avoiding common pitfalls, and benefiting from these unique and valuable alliances. *Item WING $13.95*

A WOMAN'S GUIDE TO OVERCOMING SEXUAL FEAR AND PAIN

This workbook provides a series of exercises designed to help women map the *terra incognita* of their own bodies and begin to overcome the fear or pain that blocks their sexuality.   *Item WGOS Paperback $14.95*

AFTER THE BREAKUP

A diverse sample of straight, lesbian, and bisexual women of all ages speak out about what really happens when couplehood ends and offer fresh perspectives on how to rebuild your identity and enjoy a life filled with new possibilities. *Item ATB $13.95*

FACING 30

A diverse group of women who are either teetering on the brink of thirty or have made it past the big day talk about careers, relationships, the inevitable kid question, and dashed dreams.   *Item F30 $12.95*

CLAIMING YOUR CREATIVE SELF

Shares the inspiring stories of women who were able to keep in touch with their creative spirit and let it lead them to a place in their lives where something truly magical is taking place.   *Item CYCS $15.95*

Call **toll-free 1-800-748-6273** to order. Have your Visa or Mastercard number ready. Or send a check for the titles you want to New Harbinger Publications, 5674 Shattuck Avenue, Oakland, CA 94609. Include $3.80 for the first book and 75¢ for each additional book to cover shipping and handling. (California residents please include appropriate sales tax.) Allow four to six weeks for delivery.

Prices subject to change without notice.

Some Other New Harbinger Self-Help Titles

Virtual Addiction, $12.95
After the Breakup, $13.95
Why Can't I Be the Parent I Want to Be?, $12.95
The Secret Message of Shame, $13.95
The OCD Workbook, $18.95
Tapping Your Inner Strength, $13.95
Binge No More, $14.95
When to Forgive, $12.95
Practical Dreaming, $12.95
Healthy Baby, Toxic World, $15.95
Making Hope Happen, $14.95
I'll Take Care of You, $12.95
Survivor Guilt, $14.95
Children Changed by Trauma, $13.95
Understanding Your Child's Sexual Behavior, $12.95
The Self-Esteem Companion, $10.95
The Gay and Lesbian Self-Esteem Book, $13.95
Making the Big Move, $13.95
How to Survive and Thrive in an Empty Nest, $13.95
Living Well with a Hidden Disability, $15.95
Overcoming Repetitive Motion Injuries the Rossiter Way, $15.95
What to Tell the Kids About Your Divorce, $13.95
The Divorce Book, Second Edition, $15.95
Claiming Your Creative Self: True Stories from the Everyday Lives of Women, $15.95
Six Keys to Creating the Life You Desire, $19.95
Taking Control of TMJ, $13.95
What You Need to Know About Alzheimer's, $15.95
Winning Against Relapse: A Workbook of Action Plans for Recurring Health and Emotional Problems, $14.95
Facing 30: Women Talk About Constructing a Real Life and Other Scary Rites of Passage, $12.95
The Worry Control Workbook, $15.95
Wanting What You Have: A Self-Discovery Workbook, $18.95
When Perfect Isn't Good Enough: Strategies for Coping with Perfectionism, $13.95
Earning Your Own Respect: A Handbook of Personal Responsibility, $12.95
High on Stress: A Woman's Guide to Optimizing the Stress in Her Life, $13.95
Infidelity: A Survival Guide, $13.95
Stop Walking on Eggshells, $14.95
Consumer's Guide to Psychiatric Drugs, $16.95
The Fibromyalgia Advocate: Getting the Support You Need to Cope with Fibromyalgia and Myofascial Pain, $18.95
Healing Fear: New Approaches to Overcoming Anxiety, $16.95
Working Anger: Preventing and Resolving Conflict on the Job, $12.95
Sex Smart: How Your Childhood Shaped Your Sexual Life and What to Do About It, $14.95
You Can Free Yourself From Alcohol & Drugs, $13.95
Amongst Ourselves: A Self-Help Guide to Living with Dissociative Identity Disorder, $14.95
Healthy Living with Diabetes, $13.95
Dr. Carl Robinson's Basic Baby Care, $10.95
Better Boundaries: Owning and Treasuring Your Life, $13.95
Goodbye Good Girl, $12.95
Fibromyalgia & Chronic Myofascial Pain Syndrome, $19.95
The Depression Workbook: Living With Depression and Manic Depression, $17.95
Self-Esteem, Second Edition, $13.95
Angry All the Time: An Emergency Guide to Anger Control, $12.95
When Anger Hurts, $13.95
Perimenopause, $16.95
The Relaxation & Stress Reduction Workbook, Fourth Edition, $17.95
The Anxiety & Phobia Workbook, Second Edition, $18.95
I Can't Get Over It, A Handbook for Trauma Survivors, Second Edition, $16.95
Messages: The Communication Skills Workbook, Second Edition, $15.95
Thoughts & Feelings, Second Edition, $18.95
Depression: How It Happens, How It's Healed, $14.95
The Deadly Diet, Second Edition, $14.95
The Power of Two, $15.95
Living Without Depression & Manic Depression: A Workbook for Maintaining Mood Stability, $18.95
Couple Skills: Making Your Relationship Work, $14.95
Hypnosis for Change: A Manual of Proven Techniques, Third Edition, $15.95
Letting Go of Anger: The 10 Most Common Anger Styles and What to Do About Them, $12.95
Infidelity: A Survival Guide, $13.95
When Anger Hurts Your Kids, $12.95
Don't Take It Personally, $12.95
The Addiction Workbook, $17.95

Call **toll free, 1-800-748-6273**, or log on to our online bookstore at **www.newharbinger.com** to order. Have your Visa or Mastercard number ready. Or send a check for the titles you want to New Harbinger Publications, Inc., 5674 Shattuck Ave., Oakland, CA 94609. Include $3.80 for the first book and 75¢ for each additional book, to cover shipping and handling. (California residents please include appropriate sales tax.) Allow two to five weeks for delivery.

Prices subject to change without notice.